Soft Tissue Pathology: Diagnostic Challenges

Editors

LEONA A. DOYLE
KAREN J. FRITCHIE

SURGICAL PATHOLOGY CLINICS

www.surgpath.theclinics.com

Consulting Editor
JOHN R. GOLDBLUM

September 2015 • Volume 8 • Number 3

ELSEVIER

1600 John F. Kennedy Boulevard • Suite 1800 • Philadelphia, Pennsylvania, 19103-2899

http://www.theclinics.com

SURGICAL PATHOLOGY CLINICS Volume 8, Number 3
September 2015 ISSN 1875-9181, ISBN-13: 978-0-323-40274-3

Editor: Lauren Boyle
Developmental Editor: Donald Mumford

Surgical Pathology Clinics (ISSN 1875-9181) is published quarterly by Elsevier Inc., 360 Park Avenue South, New York, NY 10010. Months of issue are March, June, September, and December. Business and Editorial Office: Elsevier Inc., 1600 John F. Kennedy Blvd., Ste. 1800, Philadelphia, PA 19103-2899. Accounting and Circulation Offices: Elsevier Inc., 3251 Riverport Lane, Maryland Heights, MO 63043. Periodicals postage paid at New York, NY and at additional mailing offices. Subscription prices are $200.00 per year (US individuals), $233.00 per year (US institutions), $100.00 per year (US students/residents), $250.00 per year (Canadian individuals), $266.00 per year (Canadian Institutions), $250.00 per year (foreign individuals), $266.00 per year (foreign institutions), and $120.00 per year (international & Canadian students/residents). Foreign air speed delivery is included in all *Clinics'* subscription prices. All prices are subject to change without notice. **POSTMASTER:** Send address changes to *Surgical Pathology Clinics*, Elsevier, 3251 Riverport Lane, Maryland Heights, MO 63043. **Customer Service: 1-800-654-2452 (US). From outside the United States, call 1-314-447-8871. Fax: 1-314-447-8029. E-mail: JournalsCustomerServiceusa@elsevier.com (for print support) and JournalsOnlineSupport-usa@elsevier.com (for online support).**

Reprints. For copies of 100 or more, of articles in this publication, please contact the Commercial Reprints Department, Elsevier Inc., 360 Park Avenue South, New York, NY 10010-1710. Tel. 212-633-3874; Fax: 212-633-3820; E-mail: reprints@elsevier.com.

Surgical Pathology Clinics of North America is covered in *MEDLINE/PubMed (Index Medicus)*.

Contributors

CONSULTING EDITOR

JOHN R. GOLDBLUM, MD
Chairman, Department of Anatomic Pathology,
Professor of Pathology; Cleveland Clinic Lerner
College of Medicine, Cleveland Clinic,
Cleveland, Ohio

EDITORS

LEONA A. DOYLE, MD
Associate Pathologist, Department of
Pathology, Brigham and Women's Hospital;
Assistant Professor of Pathology, Harvard
Medical School, Boston, Massachusetts

KAREN J. FRITCHIE, MD
Assistant Professor, Department of Laboratory
Medicine and Pathology, Mayo Clinic,
Rochester, Minnesota

AUTHORS

ALYAA AL-IBRAHEEMI, MD
Pediatric Pathology Fellow, Department of
Pathology, Boston Children's Hospital and
Harvard Medical School, Boston,
Massachusetts

STEVEN D. BILLINGS, MD
Staff Pathologist and Professor of Pathology,
Department of Pathology, Cleveland Clinic,
Cleveland, Ohio

SOO-JIN CHO, MD, PhD
Assistant Clinical Professor, Pathology, UCSF
Medical Center Mission Bay, San Francisco,
California

LEONA A. DOYLE, MD
Associate Pathologist, Department of
Pathology, Brigham and Women's Hospital;
Assistant Professor of Pathology, Harvard
Medical School, Boston, Massachusetts

SARAH M. DRY, MD
Professor, Department of Pathology and
Laboratory Medicine, David Geffen School of
Medicine, University of California, Los Angeles,
Los Angeles, California

**CHRISTOPHER D.M. FLETCHER, MD,
FRCPath**
Department of Pathology, Brigham and
Women's Hospital, Harvard Medical School,
Boston, Massachusetts

KAREN J. FRITCHIE, MD
Assistant Professor, Department of Laboratory
Medicine and Pathology, Mayo Clinic,
Rochester, Minnesota

JERAD M. GARDNER, MD
Assistant Professor, Departments of
Pathology and Dermatology, University of
Arkansas for Medical Sciences, Little Rock,
Arkansas

ANDREW HORVAI, MD, PhD
Clinical Professor, Pathology, UCSF
Medical Center Mission Bay, San Francisco,
California

AARON W. JAMES, MD
Department of Pathology and Laboratory
Medicine, David Geffen School of Medicine,
University of California, Los Angeles, Los
Angeles, California

VICKIE Y. JO, MD
Assistant Professor, Department of
Pathology, Brigham and Women's Hospital,
Harvard Medical School, Boston,
Massachusetts

JENNIFER S. KO, MD, PhD
Associate Staff Pathologist, Department of
Pathology, Cleveland Clinic, Cleveland, Ohio

HARRY KOZAKEWICH, MD
Associate Professor of Pathology, Department
of Pathology, Boston Children's Hospital and
Harvard Medical School, Boston,
Massachusetts

ADRIAN MARINO-ENRIQUEZ, MD
Instructor, Department of Pathology, Brigham
and Women's Hospital, Harvard Medical
School, Boston, Massachusetts

DEEPA T. PATIL, MD
Assistant Professor of Pathology, Staff,
Department of Pathology, Robert J.
Tomsich Pathology and Laboratory
Medicine Institute, Cleveland Clinic,
Cleveland, Ohio

ANTONIO R. PEREZ-ATAYDE, MD
Associate Professor of Pathology,
Director of Diagnostic Surgical Pathology,
Department of Pathology, Boston Children's
Hospital and Harvard Medical School,
Boston, Massachusetts

NICOLE N. RIDDLE, MD
Assistant Professor, Department of
Pathology, University of Texas Health
Science Center San Antonio, San Antonio,
Texas

BRIAN P. RUBIN, MD, PhD
Professor and Vice-Chair of Pathology,
Department of Pathology, Robert J.
Tomsich Pathology and Laboratory
Medicine Institute, Cleveland Clinic;
Department of Molecular Genetics,
Cleveland Clinic and Lerner Research
Institute, Cleveland, Ohio

INGA-MARIE SCHAEFER, MD
Department of Pathology, Brigham and
Women's Hospital, Harvard Medical School,
Boston, Massachusetts

Contents

In this article, we focus on the histologic features, differential diagnosis, and potential pitfalls in the diagnosis of epithelioid sarcoma, alveolar soft part sarcoma, clear-cell sarcoma, ossifying fibromyxoid tumor, and malignant extrarenal rhabdoid tumor. Numerous other soft tissue tumors also may have epithelioid variants or epithelioid features. Examples include epithelioid angiosarcoma, epithelioid malignant peripheral nerve sheath tumor, epithelioid gastrointestinal stromal tumor, and perivascular epithelioid cell tumor, among others.

The diagnosis of vascular tumors is a challenging area in soft tissue pathology. Epithelioid vascular tumors pose a particular challenge. Due to the epithelioid morphology of the tumor cells, they can be misdiagnosed as a variety of other entities, including metastatic carcinoma or epithelioid sarcoma. Furthermore, it can be difficult to distinguish between different epithelioid vascular tumors. This review focuses on vascular tumors characterized by epithelioid endothelial cells, including epithelioid hemangioma, cutaneous epithelioid angiomatous nodule, epithelioid hemangioendothelioma, epithelioid sarcomalike hemangioendothelioma/pseudomyogenic hemangioendothelioma, and epithelioid angiosarcoma.

The diagnostic spectrum of spindle cell neoplasms arising in the retroperitoneum is wide and, in the presence of commonly shared morphologic features, it may be challenging to establish a correct diagnosis in certain cases. Beyond seemingly undifferentiated spindle cell morphology, most neoplasms may reveal distinctive adipocytic, smooth muscle or myofibroblastic or nerve sheath differentiation and show additional diagnostic clues or characteristic molecular abnormalities. Obtaining sufficient and representative biopsy material, a thorough work-up, and extensive sampling of gross specimens followed by a combined histopathologic, immunohistochemical, and, if necessary, molecular work-up of these cases is advisable so as not to miss important diagnostic and/or prognostic indicators.

A variety of benign and malignant retroperitoneal mesenchymal lesions may have a component of adipose tissue, including entities such as lipoma, myolipoma, angiomyolipoma, solitary fibrous tumor, genital stromal tumors, and well-differentiated/dedifferentiated liposarcoma. Although definitive diagnosis is usually straightforward on the complete resection specimen, it is often more difficult to workup these lesions on small biopsy samples. This review focuses on challenging diagnostic scenarios of retroperitoneal lesions with a "fatty" component and provides major differential diagnoses for commonly encountered morphologic patterns, clinicopathologic features of the various entities, and strategy for use of ancillary techniques, such as immunohistochemistry and cytogenetic studies.

Many benign and malignant soft tissue tumors in children are challenging and their diagnosis requires knowledge of their vast diversity, histopathological complexity, and immunohistochemical, cytogenetic, and molecular characteristics. The importance of clinical and imaging features cannot be overstated. Soft tissue sarcomas account for 15% of all pediatric malignancies after leukemia/lymphoma, central nervous system tumors, neuroblastoma and Wilms tumor. This article discusses selected challenging pediatric soft tissue tumors with an update on recently described entities.

Soft tissue lesions can contain bone or cartilage matrix as an incidental, often metaplastic, phenomenon or as a diagnostic feature. The latter category includes a diverse group ranging from self-limited proliferations to benign neoplasms to aggressive malignancies. Correlating imaging findings with pathology is mandatory to confirm that a tumor producing bone or cartilage, in fact, originates from soft tissue rather than from the skeleton. The distinction can have dramatic diagnostic and therapeutic implications. This content focuses on the gross, histologic, radiographic, and clinical features of bone or cartilage-producing soft tissue lesions. Recent discoveries regarding tumor-specific genetics are discussed.

Primary myoepithelial neoplasms of soft tissue are uncommon, and have been increasingly characterized by clinicopathologic and genetic means. Tumors are classified as mixed tumor/chondroid syringoma, myoepithelioma, and myoepithelial carcinoma, and they share morphologic, immunophenotypic, and genetic features with their salivary gland counterparts. However, soft tissue myoepithelial tumors are classified as malignant based on the presence of cytologic atypia, in contrast to the criterion of invasive growth in salivary gland sites. This review discusses the clinicopathologic and morphologic characteristics, distinct variants, and currently known genetic alterations of myoepithelial neoplasms of soft tissue, skin, and bone.

Soft tissue pathology is a rapidly changing subspecialty. New entities are described relatively often, and new molecular findings for soft tissue tumors are reported in the literature almost every month. This article summarizes the major features and diagnostic approach to several recently characterized entities: superficial CD34-positive fibroblastic tumor, fibrosarcoma-like lipomatous neoplasm, angiofibroma of soft tissue, low-grade sinonasal sarcoma with neural and myogenic features, malignant gastrointestinal neuroectodermal tumor, hemosiderotic fibrolipomatous tumor, and epithelioid inflammatory myofibroblastic sarcoma. Additionally, the article also provides a summary table of recent molecular findings in soft tissue tumors.

A variety of different non-mesenchymal neoplasms may mimic sarcoma, in particular sarcomatoid carcinoma and melanoma, but also mesothelioma and rarely some lymphomas. This article reviews the key clinical and histologic features of such neoplasms in different settings, along with the use of ancillary studies to help identify the tumor types most frequently misdiagnosed as sarcoma.

Approximately 85–90% of adult gastrointestinal stromal tumors (GISTs) harbor *KIT* and *PDGFRA* mutations. The remaining cases, including the majority of pediatric GISTs, lack these mutations, and have been designated as *KIT/PDGFRA* wild-type (WT) GISTs. Nearly 15% of WT GISTs harbor *BRAF* mutations, while others arise in patients with type I neurofibromatosis. Recent work has confirmed that 20–40% of *KIT/PDGFRA* WT GISTs show loss of function of succinate dehydrogenase complex. Less than 5% of GISTs lack known molecular alterations ("quadruple-negative" GISTs). Thus, it is important to consider genotyping these tumors to help better define their clinical behavior and therapy.

The emergence of high-throughput molecular technologies has accelerated the discovery of novel diagnostic, prognostic and predictive molecular markers. Clinical implementation of these technologies is expected to transform the practice of surgical pathology. In soft tissue tumor pathology, accurate interpretation of comprehensive genomic data provides useful diagnostic and prognostic information, and informs therapeutic decisions. This article reviews recently developed molecular technologies, focusing on their application to the study of soft tissue tumors. Emphasis is made on practical issues relevant to the surgical pathologist. The concept of genomically-informed therapies is presented as an essential motivation to identify targetable molecular alterations in sarcoma.

SURGICAL PATHOLOGY CLINICS

THE CLINICS ARE AVAILABLE ONLINE!
Access your subscription at:
www.theclinics.com

Preface

Diagnostic Challenges and Recent Developments in Soft Tissue Pathology

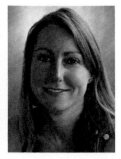 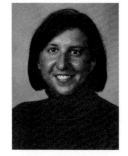

Leona A. Doyle, MD   Karen J. Fritchie, MD

Editors

This issue of *Surgical Pathology Clinics* is the second devoted to soft tissue tumors, the first presented in 2011. The current issue addresses diagnostic challenges in several common areas of soft tissue pathology, with an emphasis on providing a practical approach to such lesions on small biopsy samples and the role of ancillary immunohistochemical and molecular techniques. The diagnosis of soft tissue tumors requires both careful morphologic evaluation and clinical correlation, and articles are therefore grouped based on morphologic and clinical characteristics, such as epithelioid tumors, adipocytic and spindle cell neoplasms that arise in the retroperitoneum, chondro-osseous lesions, and diagnostically challenging pediatric soft tissue tumors. Additional articles review recent advances in the field of soft tissue pathology, describing newly characterized entities, recent molecular insights into myoepithelial tumors of soft tissue and gastrointestinal stromal tumor, as well as a comprehensive review of the myriad molecular techniques (and their utility) now employed in both clinical and research settings for the evaluation of soft tissue tumors. Finally, because many non-mesenchymal neoplasms may mimic sarcoma (and vice versa), one article reviews the pertinent clinical, morphologic, immunohistochemical, and molecular features that distinguish the most common non-mesenchymal mimics of sarcoma from different sarcoma types. It is hoped that this issue will provide practicing pathologists with the tools to effectively and efficiently evaluate challenging soft tissue tumors based on their clinical and morphologic features, along with the appropriate use of ancillary diagnostic tests, and also provide a comprehensive overview of recent developments in soft tissue pathology, including newly described tumor types, novel molecular insights into the pathogenesis of different soft tissue tumors, and the emerging role of sequencing techniques, along with existing and other novel molecular methods used in the evaluation of sarcoma.

Leona A. Doyle, MD
Department of Pathology
Brigham & Women's Hospital
75 Francis Street
Boston, MA 02115, USA

Karen J. Fritchie, MD
Mayo Clinic
Department of Anatomic Pathology
Hilton 11
200 First Street, Southwest
Rochester, MN 55905, USA

E-mail addresses:
ladoyle@partners.org (L.A. Doyle)
fritchie.karen@mayo.edu (K.J. Fritchie)

Surgical Pathology 8 (2015) ix
http://dx.doi.org/10.1016/j.path.2015.07.001
1875-9181/15/$ – see front matter © 2015 Published by Elsevier Inc.

Diagnostically Challenging Epithelioid Soft Tissue Tumors

Aaron W. James, MD, Sarah M. Dry, MD*

KEYWORDS

- Epithelioid sarcoma • Alveolar soft part sarcoma • Clear-cell sarcoma
- Ossifying fibromyxoid tumor • Malignant extrarenal rhabdoid tumor

ABSTRACT

In this article, we focus on the histologic features, differential diagnosis, and potential pitfalls in the diagnosis of epithelioid sarcoma, alveolar soft part sarcoma, clear-cell sarcoma, ossifying fibromyxoid tumor, and malignant extrarenal rhabdoid tumor. Numerous other soft tissue tumors also may have epithelioid variants or epithelioid features. Examples include epithelioid angiosarcoma, epithelioid malignant peripheral nerve sheath tumor, epithelioid gastrointestinal stromal tumor, and perivascular epithelioid cell tumor, among others.

OVERVIEW

In this article, we focus on the histologic features, differential diagnosis, and potential pitfalls in the diagnosis of epithelioid sarcoma (ES), alveolar soft part sarcoma (ASPS), clear-cell sarcoma (CCS), ossifying fibromyxoid tumor (OFMT), and malignant extrarenal rhabdoid tumor (MERT). Numerous soft tissue tumors may have epithelioid variants or epithelioid features. Examples include epithelioid angiosarcoma, epithelioid malignant peripheral nerve sheath tumor (MPNST), epithelioid gastrointestinal stromal tumor, and perivascular epithelioid cell tumor (PEComa), among others. Other articles in this special issue discuss many of these sarcomas.

EPITHELIOID SARCOMA

ES is a distinctive neoplasm of uncertain lineage of differentiation, which may be mistaken for either a benign granulomatous process or a carcinoma. First described as a distinct entity by Enzinger in 1970,[1] current understanding is of 2 types of ES, including the originally described conventional (classic-type or distal-type) ES, and the later described proximal-type ES. As we review, the 2 differ in their typical anatomic locations, histopathologic features, and prognosis. Both types are characterized by epithelioid cytomorphology, tumor necrosis, epithelial marker expression, and inactivation of the hSNF5/SMARCB1/INI1 gene. Classic-type ES typically involves young adults in the second to fourth decades of life,[2] with a male:female ratio of approximately 2:1.[2,3] It is uncommon in children and the elderly.[4] Proximal-type ES involves slightly older individuals (typically a decade older).[5,6]

GROSS FEATURES

The characteristic appearance of ES is a small indurated, ill-defined dermal and subcutaneous nodule or nodules. The flexor surface of the fingers, hand, wrist, and forearms are most commonly involved,[2] followed by other locations of the proximal and distal extremities.[1,2,7] ES rarely involves the trunk or head and neck areas. Large coalescent and variably necrotic mass lesions may also be seen to involve the tendons and aponeuroses. Tumor size varies from a few millimeters to 5 cm, whereas deep-seated lesions have been reported up to 15 cm in dimension.[1,2,8] Ulceration is a common feature, and clinical suspicion may be of an indurated ulcer or draining abscess. Proximal-type ESs are generally deep-seated tumors that involves the pelvis, perineum, and genital tract.[5,6] On cut section, ES is most often

Department of Pathology & Laboratory Medicine, David Geffen School of Medicine, University of California, Los Angeles, 10833 Le Conte Avenue, Los Angeles, CA 90077, USA
* Corresponding author. Department of Pathology & Laboratory Medicine, David Geffen School of Medicine, University of California, Los Angeles, 10833 Le Conte Avenue, CHS A3-251, Los Angeles, CA 90077.
E-mail address: sdry@mednet.ucla.edu

Surgical Pathology 8 (2015) 309–329
http://dx.doi.org/10.1016/j.path.2015.05.002
1875-9181/15/$ – see front matter Published by Elsevier Inc.

gray-white and may have yellow or brown areas owing to either necrosis or hemorrhage.

MICROSCOPIC FEATURES

Classic-type (distal-type) ES has a distinctive nodular arrangement of epithelioid to spindled tumor cells, with frequent central necrosis (Fig. 1A). The nodular pattern may vary somewhat from distinct tumor nodules in some cases to an irregular and conglomerate multinodular mass in others. Perineural and perivascular invasion are frequent findings. Ulceration is also frequent and may create diagnostic confusion

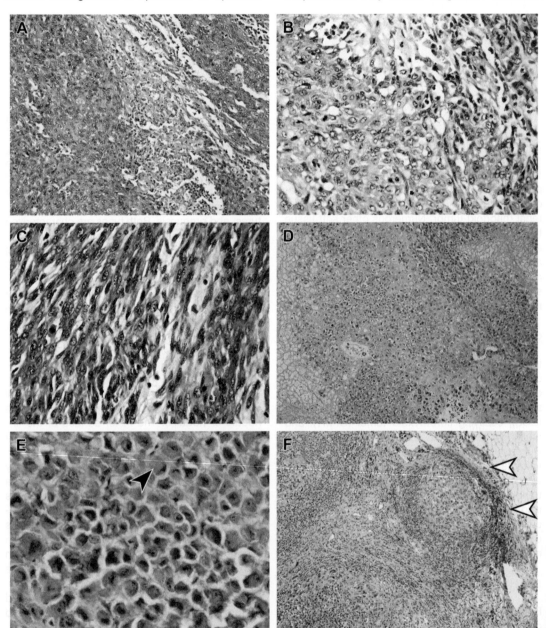

Fig. 1. Histologic appearance of ES. (A) Typical appearance of ES with nodules of epithelioid to focally spindled cells with central necrosis (×200). (B) Epithelioid tumor cells show enlarged round to ovoid nuclei. Tumor cell apoptosis and necrosis is readily identified (×400). (C) Focal spindling of tumor cells may be seen (×400). (D) Appearance of proximal-type ES typically includes larger lesions with a more confluent growth pattern composed of enlarged tumor cells (×200). (E) Cytologically, proximal-type ES demonstrates enlarged nuclei, prominent pseudoinclusions, and focal rhabdoid features (arrowhead) (×500). (F) Effacement of a lymph node with metastastic ES, arrowhead shows residual lymphoid tissue (×200).

with an ulcerated squamous cell carcinoma. Cytologically, ES tumor cells are enlarged ovoid to polygonal cells with abundant eosinophilic cytoplasm (see **Fig. 1B**). Focal to prominent spindled morphology may be seen (see **Fig. 1C**), and in some cases spindled cells may dominate.[9] Despite the variation in tumor cell appearance, a biphasic population of tumor cells is not seen. Occasionally, hemorrhage and a discohesive growth pattern may mimic angiosarcoma.[5] Calcification and ossification are seen in a minority of cases. Chronic inflammation is commonly seen, especially along the tumor periphery, again suggesting a chronic inflammatory process.

Proximal-type ES typically shows larger nodules of tumor, with confluent areas of necrosis (see **Fig. 1D**). Cytologically, proximal-type ES shows enlarged epithelioid cells with increased cytologic atypia and frequent rhabdoid features (see **Fig. 1E**).[5,6] Intracytoplasmic eosinophilic inclusions may be seen in some cases (see **Fig. 1E**). Lymph node metastasis is common in both classical and proximal-type ES (see **Fig. 1F**).

DIAGNOSIS

The diagnosis is made via recognition of the architectural and cytologic features of ES, followed by immunohistochemical stains to confirm the diagnosis and rule out benign and malignant processes with an overlapping histopathologic appearance.

Most ESs demonstrate immunoreactivity for both high-molecular weight and low-molecular weight keratins (**Fig. 2A–C**).[10] ES is generally negative for CK5/6, a helpful feature in distinguishing ES from squamous cell carcinoma.[11] Epithelial marker staining appears to be most abundant in areas of epithelioid cytomorphology. As well, significant intertumor variation exists in the approximate percentage of tumor cells with epithelial marker positivity. Approximately 50% of cases demonstrate membranous CD34 staining (see **Fig. 2D**). ERG immunoreactivity is seen in up to 40% of cases, depending on the antibody used.[12] Other vascular markers (CD31, von Willebrand factor [vWF]), melanocytic markers (S100, HMB45, MelanA), and neurofilament are negative. Loss of INI1 immunoreactivity is a consistent finding in ES (found in >90% of tumors), whereas in comparison unaffected juxtalesional tissue is positive (see **Fig. 2E, F**). The immunohistochemical profile is similar in both classic-type and proximal-type ES.[5]

DIFFERENTIAL DIAGNOSIS

The main differential is that of a benign necrotizing inflammatory process. The recognition of a nodular proliferation of atypical epithelioid cells with cytokeratin and epithelial membrane antigen (EMA) immunoreactivity aids in the diagnosis of ES. Additionally, the presence of tumor cell necrosis rather than necrobiosis is a helpful feature.[13]

Other epithelioid mesenchymal malignancies demonstrate histologic overlap with ES, although most are readily distinguished based on a combination of histopathologic appearance and immunohistochemical markers. These include epithelioid MPNST, epithelioid angiosarcoma, ES-like hemangioendothelioma, and MERT. Epithelioid MPNST may share cytologic features with ES and on occasion demonstrates EMA immunoreactivity and loss of INI1 expression, but shows strong S100 in all cases.[14] Epithelioid angiosarcoma shows a somewhat similar immunohistochemical profile to epithelioid sarcoma, including expression of cytokeratins, CD34, and ERG. In addition, a pseudoangiosarcomatous growth pattern has been described in ES, especially in proximal-type ES.[5] However, epithelioid angiosarcoma can be differentiated from ES based on immunoreactivity for endothelial markers, such as CD31, ERG, and vWF. ES-like hemangioendothelioma shares similarities with ES, including characteristic location on the extremities, cytokeratin expression, and epithelioid tumor morphology. However ES-like hemangioendothelioma demonstrates characteristic endothelial marker expression (including CD31 and FLI-1), intact INI1 expression, and an indolent clinical course.[15] MERT shares many features with proximal-type ES, including rhabdoid tumor cell morphology, cytokeratin expression, and loss of INI1 immunoreactivity.[13] However, MERT occurs primarily in children, with a wide range of anatomic sites, and uniform CD34 negativity. In fact, most diagnoses of MERT made in adults more likely represent other tumors with rhabdoid-type morphology.[16]

The differential diagnosis for ES also includes nonsarcomatous malignancies, including squamous cell carcinoma, poorly differentiated carcinoma, and melanoma. Ulcerating squamous cell carcinoma shares features of ES, including invasive eosinophilic epithelioid cells with ulceration of the skin. Keratinization is not present in ES, and dyskeratosis of the adjacent epithelium also is not seen. CK5/6 immunoreactivity is generally not seen in ES. Melanoma may have overlapping cytologic features with ES, but is

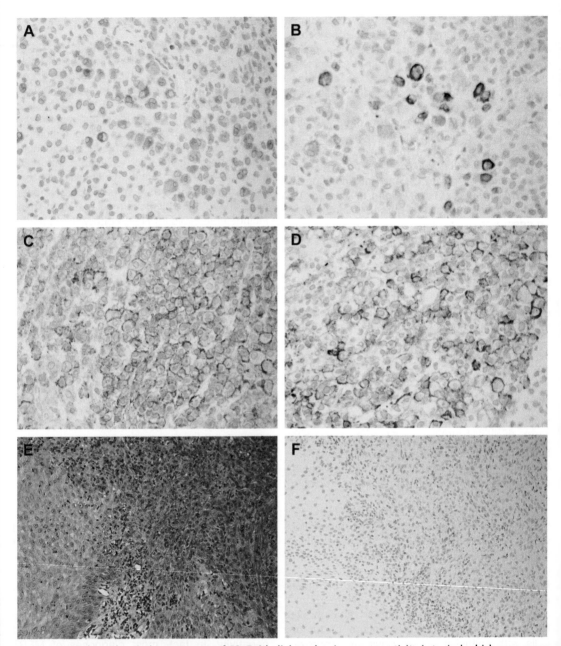

Fig. 2. Immunohistochemical appearance of ES. Epithelial marker immunoreactivity is typical which may range from patchy to diffuse, including (*A*) Pankeratin (×400), (*B*) CAM5.2 (×400), and (*C*) EMA (×400). (*D*) A typical membranous pattern of CD34 immunoreactivity is seen in approximately 50% of cases (×400). (*E, F*) Loss of INI1 immunoreactivity in tumor cells is a universal finding in ES (×200).

readily identifiable by the presence of melanocytic markers (including S100, HMB45, and Melan-A).

PROGNOSIS

ES has a high risk of local recurrence and metastasis.[1,2,7,13] Classic-type ES has an overall 5-year survival rate from 50% to 85% and a 10-year survival rate from 42% to 55%. Local recurrence occurs in up to 77% of patients, and metastases in up to 45%. Metastases are most common to the lung, lymph nodes, and soft tissue (especially the scalp), and are almost uniformly fatal. Poor prognostic indicators include male gender, proximal tumor location, large tumor size (>5 cm), increased tumor depth, high mitotic index, and the presence of hemorrhage, necrosis, or vascular invasion.

Pathologic Key Features

- Most common in the distal extremities of young adults
- Most commonly a superficial nodular growth pattern with central necrosis
- Epithelioid cells with epithelial marker expression, loss of INI1, often CD34+
- Proximal-type ES presents as a deep-seated pelvic/perineal mass with enlarged tumor cells and a worse prognosis

Differential Diagnosis

- Benign Tumor-like Lesions
  - Granuloma annulare
  - Rheumatoid nodule
- Epithelioid Mesenchymal Neoplasms
  - Epithelioid angiosarcoma
  - Epithelioid malignant peripheral nerve sheath tumor (MPNST)
  - Malignant extrarenal rhabdoid tumor (MERT)
- Spindled Mesenchymal Neoplasms
  - Clear cell sarcoma
  - Myofibroblastic sarcoma
  - Synovial sarcoma
  - Epithelioid sarcomalike hemangioendothelioma
- Nonmesenchymal Neoplasms
  - Ulcerated squamous cell carcinoma
  - Poorly differentiated carcinoma
  - Melanoma
  - Malignant mesothelioma

Pitfalls

! A prominent rhabdoid phenotype in ES may have phenotypic overlap with malignant extrarenal rhabdoid tumor, epithelioid angiosarcoma, and PEComa (perivascular epithelioid cell tumor)

! Loss of INI1 immunoreactivity, as seen in ES,[17] is also characteristic of MERT and can be seen in epithelioid MPNST, and extraskeletal myxoid chondrosarcoma[14,18]

! Regional lymph nodes are the most common site of ES metastasis and should not create diagnostic confusion with carcinomas. This feature is shared with other sarcomas, including angiosarcoma, embryonal rhabdomyosarcoma, and clear-cell sarcoma[19,20]

ALVEOLAR SOFT PART SARCOMA

First described by Christopherson and colleagues in 1952,[21] ASPS is a rare malignant translocation sarcoma most commonly found in the soft tissue. Despite its well-characterized immunohistochemical, electron microscopic, and cytogenetic features, the histogenesis of ASPS is still essentially unknown. Recent evidence has shown ASPS harbors a recurrent nonreciprocal translocation der(17)t(X;17) (p11.2;q25), involving the *TFE3* gene in almost all cases.[22]

ASPS is rare, and accounts for fewer than 1% of all soft tissue malignancies. ASPS most commonly occurs between 15 and 35 years of age,[21] although it may present as early as infancy. Female individuals are more frequently affected. The most common presentation is that of a slowly growing painless mass. Not infrequently, the primary tumor is overlooked and the initial presentation is with disseminated disease to the lung or brain.[23]

GROSS FEATURES

ASPS primarily arises from the deep soft tissue of the extremities, trunk, retroperitoneum, head, and neck.[23] The thigh and buttocks are the most commonly reported site of involvement (up to 39.5% of cases).[24] In children and infants, ASPS has an unusual tendency to involve the tongue and orbit.[25,26] ASPS rarely occurs in other locations, such as the female genital tract,[27] mediastinum,[28] lung,[29,30] gastrointestinal tract,[31] and bone.[32] Grossly, tumors are often gray-white, fleshy or friable, and generally poorly circumscribed. Necrosis and hemorrhage are characteristic.

MICROSCOPIC FEATURES

The histologic appearance of ASPS is characteristic and readily identifiable: large, epithelioid cells with abundant eosinophilic cytoplasm arranged in a characteristic nesting or pseudoalveolar pattern (Fig. 3A). Tumor cell aggregates are separated from one another by thin-walled, sinusoidal vascular channels. Less commonly, the pseudoalveolar pattern is not as easily appreciated or is absent, and the histologic appearance is that of uniform sheets of large epithelioid cells. Vascular invasion is common.[33]

Cytologically, individual tumor cells are large, rounded to polygonal, and relatively monomorphic (see Fig. 3B). They demonstrate distinct cell borders, vesicular nuclei with small nucleoli, and abundant granular eosinophilic cytoplasm. Mitoses are inconspicuous. The characteristic intracytoplasmic crystals of ASPS are rarely appreciated on hematoxylin and eosin (H&E) staining, and are more easily identified by histochemical stains (periodic acid–Schiff [PAS] with diastase)[34,35] (see Fig. 3C, D). Rare examples of more pleomorphic ASPS tumor cells have been reported.[36]

As mentioned, intracytoplasmic PAS-positive, diastase-resistant crystals and granules are observed, although the frequency of crystals varies greatly from case to case.[34,35] At times, only small PAS-positive granular material is identified, without well-formed crystals. Initial studies of these cytoplasmic granules reported protein and polysaccharide complexes.[35] Recent studies have found an accumulation of MCT1-CD147 complexes localized to the intracytoplasmic crystals of ASPS.

DIAGNOSIS

As mentioned, histochemical stains are helpful in highlighting PAS-positive, diastase-resistant intracytoplasmic crystals. However, intertumor variation in the number of crystals can be significant, and in some cases no crystals are identified: so-called "crystal-deficient" ASPS. The absence of crystals does not preclude the diagnosis of ASPS.

In an effort to ascertain the lineage of differentiation of ASPS, the immunohistochemical profile of ASPS is relatively well studied. Rare to occasional immunoreactivity for S100 and Neuron specific enolase (NSE) are seen. Although immunoreactivity for muscle markers may be present (including Muscle specific actin, desmin, myogenin, and cytoplasmic MyoD1 staining),[37] it is generally accepted that this does not indicate true skeletal muscle differentiation.[37–39] Negative stains include cytokeratins, EMA, neurofilaments, glial fibrillary acidic protein (GFAP), serotonin, and synaptophysin.[32,33] An antibody to TFE3 has been validated (a member of the characteristic

ASPL-TFE3 translocation product), although this also may be positive in pediatric renal cell carcinoma, granular cell tumor,[40] PEComa,[41] CCS,[42] and malignant melanoma.[42]

Electron microscopy is no longer routinely performed, but does show characteristic findings in ASPS. The intracytoplasmic crystals appear rhomboid or rod-shaped, with a regular lattice pattern.[35] Also seen are sparse electron-dense granules. Both the crystal and granules appear to be membrane bound.[43]

Cytogenetic analysis of ASPS has identified a nonreciprocal translocation: der(17)t(X; 17) (p11; q25) (see Fig. 3E). This unbalanced structure results in the fusion of the transcription factor E3 (TFE3) gene located at Xp11 with the novel gene at 17q25, creating the novel ASPL-TFE3 translocation.[22] Among soft tissue tumors, the ASPL-TFE3 fusion appears to be sensitive and specific. This transcriptional deregulation is not unique to ASPS, as it is also found in pediatric renal cell carcinoma (RCC), which is characterized by a balanced X;17 translocation.[40] It is currently hypothesized that the ASPL-TFE3 protein is responsible for irregular transcription of TFE3, which results in the development of ASPS because of the pathogenetic loss and/or gains of uncharacterized genes. Support for this theory has been found by ASPL-TFE3 upregulation of the MET receptor tyrosine kinase, which disrupts signaling pathways and leads to phenotypes associated with tumorigenesis.[44]

DIFFERENTIAL DIAGNOSIS

The differential diagnosis of ASPS involves a wide range of neoplasms with similar architectural or cytologic features. Most are readily differentiated by light microscopy combined with immunohistochemical stains. None share the unique unbalanced X;17 translocation of ASPS.

Soft tissue tumors with resemblance to ASPS include paraganglioma, granular cell tumor, alveolar rhabdomyosarcoma, and ES. Unlike ASPS, paragangliomas typically occur in older individuals, show strong expression of neuroendocrine markers, and contain S100-positive sustentacular cells. Granular cell tumors share overlap with ASPS, including abundant eosinophilic granular cytoplasm with PAS-D–positive granules, as well as TFE3 immunoreactivity. However, granular cell tumors are strongly positive for S100, inhibin, and SOX10,[45] and lack the characteristic vascularity of ASPS. Due to the alveolar architecture and occasional staining for muscle markers, a diagnosis of alveolar rhabdomyosarcoma may be considered. However, the cytology of ASPS differs significantly from alveolar rhabdomyosarcoma, with ASPS

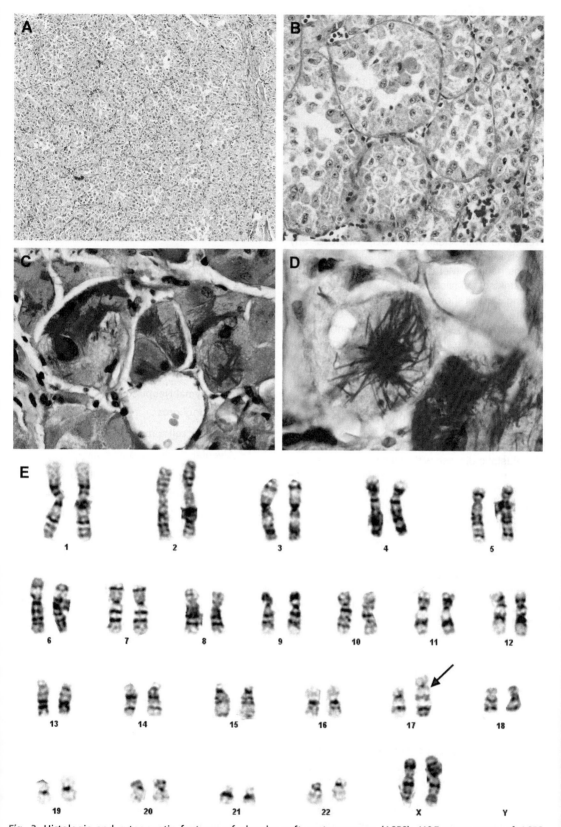

Fig. 3. Histologic and cytogenetic features of alveolar soft parts sarcoma (ASPS). H&E appearance of ASPS, demonstrating a characteristic pseudoalveolar pattern of cells, including nests of relatively uniform cells with large round or polygonal shapes and fibrils that define and separate these nests of cells. Shown at ×100 (*A*) and ×400 (*B*). (*C, D*) Representative images of PAS-D staining, highlighting intracytoplasmic rod-shaped crystals (×1000). (*E*) Karyotype in ASPS, demonstrating the unbalanced translocation der(17)t(X; 17) (p11; q25) (*arrow*).

tumor cells demonstrating larger eosinophilic polygonal with abundant granular cytoplasm, whereas alveolar rhabdomyosarcoma is composed of small round blue cells with small amounts of eosinophilic cytoplasm. ES may be distinguished based on the more typical location on the distal extremity, presence of necrosis, lack of pseudoalveolar pattern, immunoreactivity for epithelial markers, and the loss of INI1 expression. Importantly, none of the soft tissue tumors listed demonstrate the characteristic cytogenetic aberrancy of ASPS.

Metastatic carcinomas can be in the differential diagnosis of ASPS. The most obvious histologic overlap is with clear-cell RCC, whereas any epithelial lesion with clear-cell change could also be entertained. Metastatic clear-cell RCC may look strikingly similar to ASPS with routine H&E staining, but will show epithelial marker immunoreactivity that lacks characteristic PAS-D–positive crystals, and does not harbor the unbalanced X;17 translocation. Importantly, a subset of pediatric RCCs show a X;17 translocation, which is typically balanced.[46] These RCCs demonstrate papillary architecture, clear to eosinophilic cytoplasm, and psammoma bodies.[47] Fluorescence in situ hybridization (FISH) probes to differentiate balanced versus unbalanced X;17 translocations have been devised, and may be of use in cases of metastatic disease with unknown primary.[46]

Malignant melanomas with epithelioid morphology can have some overlap with ASPS, but can be differentiated by immunoreactivity for melanocytic markers and lack of PAS-D–positive crystals.

PROGNOSIS

ASPS has a relatively slow growth, but frequently metastasizes and has a poor long-term prognosis. Survival rates decrease substantially with time, from 77% survival at 2 years to only 15% survival at 20 years.[24] Patients presenting with localized disease have a greater disease-free survival (71% at 5 years), in comparison to those presenting with metastasis, (20% at 5 years).[23] Common sites of metastases include the lung, brain, and bone.[23,24] As compared with other sarcomas, ASPS has a predilection for brain metastases.[48,49]

Prognostic factors in ASPS include age at diagnosis, tumor size, and the presence of metastases.[24,50] Relatively improved prognosis in children may reflect early clinical detection and total resection.[51] Treatments for ASPS are generally not promising. Systemic chemotherapy generally meets with limited success, most likely owing to the typical slow growth of ASPS tumor cells.[49] Most patients are treated with radical surgical

Pathologic Key Features

- Most common in the proximal lower extremities of young adults
- Pseudoalveolar growth pattern of epithelioid tumor cells with eosinophilic cytoplasm
- PAS-positive, diastase-resistant intracytoplasmic crystals and granules
- TFE3 immunoreactivity, with occasional expression of muscle markers, S100, and NSE
- Unbalanced translocation involving x;17 and the *APSL-TFE3* fusion product

Differential Diagnosis

- Mesenchymal Neoplasms
  - Paraganglioma
  - Granular cell tumor
  - Alveolar rhabdomyosarcoma
  - Other sarcomas with epithelioid change
- Nonmesenchymal Neoplasms
  - Clear-cell renal cell carcinoma (RCC)
  - Pediatric RCC (Xp11 translocation RCC)
  - Other carcinomas with clear cell change

Pitfalls

! Immunoreactivity for muscle markers can be seen in ASPS, and should not be confused with sarcomas with true skeletal muscle differentiation

! Metastases to the lung and brain are common in both clear-cell renal cell carcinoma (RCC) and ASPS

! TFE3 immunoreactivity is not specific for ASPS, and can be seen in granular cell tumor, PEComa, clear cell sarcoma, and pediatric RCC among others

! TFE3 gene rearrangements can be seen in pediatric RCC and PEComa

excision of primary and metastatic lesions combined with chemoradiation.

CLEAR-CELL SARCOMA

CCS of soft tissue is a translocation sarcoma of young adults with melanocytic differentiation and a tendency to involve the tendons and aponeuroses.[52] Most tumors arise in patients 20 to 40 years old, with a slight female predominance. CCS has a striking tendency to involve the extremities, most often the foot, ankle, or knee. Melanocytic marker expression and the presence of melanosomes are defining characteristics of CCS.[53–55] Chung and Enzinger[56] proposed the term "malignant melanoma of soft parts," although even at this time it was clearly recognized that CCS is clinically distinct from melanoma. With current molecular genetics, melanocytic differentiation in CCS is thought to stem from the transcriptional activity of the fusion gene products that typify the lesion: *EWSR1-ATF1* and *EWSR1-CREB*.[57–59]

GROSS FEATURES

As mentioned, the vast majority of CCSs affect the extremities (>90%), with the foot and ankle being the most common locations of involvement. Most CCSs are deep-seated, with involvement of the tendons or aponeuroses. CCS does not typically infiltrate superficially (infrequently into the subcutis and very rarely into the epidermis), a feature that helps differentiate this from true nevocytic/melanocytic proliferations. Tumors are usually small (2–6 cm). The cut surfaces demonstrate lobulated gray-white mass lesions. Necrosis, cystic change, and pigment can be rarely seen macroscopically.

MICROSCOPIC FEATURES

CCS is a proliferation of epithelioid to spindled cells with clear to eosinophilic cytoplasm arranged in a nested to fascicular growth pattern (**Fig. 4**). Nests and short fascicles of tumor cells are typically separated by dense fibrous septa, sometimes with a vague organoid or neuroendocrinelike architectural pattern (see **Fig. 4**A). Other cytologic features include vesicular nuclei and prominent nucleoli (see **Fig. 4**B). Melanin pigment is detectable in approximately 50% of cases, although most often histochemical detection is required for better visualization (eg, Fontana staining). Scattered wreathlike multinucleated giant cells are often seen, which is a characteristic feature of CCS (see **Fig. 4**C). Cytologic atypia is usually mild. Rarely, CCS may demonstrate more marked cytologic pleomorphism and brisk mitotic activity, findings that are more frequent in recurrent or metastatic disease.[60] Mitoses are usually low (usually <4 per 10 high-power fields [HPFs]). Necrosis may be seen but is an uncommon finding.

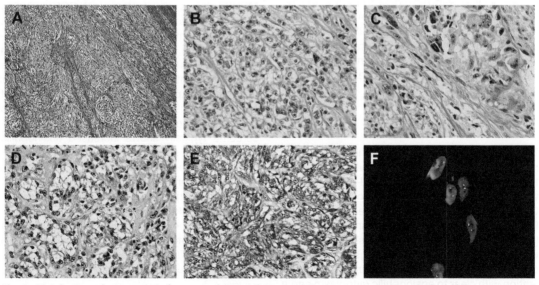

Fig. 4. Histologic and cytogenetic features of CCS. (*A*) Nests of clear to eosinophilic spindled cells are observed, separated by intervening fibrous septa (×100). (*B*) Tumor shows demonstrate ovoid nuclei with pinpoint nucleoli, clear to eosinophilic cytoplasm and well-defined cytoplasmic borders (×400). (*C*) Multinucleated giant cells are usually identified (×400). (*D*) S100 immunohistochemical staining (×400). (*E*) HMB45 immunohistochemical staining (×400). (*F*) Break-apart FISH probe for the EWSR1 locus confirms rearrangement in the *EWSR1* gene (separation of gene and red signals confirms monoallelic gene rearrangement).

DIAGNOSIS

The diagnosis of CCS is first suggested by the architectural and cytologic features previously described, including a spindled to epithelioid proliferation of cells in a nested and fascicular growth pattern. Other helpful diagnostic features include the presence of melanin pigment (as detected by histochemical or immunohistochemical stains), foci of wreathlike multinucleated giant cells, and presence of fibrous septa that separate tumor nests. The history or gross appearance of a lesion involving the tendon or aponeuroses would favor CCS. Conversely, the presence of an intraepithelial tumor component would strongly argue against a diagnosis of CCS.

The immunophenotype of CCS is notable for expression of melanocytic markers in nearly all cases. This includes S100 protein (see **Fig. 4**D), HMB45 (see **Fig. 4**E), MelanA, and microphthalmia-associated transcription factor. Immunoreactivity for NSE, synaptophysin, and CD57 have been described, as well as occasional positivity for cytokeratins or actin.

Electron microscopy, although not usually performed, demonstrates various stages of melanosomes.[61,62] However, the detection of melanosomes is generally not diagnostically useful, as the differential typically includes other tumors with melanocytic differentiation.

As mentioned, recurrent cytogenetic aberrancies are the hallmark of CCS,[57,58,63,64] and most tumors are associated with reciprocal t(12;22) (q13;q12) translocation resulting in EWSR1-ATF1 fusions. A small subset bears the EWSR1-CREB1 fusion, resulting from a t(2;22) (q33;q12) translocation. In the appropriate histopathologic context, a positive FISH for EWSR1 rearrangement is essentially diagnostic of CCS (see **Fig. 4**F).

DIFFERENTIAL DIAGNOSIS

The main differential includes other benign and malignant tumors with melanocytic differentiation. Cellular blue nevi are dermal-based lesions with smaller pinpoint nucleoli in comparison with CCS and do not harbor EWSR1 rearrangements. Paragangliomalike dermal melanocytic tumor (PDMT) is a very rare entity that shares features with CCS, including the histologic appearance of a monomorphic, low-grade, spindle-cell proliferation with clear to eosinophilic cytoplasm and a nested architecture. Unlike CCS, PDMT is typically dermal-based, lacks melanin pigment, and does not demonstrate translocations involving EWSR1.[65] Malignant melanoma should be suspected in the setting of a personal clinical history, significant cytologic atypia/pleomorphism, high mitotic activity, or cytogenetic studies demonstrating aneuploidy rather than the specific translocations of involving EWSR1.

CCS-like tumor of the gastrointestinal tract (CCSLTGT) is a very rare entity with histologic and genetic overlap with CCS of soft tissue. CCSLTGT demonstrates identical cytogenetic aberrancies as CCS, including EWSR1-ATF1 and EWSR1-CREB1 fusion genes (although their relative frequencies differ).[66] In fact, it is unclear if CCSLTGT is an unusual and rare variant of CCS or a distinct entity altogether.[67] However, clear differences between the 2 entities exist. First and foremost, CCSLTGT is defined by its visceral location in comparison with CCS, which involves tendons and aponeuroses of the distal extremities. CCSLTGT expresses S100, but most are negative for other melanocytic markers and have little or no melanin production.[66] In addition, a large fraction of CCSLTGT demonstrate a prominent component of osteoclastic giant cells.[68] Finally, it appears that CCSLTGT demonstrates a relatively poorer prognosis with frequent lymph node and liver metastases.[68,69]

Other mesenchymal spindled neoplasms share some overlap with CCS, including MPNST, leiomyosarcoma, fibrosarcoma, and synovial sarcoma. However, the histologic appearance in conjunction with immunophenotype should readily distinguish these entities from CCS. Although MPNST shares some features with CCS, including melanin production and S100 immunoreactivity, tumor cells demonstrate increased cytologic pleomorphism and increased mitoses in comparison with CCS. As well, MPNST does not feature neoplastic giant cells, generally shows focal rather than diffuse expression of S100 protein, does not express other melanocytic markers, and lacks the cytogenetic aberrations of CCS.[13] Leiomyosarcoma typically shows increased eosinophilic cytoplasm and smooth muscle marker immunoreactivity, whereas CCS does not. Monophasic synovial sarcoma lacks the characteristic clear cytoplasm seen in CCS, and shows immunoreactivity to cytokeratins and EMA. Cytogenetic studies also help distinguish synovial sarcoma from CCS. With the exception of S100 protein seen in MPNST, all of these tumors are typically negative for melanocytic markers.

PROGNOSIS

CCS is a rare entity, and therefore clinical data are relatively limited by small sample size. However in aggregate, the clinical behavior of CCS is that of a high-grade sarcoma.[61,70–72] Local recurrence rates range from 14% to 39%. Metastases to lymph nodes, lungs, or bone occur in 30% to 50% of cases. Indicators of poor prognosis include large tumor size (>5 cm), and the presence of necrosis.[61,70] Surgical excision is the primary modality of treatment with or without radiotherapy, whereas chemotherapy has little proven efficacy.[73] Given the relatively frequent occurrence of lymph node metastasis, sentinel lymph node biopsy may have some role in the management of CCS.[74] Late metastatic spread is typical for CCS, and indefinite clinical follow-up is generally recommended.

Pathologic Key Features

- Most common in the distal lower extremities of young adults, in association with tendon or aponeuroses

- Compact nests and fascicles of spindled to epithelioid cells with clear cytoplasm

- Multinucleated tumor giant cells are a distinguishing feature

- Melanocytic markers are universally present, whereas melanin pigment may be present (~50%)

- Characteristic *EWSR1* translocations, most commonly *EWSR1-ATF1* fusion resulting from t(12;22)

Differential Diagnosis

- Melanocytic Neoplasms
  - Cellular blue nevus
  - Paragangliomalike dermal melanocytic tumor
  - Malignant melanoma
- Spindled Mesenchymal Neoplasms
  - Clear cell sarcoma-like tumor of the gastrointestinal tract (CCSLTGT)
  - Malignant peripheral nerve sheath tumor (MPNST)
  - Monophasic synovial sarcoma
  - Leiomyosarcoma

Pitfalls

! CCS is only one of many tumors with melanin and melanocytic differentiation (see differential diagnosis table)

! A diagnosis of CCS should be cautioned in the context of a high mitotic index, significant cytologic pleomorphism, or aneuploidy

! Although histologically distinct, CCS shares the same cytogenetic translocation with angiomatoid fibrous histiocytoma

! Clear cell sarcoma-like of the gastrointestinal tract (CCSLTGT) demonstrates the same cytogenetic aberrancies as CCS of soft tissue, but with a more aggressive clinical course

OSSIFYING FIBROMYXOID TUMOR

OFMT is a soft tissue tumor of uncertain mesenchymal lineage that most often arises in the subcutaneous tissue of the extremities (70% of cases) in adult men (mean age approximately 50 years). Less common sites include the trunk, head and neck, and deep sites such as the retroperitoneum or mediastinum.[75–78] Some of these tumors may be long-standing; in one series, tumors had been present for more than 10 years before initial excision in approximately 10% of patients.[75]

The original description of OFMT by Enzinger and colleagues[76] in 1989 emphasized bland morphology; however, subsequent reports described OFMTs with atypical or frankly malignant histologic features.[77–81] Although most OFMTs pursue a benign clinical course, these are similar to solitary fibrous tumors in that rare histologically bland tumors can recur or metastasize and not all OFMTs with atypical or malignant features are clinically aggressive.

A variety of cytogenetic abnormalities have been described.[77,82–84] Recent work has identified different rearrangements of the PHF1 gene on chromosome 6p21 in approximately 50% of typical, atypical, and malignant OFMTs.[85,86]

GROSS FEATURES

OFMTs usually measure 3 to 5 cm, although tumors larger than 20 cm have been reported. Grossly, tumors typically are well circumscribed and lobulated or multinodular and surrounded by a thick fibrous pseudocapsule. Cut section shows a tan-white, gritty tumor, occasionally with a grossly visible rim of bone.[75–78]

MICROSCOPIC FEATURES

Characteristic microscopic features are a well-circumscribed, often multinodular tumor, a thick fibrous pseudocapsule (Fig. 5A), an incomplete peripheral rim of mature lamellar bone (see Fig. 5B), and uniform epithelioid tumor cells arranged in cords and nests in a fibromyxoid matrix (see Fig. 5C). A rim of bone is present in approximately 70% of all cases. The bone may be just below or inside of the fibrous pseudocapsule and at times extends into the tumor itself (see Fig. 5D). Intratumoral calcification may be seen and rarely cartilage is present. Lesional cells are uniform and epithelioid, round, or ovoid and usually are present in cords or nests and rarely in sheets. The background stroma may be predominantly collagenous or myxoid, but most OFMTs show a fibromyxoid matrix. Mitoses are very rare in typical OFMTs, less than 2 per 50 HPFs (see later in this article). Satellite tumor nodules may be present and often show a fibrous pseudocapsule as well.[75–78,80]

Various atypical or malignant histologic features have been described in OFMTs.[77–81] In a series of 70 cases of OFMTs, Folpe and Weiss[77] proposed criteria for malignant OFMTs, which included increased cellularity or marked nuclear pleomorphism AND increased mitoses (>2/50 HPFs). Their article defines atypical OFMTs as showing any atypical feature without meeting criteria for malignant OFMT and note that atypical/malignant OFMTs retain many classic features, such as a lobulated/multinodular architecture, cellular arrangement in cords or nests, and a fibromyxoid matrix.[77] The existence of atypical/malignant histologic features in OFMTs and their prognostic significance remains controversial.[75] This is discussed further, later in this article.

OFMTs are positive for S100 (60%–90%+ of cases). S100 staining commonly is patchy in distribution and is less diffuse and weaker than seen in schwannomas. S100 staining is described as diminished in regions of OFMTs that display atypical or malignant features. Reported cases have also showed positive staining for desmin (7%–40% of cases), keratins (10% of cases), SMA (5%), and GFAP (0%–7%).[75–77] One recent large series reported loss of INI1 (SMARCB1) in a mosaic

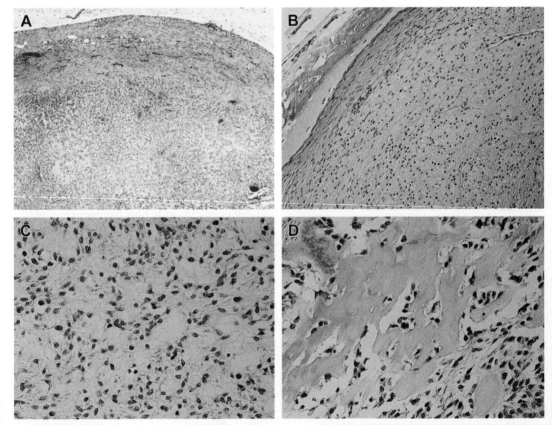

Fig. 5. Histologic features of OMFT. (A) A well-circumscribed tumor with a thick fibrous pseudocapsule (×100). (B) A peripheral rim of lamellar bone is often seen (×200). (C) Lesional cells are uniform, epithelioid, present in cords in a fibromyxoid matrix (×400). (D) In this tumor, lamellar bone was also present within the tumor (×400).

pattern in 70% of cases, which correlated with hemizygous loss of the SMARCB1 locus by FISH.[78]

DIAGNOSIS

The diagnosis of OFMT is straightforward when all the classic features are present. The peripheral shell of mature lamellar bone, in combination with uniform, small, bland cells in nests and cords in a fibromyxoid matrix is particularly helpful. Bone is more commonly seen in typical OFMTs (approximately 75% of cases) compared with atypical/malignant cases (50% of cases). Woven bone or osteoid has been reported in malignant OFMTs and may cause confusion with osteosarcoma.[77,78] Other helpful diagnostic features include the thick fibrous pseudocapsule and the overwhelming tendency to arise in subcutaneous tissues. More deeply seated tumors may be seen within skeletal muscle or adherent to tendons or fascia.

It is unusual for an OFMT to show purely malignant histology. The diagnosis of malignant OFMT is facilitated by areas of typical OFMT within the same tumor, or a history of OFMT at the same site. Atypical/malignant areas have been described to be focal or diffuse and may be discrete foci or merge gradually with more typical OFMT areas.[75–77]

Atypical and malignant OFMTs remain somewhat controversial. Miettinen and colleagues[75] examined a series of 104 OFMTs using very strict criteria for inclusion. Tumors had to show minimal cellular atypia, mainly epithelioid morphology, be lobulated, and have cells in cords and nests in a myxocollagenous matrix. Peripheral metaplastic bone was seen in a subset of cases, but not required. Tumors were not included in the study cohort if they showed high nuclear grade, sheets of cells, extensive spindled morphology, or showed no or minimal extracellular matrix. Using these criteria, no metastases were seen, even in cases with numerous mitoses (mitoses ranged from 0–41 per 50 HPFs). These investigators expressed concern that some previously reported cases of atypical or malignant OFMT may represent other histologically similar tumors in the differential diagnosis (see later in this article).[75]

As mentioned, rearrangements of the PHF1 gene recently have been reported in up to half of all OFMTs.[85,86] A FISH test for rearrangements of the PHF1 gene is commercially available and may be helpful in challenging diagnostic situations.

DIFFERENTIAL DIAGNOSIS

Myoepithelioma/mixed tumor of soft tissues/chondroid syringoma can show many overlapping features with OFMT, including a well-circumscribed mass of low-grade epithelioid cells arranged in cords and nests in a myxoid matrix and location in the dermis/subcutaneous tissues. Bone may be present in approximately 5% of mixed tumors, but usually is not present at the periphery. In contrast to OFMT, mixed tumors often have a myxochondroid or chondroid matrix, 15% to 20% show epithelial (ductal) elements, spindled cells are commonly present, and cartilage also may be seen. Mixed tumors lack the well-defined, fibrous pseudocapsule seen in OFMT, and nests of cells frequently extend into adjacent soft tissues. Unlike OFMT, mixed tumors express epithelial markers (EMA or keratins) in virtually all cases and more than 85% of cases are positive for S100 and calponin as well. OFMTs only rarely coexpress S100 and epithelial markers, and calponin staining has not been reported. Finally, mixed tumors contain either EWSR1 or PLAG1 gene rearrangements.[87–89]

Sclerosing epithelioid fibrosarcoma (SEF) is a clinically aggressive, deep-seated tumor composed of relatively uniform epithelioid cells with scant, cleared out cytoplasm within a densely hyalinized, collagenous stroma. SEF has infiltrative borders and does not typically show a myxochondroid matrix. Mitoses are usually infrequent. Lamellar bone is not seen, although tumoral calcifications may be present. Most cases show at least focal areas with typical fibrosarcoma or low-grade fibromyxoid sarcoma morphology, which can aid in the diagnosis. There is genetic evidence to suggest SEF is related to low-grade fibromyxoid sarcoma, in addition to frequent reports of morphologic overlap between these tumors. EMA is positive in approximately 50% of cases, whereas S100 is only rarely positive. Recently, strong, diffuse MUC4 staining was reported in approximately 80% of SEFs, with only focal staining in 30% of OFMTs.[90] At least half of all patients develop local or distant recurrences, which may not appear for more than 5 years.[90–93]

Low-grade fibromyxoid sarcoma is a deep-seated, infiltrative tumor with a predilection for the lower limb girdle. This tumor primarily is composed of spindled to ovoid cells present in whorls or sheets within a background matrix that varies from myxoid to collagenous. As noted previously, areas of SEF may be admixed with areas of low-grade fibromyxoid sarcoma. Large, rosettelike structures with central eosinophilic collagen rimmed by uniform epithelioid, round, or ovoid cells also can be seen. MUC4 is reported positive in the vast majority of cases, whereas other markers (including S100) are negative. This tumor is characterized by a 7;16 translocation involving the FUS and CREB3L2 genes (more rarely the CREB3L1 gene), which can be identified by commercial FISH probes.[94–99]

Soft tissue masses that produce bone also may be in the differential diagnosis. Although myositis ossificans also shows a peripheral rim of bone, the central lesional cells are spindled and strongly resemble nodular fasciitis, so this generally does not present a diagnostic challenge. Extraskeletal osteosarcoma typically shows features of a high-grade pleomorphic sarcoma with malignant osteoid, and cartilage is often present as well.

PROGNOSIS

OFMTs currently are considered a tumor of intermediate malignant potential.[89] As noted previously, the clinical behavior of OFMTs is difficult to predict. Taking all OFMTs together (histologically typical, atypical, and malignant), local recurrence rates are reported to range from 18% to 22% and distant metastases from 0% to 16%. Histologically typical OFMTs may recur (up to 27%) or metastasize (0%–25%), although these numbers may be somewhat inflated due to consultation bias. Interestingly, atypical OFMTs have similar rates of recurrence and metastasis as typical OFMTs. Malignant OFMTs in the large series reported by Folpe and Weiss[77] showed a greater propensity for both local recurrences (86%) and metastasis (86%). Recurrences have been reported to occur decades after the initial presentation, including 1 patient who experienced 3 local recurrences over 57 years.[75–77]

Miettinen and colleagues,[75] using a strict, classic definition of OFMT, did not find any distant metastases in a large series of 104 patients with OFMTs. Approximately 40% of the tumors in their series showed more than 2 mitoses per 50 HPFs, thus meeting criteria for "malignant" OFMT as proposed by Folpe and Weiss.[77] This study did confirm that mitoses greater than 2 per 50 HPFs was associated with an increased likelihood of local recurrence. Although retaining the term "malignant OFMT," these investigators expressed concern that OFMTs with obvious histologic features of malignancy are more likely to represent other tumors in the differential diagnosis with known metastatic potential, such as malignant mixed tumor/myoepithelioma of soft tissue, sclerosing fibrosarcoma, low-grade fibromyxoid sarcoma, and extraskeletal osteosarcoma.[75]

It is important to remember that not all OFMTs with atypical or malignant features follow an aggressive clinical course, and entirely typical OFMTs have been reported to recur or metastasize. Local or distant recurrences may occur years or even decades after primary resection. Elevated mitoses (>2 per 50 HPFs) in several series are the only consistent feature associated with recurrences or metastases.[75,77]

Pathologic Key Features

- Peripheral rim of lamellar bone in 70% of cases
- Uniform cells, which may be round, ovoid, or spindled and have scant cytoplasm
- Most (70%) located in subcutaneous tissue
- Grossly well circumscribed, multinodular/lobulated, with thick fibrous pseudocapsule
- Malignant features are increased cellularity or marked nuclear pleomorphism AND mitoses greater than 2 per 50 HPFs
- Atypical features are anything other than typical OFMT that does not meet criteria for malignant OFMT

Differential Diagnosis

- Sclerosing epithelioid fibrosarcoma
- Low-grade fibromyxoid sarcoma
- Myoepithelioma/mixed tumor/chondroid syringoma
- Extraskeletal osteosarcoma

Pitfalls

! A diagnosis of OFMT should be cautioned in the context of marked pleomorphism, sheets of tumor cells, absence of S100 staining, or infiltrative margins.

! Although characteristic, the presence of lamellar bone is not required for a diagnosis of OFMT.

! Positivity in lesional cells for epithelial markers in addition to S100 or positivity for MUC4 should raise consideration of myoepithelioma/mixed tumor/chondroid syringoma, low-grade fibromyxoid sarcoma, or sclerosing epithelioid fibrosarcoma.

! Although mitoses greater than 2 per 50 HPFs is associated with local recurrences, and in some series distant metastases, prognosis currently cannot be accurately predicted by histologic features alone.

MALIGNANT EXTRARENAL RHABDOID TUMOR

Malignant rhabdoid tumors (MRTs) were first identified among tumors from the First National Wilms Tumor Study. In 1978, Beckwith and Palmer described a "rhabdomyosarcomatoid variant of Wilm's tumor" in the kidney; however, ensuing studies established MRT as a distinct clinicopathologic entity.[100,101] Tumors with an identical rhabdoid morphology subsequently were identified throughout the body, particularly in the central nervous system (CNS), where they are called "atypical teratoid/rhabdoid tumor." Renal and CNS MRTs are tumors of infancy and childhood; approximately 50% of renal MRTs arise in infants younger than 1 year, with virtually all CNS and renal tumors present by the age of 5 years.[101,102] Tumors reported as soft tissue MRTs have spanned a much wider age range, however, it is not certain if all reported adult cases are bona fide MRTs (see later in this article).

More recently, mutations in or deletions of the SMARCB1/INI1 gene on chromosome 22q have been found in the vast majority of MRTs at renal and extrarenal locations. This corresponds to loss of INI1 staining by immunohistochemistry.[102–108] A subset of patients with MRT have germline SMARCB1/INI1 mutations/deletions; these patients tend to develop widespread MRTs as infants and succumb rapidly.[107,109] However, not all patients with germline INI1 mutations develop MRTs,[102] and germline mutations also may be seen in patients with schwannomatosis.[110,111]

MERTs of soft tissue have been described at most anatomic sites, with a predilection for deep axial locations, including the trunk, neck, and paraspinal region. These are rare tumors.[112] Study of MERT has been complicated because many diverse tumors, including carcinomas, melanomas, different sarcomas, and mesotheliomas may show rhabdoid morphology.[112–114] Some have used the term "composite extrarenal rhabdoid tumor" or CERT, to describe a tumor consisting of a distinct "parent" neoplasm (such as a mesothelioma or a melanoma or a rhabdomyosarcoma) with marked rhabdoid change.[115] CERTs are not true MERTs, as is supported by an absence of SMARCB1/INI1 mutations by FISH and/or intact INI1 expression by immunohistochemistry in cases of CERT.[116,117] Overall, it is believed that many published examples of MERT in adults in fact represent CERT, particularly in cases reported before the widespread availability of immunohistochemistry or molecular testing.

Currently, the diagnosis of soft tissue MERT is restricted to tumors with classic MRT histology, including a predominant rhabdoid morphology, without any other evident lines of differentiation. SMARCB1/INI1 mutations/deletions should be present in the vast majority of soft tissue MERTs.[89]

GROSS FEATURES

MERTs average 5 to 7 cm in maximal diameter, although examples up to 25 cm have been reported.[112] Renal MRTs are slightly larger on average (9 cm).[101] The cut surface is fleshy, gray-tan, and soft. Foci of necrosis and hemorrhage are often present.[101,112]

MICROSCOPIC FEATURES

MRTs are characterized by large, polygonal to epithelioid cells with eccentric and vacuolated nuclei, a large prominent nucleolus, and paranuclear cytoplasmic inclusions (**Fig. 6**A–C). Tumor cells are present in discohesive sheets or clusters, although may show nests as well. A high mitotic rate is typical. The cytoplasmic inclusions are PAS positive, diastase resistant, and also may stain positive for vimentin, cytokeratins, and EMA.[101,112] By electron microscopy, the paranuclear inclusions

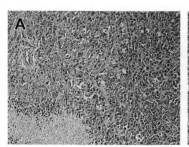 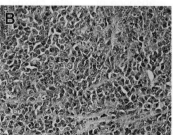 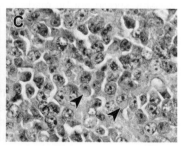

Fig. 6. Histologic features of MERT. (*A*) Sheets of large, polygonal, epithelioid tumor cells with necrosis (×200). (*B*) Higher power demonstrates the rhabdoid morphology and large, prominent nucleolus (×400). (*C*) High magnification demonstrates intracytoplasmic inclusions (*arrowheads*, ×1000).

have been demonstrated to consist of intermediate filaments 6 to 10 nm in diameter present in whorls and compact bundles.[118]

INI1 is consistently lost by immunohistochemistry, which can aid in the differential diagnosis.[103,108] Although ES also shows INI1 loss, INI1 is present in other sarcomas that can show rhabdoid morphology, such as rhabdomyosarcoma, Ewing sarcoma, desmoplastic small round cell sarcoma, clear-cell sarcoma, and Wilms tumor.[103] Although INI1 may be lost in some salivary mixed tumors/myoepitheliomas, this has only very rarely been reported in the large number of other tumors that may be in the differential diagnosis.[14] MERTs, in addition to being positive for vimentin, cytokeratins, and EMA, also have less frequently been reported to be positive for muscle actins, synaptophysin, S100, CD57, and CD99.[101,112]

DIAGNOSIS

In infants and children, this diagnosis usually is straightforward, particularly in the setting of classic histology and the absence of INI1 staining. In adults, care is required to exclude the more common possibility of a carcinoma, melanoma, mesothelioma, or other sarcoma with a prominent rhabdoid appearance (so-called "CERT").

As noted, loss of INI1 staining is very helpful, as this is characteristic of MERT and with the exception of ES and salivary mixed tumor/myoepithelioma, not reported in other tumors in the differential diagnosis. Additional immunohistochemistry should be interpreted with caution, as other tumors in the differential diagnosis may show positive staining for immunostains reported to be positive in MERT, including cytokeratins, EMA, S100, muscle actins, and CD99.

Extensive sectioning may be required to demonstrate the underlying primary tumor in a CERT. If INI1 is intact by immunohistochemistry, and there is no molecular evidence of *SMARCB1/INI1* gene mutation/deletion, a diagnosis of MERT probably should not be made in the absence of expert soft tissue pathologist consultation and confirmation.

DIFFERENTIAL DIAGNOSIS

As noted previously, the differential diagnosis is broad, particularly in adults, because of the diverse tumor types that can show rhabdoid morphology. In a pediatric kidney tumor, the differential diagnosis would include Wilms tumor, congenital mesonephric nephroma, and RCC, whereas in the same location in adults, a renal clear cell carcinoma or urothelial carcinoma would be more likely.[101,114]

Many other types of sarcoma have been reported to show rhabdoid morphology and are in the differential diagnosis. These include rhabdomyosarcoma, ES, extraskeletal myxoid chondrosarcoma, epithelioid MPNST, leiomyosarcoma, synovial sarcoma, and desmoplastic small round cell tumor (DSRCT). These tumors, other than rhabdomyosarcoma, are all very rare in children younger than 5 years. With the exception of ES and some examples of extraskeletal myxoid chondrosarcoma and epithelioid MPNST, INI1 has not been reported to be lost in other forms of sarcoma, and thus represents a key stain to be performed whenever MERT is being considered.[103,108,119] As noted previously, other immunostains reported positive in MERT are frequently positive in tumors in the differential diagnosis and thus are less helpful. Rhabdomyosarcomas are positive for myogenin, which has not been reported in MERT. Although rare rhabdoid variants of rhabdomyosarcoma have been reported, most rhabdomyosarcomas show very different cytomorphology from MERT, being composed of small blue cells with scant cytoplasm.

FISH or other molecular studies can be very helpful for confirming the diagnosis of synovial sarcoma (t[X;18], involving the *SYT* and one of the *SSX* genes), DSRCT (t[11;22], involving the *EWSR1* and *WT1* genes), or alveolar rhabdomyosarcoma (t[2;13] or t[1;13], involving the *FOXO1* and either *PAX3* or *PAX7* genes). The differential diagnosis of MERT and ES was discussed previously, in the section on ES.

Extraskeletal myxoid chondrosarcoma typically shows different morphology from MERT, with multiple lobules of ovoid tumor cells within a myxoid stroma in cords, strands, or pseudoacini. Some tumors are hypercellular and are referred to as the "cellular variant of extracellular myxoid chondrosarcoma" and others may show prominent rhabdoid features; these latter 2 variants can be confused with MERT. Typical features of extraskeletal myxoid chondrosarcoma are often seen in other sections. In diagnostically challenging cases, FISH for *EWSR1* or *NR4A3* can be helpful, as the vast majority of extraskeletal myxoid chondrosarcomas show a translocation involving these genes.

Epithelioid MPNST comprises fewer than 5% of all MPNSTs and often involves major nerves. This usually has a marked nested growth pattern, unlike the discohesive sheets seen in MERT. S100 stain is characteristically strongly and diffusely positive, which has not been reported in MERT.

PROGNOSIS

MRTs of the kidney arise in infancy or childhood with a predilection for males; in one large study, approximately 50% occurred in infants younger than 1 year and only 3% in patients older than 5 years.[101] These are highly aggressive neoplasms that result in death in most patients shortly after initial diagnosis. Lesions that present with widespread metastatic disease are particularly aggressive.[101] Atypical teratoid/rhabdoid tumors of the central nervous system also present predominantly in infants or young children and are similarly aggressive.[120] The only series of soft tissue MERTs is a 1989 article from the armed forces institute of pathology (AFIP). This study found an average age of diagnosis of 13 years (range 6 months–56 years) and 60% of patients died of disease, usually within 2 years of diagnosis.[112] These tumors have not responded to traditional therapies and, regardless of anatomic location, are all considered highly aggressive tumors.

Pathologic Key Features

- Large epithelioid cells with rhabdoid morphology, abundant eosinophilic cytoplasm, and eccentric, vesicular nuclei with prominent nucleoli

- Juxta-nuclear hyaline, PAS-positive eosinophilic globules/inclusions

- INI1 loss by immunohistochemistry (IHC) (corresponding to mutation or homozygous deletion of the *SMARCB1* gene) is characteristically seen

Differential Diagnosis

- Carcinoma with rhabdoid features

- Melanoma with rhabdoid features

- Meningioma with rhabdoid features

- Mesothelioma with rhabdoid features

- Various sarcomas, including epithelioid sarcoma, epithelioid MPNST, and rhabdomyosarcoma

Pitfalls

! Cells with rhabdoid morphology may be seen in a wide array of tumors, including carcinomas, melanomas, mesothelioma, various sarcomas, and meningioma.

! Extensive sectioning may be required to identify a distinct primary tumor (eg, a renal cell carcinoma) in a tumor with extensive rhabdoid morphology.

! Both MERT and carcinomas are positive for cytokeratins and EMA.

! Loss of INI1 staining is also seen in epithelioid sarcoma and in some cases of epithelioid MPNST and extraskeletal myxoid chondrosarcoma.

ACKNOWLEDGMENTS

The authors thank G. Asatrian, A.S. James, and G. LaChaud for their excellent technical assistance.

REFERENCES

1. Enzinger FM. Epithelioid sarcoma. A sarcoma simulating a granuloma or a carcinoma. Cancer 1970; 26:1029–41.
2. Chase DR, Enzinger FM. Epithelioid sarcoma. Diagnosis, prognostic indicators, and treatment. Am J Surg Pathol 1985;9:241–63.
3. Prat J, Woodruff JM, Marcove RC. Epithelioid sarcoma: an analysis of 22 cases indicating the prognostic significance of vascular invasion and regional lymph node metastasis. Cancer 1978;41: 1472–87.
4. Kodet R, Smelhaus V, Newton WA Jr, et al. Epithelioid sarcoma in childhood: an immunohistochemical, electron microscopic, and clinicopathologic study of 11 cases under 15 years of age and review of the literature. Pediatr Pathol 1994;14:433–51.
5. Guillou L, Wadden C, Coindre JM, et al. "Proximal-type" epithelioid sarcoma, a distinctive aggressive neoplasm showing rhabdoid features. Clinicopathologic, immunohistochemical, and ultrastructural study of a series. Am J Surg Pathol 1997;21:130–46.
6. Hasegawa T, Matsuno Y, Shimoda T, et al. Proximal-type epithelioid sarcoma: a clinicopathologic study of 20 cases. Mod Pathol 2001;14:655–63.
7. Chbani L, Guillou L, Terrier P, et al. Epithelioid sarcoma: a clinicopathologic and immunohistochemical analysis of 106 cases from the French sarcoma group. Am J Clin Pathol 2009;131:222–7.

8. Fisher C. Epithelioid sarcoma of Enzinger. Adv Anat Pathol 2006;13:114–21.

9. Mirra JM, Kessler S, Bhuta S, et al. The fibroma-like variant of epithelioid sarcoma. A fibrohistiocytic/myoid cell lesion often confused with benign and malignant spindle cell tumors. Cancer 1992;69:1382–95.

10. Miettinen M, Fanburg-Smith JC, Virolainen M, et al. Epithelioid sarcoma: an immunohistochemical analysis of 112 classical and variant cases and a discussion of the differential diagnosis. Hum Pathol 1999;30:934–42.

11. Lin L, Skacel M, Sigel JE, et al. Epithelioid sarcoma: an immunohistochemical analysis evaluating the utility of cytokeratin 5/6 in distinguishing superficial epithelioid sarcoma from spindled squamous cell carcinoma. J Cutan Pathol 2003;30:114–7.

12. Miettinen M, Wang Z, Sarlomo-Rikala M, et al. ERG expression in epithelioid sarcoma: a diagnostic pitfall. Am J Surg Pathol 2013;37:1580–5.

13. Folpe AL. Selected topics in the pathology of epithelioid soft tissue tumors. Mod Pathol 2014;27(Suppl 1):S64–79.

14. Hollmann TJ, Hornick JL. INI1-deficient tumors: diagnostic features and molecular genetics. Am J Surg Pathol 2011;35:e47–63.

15. Hornick JL, Fletcher CD. Pseudomyogenic hemangioendothelioma: a distinctive, often multicentric tumor with indolent behavior. Am J Surg Pathol 2011;35:190–201.

16. Ogino S, Ro TY, Redline RW. Malignant rhabdoid tumor: a phenotype? An entity?–A controversy revisited. Adv Anat Pathol 2000;7:181–90.

17. Hornick JL, Dal Cin P, Fletcher CD. Loss of INI1 expression is characteristic of both conventional and proximal-type epithelioid sarcoma. Am J Surg Pathol 2009;33:542–50.

18. Kohashi K, Oda Y, Yamamoto H, et al. SMARCB1/INI1 protein expression in round cell soft tissue sarcomas associated with chromosomal translocations involving EWS: a special reference to SMARCB1/INI1 negative variant extraskeletal myxoid chondrosarcoma. Am J Surg Pathol 2008;32:1168–74.

19. Riad S, Griffin AM, Liberman B, et al. Lymph node metastasis in soft tissue sarcoma in an extremity. Clin Orthop Relat Res 2004;(426):129–34.

20. Fong Y, Coit DG, Woodruff JM, et al. Lymph node metastasis from soft tissue sarcoma in adults. Analysis of data from a prospective database of 1772 sarcoma patients. Ann Surg 1993;217:72–7.

21. Christopherson WM, Foote FW Jr, Stewart FW. Alveolar soft-part sarcomas; structurally characteristic tumors of uncertain histogenesis. Cancer 1952;5:100–11.

22. Ladanyi M, Lui MY, Antonescu CR, et al. The der(17)t(X;17)(p11;q25) of human alveolar soft part sarcoma fuses the TFE3 transcription factor gene to ASPL, a novel gene at 17q25. Oncogene 2001;20:48–57.

23. Portera CA Jr, Ho V, Patel SR, et al. Alveolar soft part sarcoma: clinical course and patterns of metastasis in 70 patients treated at a single institution. Cancer 2001;91:585–91.

24. Lieberman PH, Brennan MF, Kimmel M, et al. Alveolar soft-part sarcoma. A clinico-pathologic study of half a century. Cancer 1989;63:1–13.

25. Fanburg-Smith JC, Miettinen M, Folpe AL, et al. Lingual alveolar soft part sarcoma; 14 cases: novel clinical and morphological observations. Histopathology 2004;45:526–37.

26. Font RL, Jurco S 3rd, Zimmerman LE. Alveolar soft-part sarcoma of the orbit: a clinicopathologic analysis of seventeen cases and a review of the literature. Hum Pathol 1982;13:569–79.

27. Zhang LL, Tang Q, Wang Z, et al. Alveolar soft part sarcoma of the uterine corpus with pelvic lymph node metastasis: case report and literature review. Int J Clin Exp Pathol 2012;5:715–9.

28. Flieder DB, Moran CA, Suster S. Primary alveolar soft-part sarcoma of the mediastinum: a clinicopathological and immunohistochemical study of two cases. Histopathology 1997;31:469–73.

29. Trabelsi A, Ben Abdelkrim S, Taher Yacoubi M, et al. Primary alveolar soft part sarcoma of the lung. Rev Mal Respir 2009;26:329–32 [in French].

30. Kim YD, Lee CH, Lee MK, et al. Primary alveolar soft part sarcoma of the lung. J Korean Med Sci 2007;22:369–72.

31. Yaziji H, Ranaldi R, Verdolini R, et al. Primary alveolar soft part sarcoma of the stomach: a case report and review. Pathol Res Pract 2000;196:519–25.

32. Das KK, Singh RK, Jaiswal S, et al. Alveolar soft part sarcoma of the frontal calvarium and adjacent frontal lobe. J Pediatr Neurosci 2012;7:36–9.

33. Setsu N, Yoshida A, Takahashi F, et al. Histological analysis suggests an invasion-independent metastatic mechanism in alveolar soft part sarcoma. Hum Pathol 2014;45:137–42.

34. Khanna P, Paidas CN, Gilbert-Barness E. Alveolar soft part sarcoma: clinical, histopathological, molecular, and ultrastructural aspects. Fetal Pediatr Pathol 2008;27:31–40.

35. Shipkey FH, Lieberman PH, Foote FW Jr, et al. Ultrastructure of alveolar soft part sarcoma. Cancer 1964;17:821–30.

36. Evans HL. Alveolar soft-part sarcoma. A study of 13 typical examples and one with a histologically atypical component. Cancer 1985;55:912–7.

37. Folpe AL. MyoD1 and myogenin expression in human neoplasia: a review and update. Adv Anat Pathol 2002;9:198–203.

38. Wang NP, Bacchi CE, Jiang JJ, et al. Does alveolar soft-part sarcoma exhibit skeletal muscle

differentiation? An immunocytochemical and biochemical study of myogenic regulatory protein expression. Mod Pathol 1996;9:496–506.

39. Gomez JA, Amin MB, Ro JY, et al. Immunohistochemical profile of myogenin and MyoD1 does not support skeletal muscle lineage in alveolar soft part sarcoma. Arch Pathol Lab Med 1999; 123:503–7.

40. Argani P, Lal P, Hutchinson B, et al. Aberrant nuclear immunoreactivity for TFE3 in neoplasms with TFE3 gene fusions: a sensitive and specific immunohistochemical assay. Am J Surg Pathol 2003;27: 750–61.

41. Schoolmeester JK, Howitt BE, Hirsch MS, et al. Perivascular epithelioid cell neoplasm (PEComa) of the gynecologic tract: clinicopathologic and immunohistochemical characterization of 16 cases. Am J Surg Pathol 2014;38:176–88.

42. Dickson BC, Brooks JS, Pasha TL, et al. TFE3 expression in tumors of the microphthalmia-associated transcription factor (MiTF) family. Int J Surg Pathol 2011;19:26–30.

43. Ordonez NG, Ro JY, Mackay B. Alveolar soft part sarcoma. An ultrastructural and immunocytochemical investigation of its histogenesis. Cancer 1989; 63:1721–36.

44. Tsuda M, Davis IJ, Argani P, et al. TFE3 fusions activate MET signaling by transcriptional up-regulation, defining another class of tumors as candidates for therapeutic MET inhibition. Cancer Res 2007;67: 919–29.

45. Chamberlain BK, McClain CM, Gonzalez RS, et al. Alveolar soft part sarcoma and granular cell tumor: an immunohistochemical comparison study. Hum Pathol 2014;45:1039–44.

46. Hodge JC, Pearce KE, Wang X, et al. Molecular cytogenetic analysis for TFE3 rearrangement in Xp11.2 renal cell carcinoma and alveolar soft part sarcoma: validation and clinical experience with 75 cases. Mod Pathol 2014;27:113–27.

47. Armah HB, Parwani AV. Xp11.2 translocation renal cell carcinoma. Arch Pathol Lab Med 2010;134: 124–9.

48. Ogose A, Morita T, Hotta T, et al. Brain metastases in musculoskeletal sarcomas. Jpn J Clin Oncol 1999;29:245–7.

49. Reichardt P, Lindner T, Pink D, et al. Chemotherapy in alveolar soft part sarcomas. What do we know? Eur J Cancer 2003;39:1511–6.

50. Ogose A, Yazawa Y, Ueda T, et al. Alveolar soft part sarcoma in Japan: multi-institutional study of 57 patients from the Japanese Musculoskeletal Oncology Group. Oncology 2003;65:7–13.

51. Orbach D, Brennan B, Casanova M, et al. Paediatric and adolescent alveolar soft part sarcoma: a joint series from European cooperative groups. Pediatr Blood Cancer 2013;60:1826–32.

52. Enzinger FM. Clear-cell sarcoma of tendons and aponeuroses. An analysis of 21 cases. Cancer 1965;18:1163–74.

53. Bearman RM, Noe J, Kempson RL. Clear cell sarcoma with melanin pigment. Cancer 1975;36: 977–84.

54. Ekfors TO, Rantakokko V. Clear cell sarcoma of tendons and aponeuroses: malignant melanoma of soft tissues? Report of four cases. Pathol Res Pract 1979;165:422–8.

55. Hoffman GJ, Carter D. Clear cell sarcoma of tendons and aponeuroses with melanin. Arch Pathol 1973;95:22–5.

56. Chung EB, Enzinger FM. Malignant melanoma of soft parts. A reassessment of clear cell sarcoma. Am J Surg Pathol 1983;7:405–13.

57. Bridge JA, Borek DA, Neff JR, et al. Chromosomal abnormalities in clear cell sarcoma. Implications for histogenesis. Am J Clin Pathol 1990;93:26–31.

58. Bridge JA, Sreekantaiah C, Neff JR, et al. Cytogenetic findings in clear cell sarcoma of tendons and aponeuroses. Malignant melanoma of soft parts. Cancer Genet Cytogenet 1991;52:101–6.

59. Zucman J, Delattre O, Desmaze C, et al. EWS and ATF-1 gene fusion induced by t(12;22) translocation in malignant melanoma of soft parts. Nat Genet 1993;4:341–5.

60. Hisaoka M, Ishida T, Kuo TT, et al. Clear cell sarcoma of soft tissue: a clinicopathologic, immunohistochemical, and molecular analysis of 33 cases. Am J Surg Pathol 2008;32:452–60.

61. Sara AS, Evans HL, Benjamin RS. Malignant melanoma of soft parts (clear cell sarcoma). A study of 17 cases, with emphasis on prognostic factors. Cancer 1990;65:367–74.

62. Kubo T. Clear-cell sarcoma of patellar tendon studied by electron microscopy. Cancer 1969;24:948–53.

63. Reeves BR, Fletcher CD, Gusterson BA. Translocation t(12;22)(q13;q13) is a nonrandom rearrangement in clear cell sarcoma. Cancer Genet Cytogenet 1992;64:101–3.

64. Fisher C. The diversity of soft tissue tumours with EWSR1 gene rearrangements: a review. Histopathology 2014;64:134–50.

65. Deyrup AT, Althof P, Zhou M, et al. Paraganglioma-like dermal melanocytic tumor: a unique entity distinct from cellular blue nevus, clear cell sarcoma, and cutaneous melanoma. Am J Surg Pathol 2004;28:1579–86.

66. Antonescu CR, Nafa K, Segal NH, et al. EWS-CREB1: a recurrent variant fusion in clear cell sarcoma–association with gastrointestinal location and absence of melanocytic differentiation. Clin Cancer Res 2006;12:5356–62.

67. Kosemehmetoglu K, Folpe AL. Clear cell sarcoma of tendons and aponeuroses, and osteoclast-rich tumour of the gastrointestinal tract with features

resembling clear cell sarcoma of soft parts: a review and update. J Clin Pathol 2010;63:416–23.

68. Yegen G, Gulluoglu M, Mete O, et al. Clear cell sarcoma-like tumor of the gastrointestinal tract: a case report and review of the literature. Int J Surg Pathol 2014;23(1):61–7.

69. Covinsky M, Gong S, Rajaram V, et al. EWS-ATF1 fusion transcripts in gastrointestinal tumors previously diagnosed as malignant melanoma. Hum Pathol 2005;36:74–81.

70. Lucas DR, Nascimento AG, Sim FH. Clear cell sarcoma of soft tissues. Mayo Clinic experience with 35 cases. Am J Surg Pathol 1992;16:1197–204.

71. Ferrari A, Casanova M, Bisogno G, et al. Clear cell sarcoma of tendons and aponeuroses in pediatric patients: a report from the Italian and German Soft Tissue Sarcoma Cooperative Group. Cancer 2002;94:3269–76.

72. Hocar O, Le Cesne A, Berissi S, et al. Clear cell sarcoma (malignant melanoma) of soft parts: a clinicopathologic study of 52 cases. Dermatol Res Pract 2012;2012:984096.

73. Bianchi G, Charoenlap C, Cocchi S, et al. Clear cell sarcoma of soft tissue: a retrospective review and analysis of 31 cases treated at Istituto Ortopedico Rizzoli. Eur J Surg Oncol 2014;40:505–10.

74. Picciotto F, Zaccagna A, Derosa G, et al. Clear cell sarcoma (malignant melanoma of soft parts) and sentinel lymph node biopsy. Eur J Dermatol 2005;15:46–8.

75. Miettinen M, Finnell V, Fetsch JF. Ossifying fibromyxoid tumor of soft parts–a clinicopathologic and immunohistochemical study of 104 cases with long-term follow-up and a critical review of the literature. Am J Surg Pathol 2008;32:996–1005.

76. Enzinger FM, Weiss SW, Liang CY. Ossifying fibromyxoid tumor of soft parts. A clinicopathological analysis of 59 cases. Am J Surg Pathol 1989;13:817–27.

77. Folpe AL, Weiss SW. Ossifying fibromyxoid tumor of soft parts: a clinicopathologic study of 70 cases with emphasis on atypical and malignant variants. Am J Surg Pathol 2003;27:421–31.

78. Graham RP, Dry S, Li X, et al. Ossifying fibromyxoid tumor of soft parts: a clinicopathologic, proteomic, and genomic study. Am J Surg Pathol 2011;35:1615–25.

79. Kilpatrick SE, Ward WG, Mozes M, et al. Atypical and malignant variants of ossifying fibromyxoid tumor. Clinicopathologic analysis of six cases. Am J Surg Pathol 1995;19:1039–46.

80. Zamecnik M, Michal M, Simpson RH, et al. Ossifying fibromyxoid tumor of soft parts: a report of 17 cases with emphasis on unusual histological features. Ann Diagn Pathol 1997;1:73–81.

81. Williams SB, Ellis GL, Meis JM, et al. Ossifying fibromyxoid tumour (of soft parts) of the head and neck: a clinicopathological and immunohistochemical study of nine cases. J Laryngol otology 1993;107:75–80.

82. Kawashima H, Ogose A, Umezu H, et al. Ossifying fibromyxoid tumor of soft parts with clonal chromosomal aberrations. Cancer Genet Cytogenet 2007;176:156–60.

83. Nishio J, Iwasaki H, Ohjimi Y, et al. Ossifying fibromyxoid tumor of soft parts. Cytogenetic findings. Cancer Genet Cytogenet 2002;133:124–8.

84. Sovani V, Velagaleti GV, Filipowicz E, et al. Ossifying fibromyxoid tumor of soft parts: report of a case with novel cytogenetic findings. Cancer Genet Cytogenet 2001;127:1–6.

85. Gebre-Medhin S, Nord KH, Moller E, et al. Recurrent rearrangement of the PHF1 gene in ossifying fibromyxoid tumors. Am J Pathol 2012;181:1069–77.

86. Graham RP, Weiss SW, Sukov WR, et al. PHF1 rearrangements in ossifying fibromyxoid tumors of soft parts: a fluorescence in situ hybridization study of 41 cases with emphasis on the malignant variant. Am J Surg Pathol 2013;37:1751–5.

87. Hornick JL, Fletcher CD. Myoepithelial tumors of soft tissue: a clinicopathologic and immunohistochemical study of 101 cases with evaluation of prognostic parameters. Am J Surg Pathol 2003;27:1183–96.

88. Fletcher CDM, editor. Diagnostic histopathology of tumors. Edinburgh (United Kingdom); New York: Churchill Livingstone; 2007. p. 1992.

89. Goldblum JR, Folpe AL, Weiss SW, et al, editors. Enzinger and Weiss's soft tissue tumors. Philadelphia: Saunders/Elsevier; 2014. p. xiv 1155.

90. Doyle LA, Wang WL, Dal Cin P, et al. MUC4 is a sensitive and extremely useful marker for sclerosing epithelioid fibrosarcoma: association with FUS gene rearrangement. Am J Surg Pathol 2012;36:1444–51.

91. Antonescu CR, Tschernyavsky SJ, Decuseara R, et al. Prognostic impact of P53 status, TLS-CHOP fusion transcript structure, and histological grade in myxoid liposarcoma: a molecular and clinicopathologic study of 82 cases. Clin Cancer Res 2001;7:3977–87.

92. Guillou L, Benhattar J, Gengler C, et al. Translocation-positive low-grade fibromyxoid sarcoma: clinicopathologic and molecular analysis of a series expanding the morphologic spectrum and suggesting potential relationship to sclerosing epithelioid fibrosarcoma: a study from the French Sarcoma Group. Am J Surg Pathol 2007;31:1387–402.

93. Meis-Kindblom JM, Kindblom LG, Enzinger FM. Sclerosing epithelioid fibrosarcoma. A variant of fibrosarcoma simulating carcinoma. Am J Surg Pathol 1995;19:979–93.

94. Evans HL. Low-grade fibromyxoid sarcoma. A report of 12 cases. Am J Surg Pathol 1993;17:595–600.

95. Evans HL. Low-grade fibromyxoid sarcoma: a clinicopathologic study of 33 cases with long-term follow-up. Am J Surg Pathol 2011;35:1450–62.

96. Doyle LA, Moller E, Dal Cin P, et al. MUC4 is a highly sensitive and specific marker for low-grade fibromyxoid sarcoma. Am J Surg Pathol 2011;35:733–41.

97. Folpe AL, Lane KL, Paull G, et al. Low-grade fibromyxoid sarcoma and hyalinizing spindle cell tumor with giant rosettes: a clinicopathologic study of 73 cases supporting their identity and assessing the impact of high-grade areas. Am J Surg Pathol 2000;24:1353–60.

98. Reid R, de Silva MV, Paterson L, et al. Low-grade fibromyxoid sarcoma and hyalinizing spindle cell tumor with giant rosettes share a common t(7;16)(q34;p11) translocation. Am J Surg Pathol 2003;27:1229–36.

99. Mertens F, Fletcher CD, Antonescu CR, et al. Clinicopathologic and molecular genetic characterization of low-grade fibromyxoid sarcoma, and cloning of a novel FUS/CREB3L1 fusion gene. Laboratory Investigation 2005;85:408–15.

100. Beckwith JB, Palmer NF. Histopathology and prognosis of Wilms tumors: results from the First National Wilms' Tumor Study. Cancer 1978;41:1937–48.

101. Weeks DA, Beckwith JB, Mierau GW, et al. Rhabdoid tumor of kidney. A report of 111 cases from the National Wilms' Tumor Study Pathology Center. Am J Surg Pathol 1989;13:439–58.

102. Biegel JA. Molecular genetics of atypical teratoid/rhabdoid tumor. Neurosurg Focus 2006;20:E11.

103. Hoot AC, Russo P, Judkins AR, et al. Immunohistochemical analysis of hSNF5/INI1 distinguishes renal and extra-renal malignant rhabdoid tumors from other pediatric soft tissue tumors. Am J Surg Pathol 2004;28:1485–91.

104. Jackson EM, Shaikh TH, Gururangan S, et al. High-density single nucleotide polymorphism array analysis in patients with germline deletions of 22q11.2 and malignant rhabdoid tumor. Hum Genet 2007;122:117–27.

105. Kohashi K, Oda Y, Yamamoto H, et al. Highly aggressive behavior of malignant rhabdoid tumor: a special reference to SMARCB1/INI1 gene alterations using molecular genetic analysis including quantitative real-time PCR. J Cancer Res Clin Oncol 2007;133:817–24.

106. Judkins AR, Mauger J, Ht A, et al. Immunohistochemical analysis of hSNF5/INI1 in pediatric CNS neoplasms. Am J Surg Pathol 2004;28:644–50.

107. Biegel JA, Tan L, Zhang F, et al. Alterations of the hSNF5/INI1 gene in central nervous system atypical teratoid/rhabdoid tumors and renal and extrarenal rhabdoid tumors. Clin Cancer Res 2002;8:3461–7.

108. Sigauke E, Rakheja D, Maddox DL, et al. Absence of expression of SMARCB1/INI1 in malignant rhabdoid tumors of the central nervous system, kidneys and soft tissue: an immunohistochemical study with implications for diagnosis. Mod Pathol 2006;19:717–25.

109. Jackson EM, Sievert AJ, Gai X, et al. Genomic analysis using high-density single nucleotide polymorphism-based oligonucleotide arrays and multiplex ligation-dependent probe amplification provides a comprehensive analysis of INI1/SMARCB1 in malignant rhabdoid tumors. Clin Cancer Res 2009;15:1923–30.

110. Boyd C, Smith MJ, Kluwe L, et al. Alterations in the SMARCB1 (INI1) tumor suppressor gene in familial schwannomatosis. Clin Genet 2008;74:358–66.

111. Hadfield KD, Newman WG, Bowers NL, et al. Molecular characterisation of SMARCB1 and NF2 in familial and sporadic schwannomatosis. J Med Genet 2008;45:332–9.

112. Fanburg-Smith JC, Hengge M, Hengge UR, et al. Extrarenal rhabdoid tumors of soft tissue: a clinicopathologic and immunohistochemical study of 18 cases. Ann Diagn Pathol 1998;2:351–62.

113. Parham DM, Weeks DA, Beckwith JB. The clinicopathologic spectrum of putative extrarenal rhabdoid tumors. An analysis of 42 cases studied with immunohistochemistry or electron microscopy. Am J Surg Pathol 1994;18:1010–29.

114. Weeks DA, Beckwith JB, Mierau GW, et al. Renal neoplasms mimicking rhabdoid tumor of kidney. A report from the National Wilms' Tumor Study Pathology Center. Am J Surg Pathol 1991;15:1042–54.

115. Wick MR, Ritter JH, Dehner LP. Malignant rhabdoid tumors: a clinicopathologic review and conceptual discussion. Semin Diagn Pathol 1995;12:233–48.

116. Fuller CE, Pfeifer J, Humphrey P, et al. Chromosome 22q dosage in composite extrarenal rhabdoid tumors: clonal evolution or a phenotypic mimic? Hum Pathol 2001;32:1102–8.

117. Perry A, Fuller CE, Judkins AR, et al. INI1 expression is retained in composite rhabdoid tumors, including rhabdoid meningiomas. Mod Pathol 2005;18:951–8.

118. Haas JE, Palmer NF, Weinberg AG, et al. Ultrastructure of malignant rhabdoid tumor of the kidney. A distinctive renal tumor of children. Hum Pathol 1981;12:646–57.

119. Jo VY, Fletcher CD. Epithelioid malignant peripheral nerve sheath tumor: clinicopathologic analysis of 63 cases. Am J Surg Pathol 2015;39(5):673–82.

120. Bikowska B, Grajkowska W, Jozwiak J. Atypical teratoid/rhabdoid tumor: short clinical description and insight into possible mechanism of the disease. Eur J Neurol 2011;18:813–8.

Diagnostically Challenging Epithelioid Vascular Tumors

Jennifer S. Ko, MD, PhD, Steven D. Billings, MD*

KEYWORDS

- Epithelioid hemangioma • Intravascular epithelioid hemangioma
- Cutaneous epithelioid angiomatous nodule • Epithelioid hemangioendothelioma
- Epithelioid sarcoma-like hemangioendothelioma • Pseudomyogenic hemangioendothelioma
- Epithelioid angiosarcoma

ABSTRACT

The diagnosis of vascular tumors is a challenging area in soft tissue pathology. Epithelioid vascular tumors pose a particular challenge. Due to the epithelioid morphology of the tumor cells, they can be misdiagnosed as a variety of other entities, including metastatic carcinoma or epithelioid sarcoma. Furthermore, it can be difficult to distinguish between different epithelioid vascular tumors. This review focuses on vascular tumors characterized by epithelioid endothelial cells, including epithelioid hemangioma, cutaneous epithelioid angiomatous nodule, epithelioid hemangioendothelioma, epithelioid sarcomalike hemangioendothelioma/pseudomyogenic hemangioendothelioma, and epithelioid angiosarcoma.

OVERVIEW

Epithelioid vascular tumors can be particularly diagnostically challenging. The epithelioid cytomorphology is, by nature, somewhat generic and elicits a broad differential diagnosis that often includes carcinoma and melanoma. Furthermore, in many epithelioid vascular tumors, the vascular nature of the neoplasm is difficult to recognize. A range of histologic overlap also exists between different epithelioid vascular tumors, and immunohistochemical markers generally do not help in classifying the different entities. This review focuses on the unique clinicopathologic and molecular features of the most common benign (epithelioid hemangioma and cutaneous epithelioid angiomatous nodule), intermediate (epithelioid hemangioendothelioma and epithelioid sarcoma-like hemangioendothelioma/pseudomyogenic hemangioendothelioma) and malignant (epithelioid angiosarcoma) epithelioid vascular neoplasms.

EPITHELIOID HEMANGIOMA

Epithelioid hemangioma was initially described in 1969 by Wells and Whimster as epithelioid angiomatous hyperplasia with eosinophilia.[1] Epithelioid hemangiomas most commonly present on the head and neck, often in a periauricular location, in middle-aged adults with a female predominance.[2,3] However, a wide range of cutaneous locations may be involved.[4–9] They clinically and grossly appear as small erythematous nodules or plaques, commonly with ulceration or excoriation, and commonly as multiple coalescing lesions. As such, epithelioid hemangiomas are often clinically mistaken for a cyst, capillary hemangioma, or pyogenic granuloma.

Epithelioid hemangioma rarely arises as a purely intravascular tumor. Intravascular epithelioid hemangioma was originally described by Rosai and Ackerman[10] under the name intravascular atypical vascular proliferation. Epithelioid hemangioma also occurs in bone, where it mostly affects long tubular bones and can be multifocal in up to 25% of cases, causing concern for malignancy.[9,11–15]

Histologically, conventional epithelioid hemangiomas are circumscribed, dermal, or subcutaneous, lobular proliferations of well-formed capillaries

Department of Pathology, Cleveland Clinic, 9500 Euclid Avenue, Cleveland, OH 44195, USA
* Corresponding author. Department of Pathology, Cleveland Clinic, 9500 Euclid Avenue, L25, Cleveland, OH 44195.
E-mail address: billins@ccf.org

Surgical Pathology 8 (2015) 331–351
http://dx.doi.org/10.1016/j.path.2015.05.001
1875-9181/15/$ – see front matter © 2015 Elsevier Inc. All rights reserved.

surrounding a larger central vessel. The proliferation is associated with an inflammatory infiltrate of lymphocytes, sometimes with germinal center formation, with admixed eosinophils, histiocytes, and plasma cells (Fig. 1A). Rare giant cells also have been described.[16] In some cases, the brisk nature of the infiltrate can obscure the underlying vascular proliferation at low magnification. The involved capillaries have retained lumina and are lined by epithelioid endothelial cells, which variably hobnail into luminal spaces (see Fig. 1B). Mitotic activity may be seen, but atypical mitotic figures are absent.

Epithelioid hemangiomas also may have relatively solid areas, a diagnostic pitfall. Solid areas may be more common in tumors at certain sites. For instance, intravascular epithelioid hemangiomas tend to be more solid with less obvious vasoformation (Fig. 2A). Intravascular forms also have a less prominent inflammatory infiltrate,

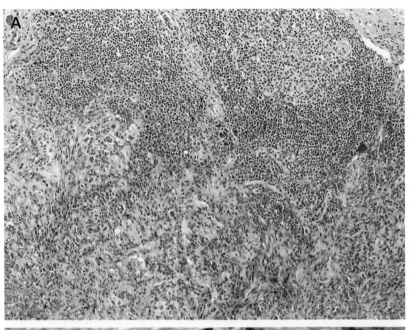

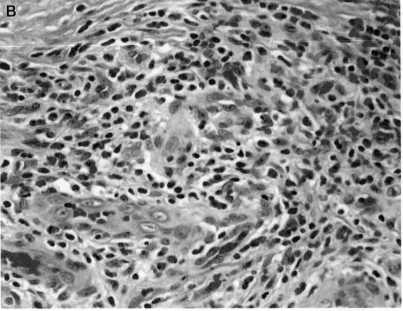

Fig. 1. (A) Epithelioid hemangioma. This tumor is composed of a lobular proliferation of capillaries lined by plump epithelioid endothelial cells with abundant eosinophilic cytoplasm. Typically present is an inflammatory infiltrate with lymphoid aggregates, often with germinal center formation and admixed eosinophils. (B) Epithelioid hemangioma. This high-power image of epithelioid hemangioma illustrates the plump endothelial cells lining the capillaries and numerous admixed eosinophils (Hematoxylin-eosin, original magnification [A] ×100; [B] ×400).

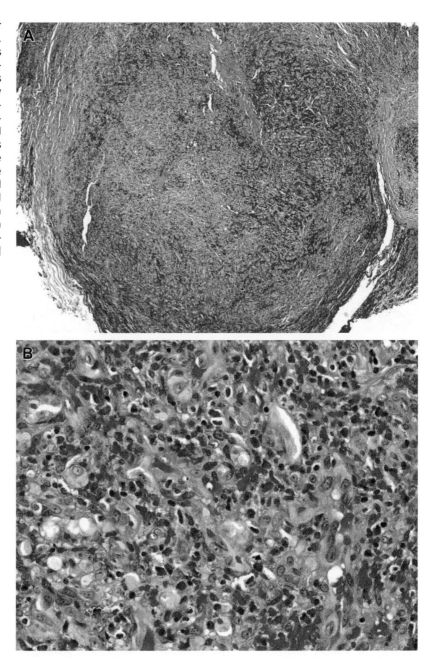

Fig. 2. (*A*) Intravascular epithelioid hemangioma. Intravascular variants are well-circumscribed lesions and have a less prominent inflammatory component. (*B*) Intravascular epithelioid hemangioma. Well-defined vascular channels are less conspicuous, but the endothelial cells have the characteristic epithelioid morphology. Admixed eosinophils are present in association with the lesion (Hematoxylin-eosin, original magnification [*A*] ×40; [*B*] ×200).

though scattered admixed eosinophils are often present (see **Fig. 2**B). Other particular sites with variant histologic features include epithelioid hemangiomas of the penis, which may have a more solid growth pattern, necrosis, and less conspicuous inflammation.[7] It is possible that some of these tumors are pathologically distinct (see later in this article). Epithelioid hemangiomas of bone also may have areas with more solid growth and less inflammation[17] (**Fig. 3**). The tumor cells are positive for vascular markers, including D2-40, but immunoreactivity for keratins and EMA may be seen[18] and is another potential diagnostic pitfall.

The pathogenesis of epithelioid hemangioma is obscure. It has traditionally been thought to possibly represent an unusual reactive process to various stimuli following trauma, infections, arteriovenous shunting, or hyperestrogenemia.[19] More recently, a subset of cases have been shown

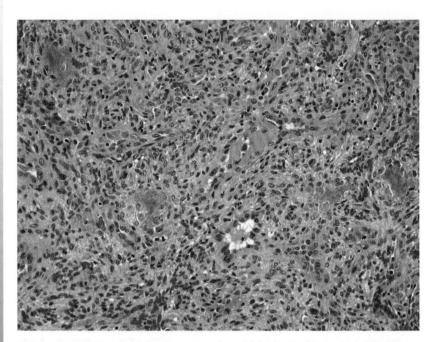

Fig. 3. Epithelioid hemangioma of bone. In this osseous epithelioid hemangioma, the tumor is relatively solid with less obvious multicellular vascular channels (Hematoxylin-eosin, original magnification ×100).

to have a recurring cytogenetic abnormality consisting of a *ZFP36-FOSB* fusion.[20] The epithelioid hemangiomas with this finding were more common on the penis and had atypical features, including solid growth, less inflammation, and necrosis. Conventional epithelioid hemangiomas were not found to have this cytogenetic abnormality, suggesting that what has been collectively described as epithelioid hemangioma may represent a molecularly diverse group of tumors with morphologic overlap.

The differential diagnosis is varied. Epithelioid hemangioma has some overlapping features with Kimura disease. Epithelioid hemangioma has a more prominent vascular proliferation with epithelioid endothelial cells and lacks the associated peripheral eosinophilia and lymphadenopathy of Kimura disease.[21–23] The vascular component of Kimura disease has relatively flattened, attenuated endothelial cells compared with the plumper, often "tomb-stoning" endothelial cells in epithelioid hemangioma.[20,24] The distinct clinical presentation of Kimura disease, including Asian men with lymphadenopathy, peripheral eosinophilia, increased serum immunoglobulin E (IgE), and possibly proteinuria and nephrotic syndrome, also is useful when clinical information is available.

Another reactive skin disease to recently enter into the differential diagnosis with epithelioid hemangioma includes certain manifestations of IgG4-related skin disease,[25–27] especially considering that this disease occurred as periauricular, erythematous nodules and plaques in 9 of 10 patients included in the largest reported series.[27] Histologic findings in this setting show a nodular dermal and subcutaneous inflammatory infiltrate of lymphocytes and plasma cells with numerous eosinophils and lymphoid follicles. Importantly, affected patients usually have extracutaneous disease manifestations, and cutaneous biopsy specimens show 50 or more IgG4+ plasma cells per high power field (HPF), with a ratio of IgG4/IgG plasma cells of 0.6 to 1.0. Conspicuous capillary proliferation is not seen.

Although rarely encountered, bacillary angiomatosis also is in the differential diagnosis. Bacillary angiomatosis, caused by infection with *Bartonella henselae* or *Bartonella quintana*, occurs in immunocompromised patients, especially in the setting of AIDS. It also is characterized by a proliferation of capillaries with epithelioid endothelial cells but with a different inflammatory background of lymphocytes, neutrophils, and histiocytes rather than distinct lymphoid aggregates and eosinophils (**Fig. 4**). Also present in bacillary angiomatosis are collections of amphophilic granular material, representing the infectious microorganisms that can be highlighted with a Warthin-Starry stain.

In cases with a prominent inflammatory infiltrate, the possibility of primary cutaneous follicle center-cell lymphoma is a potential consideration in the

Fig. 4. Bacillary angiomatosis. This potential mimic of epithelioid hemangioma also consists of a proliferation of vessels lined by epithelioid endothelial cells, but neutrophils are a conspicuous component of the associated inflammatory infiltrate (Hematoxylin-eosin, original magnification ×100). (*Courtesy of* Dr Karen Fritchie, MD, Mayo Clinic, Rochester, MN.)

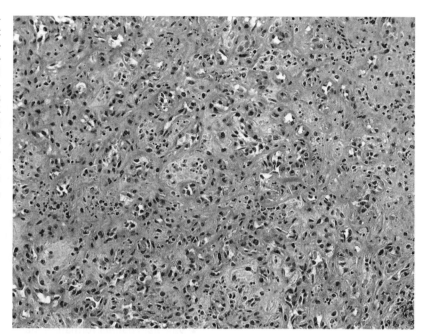

differential diagnosis. Primary cutaneous B-cell lymphomas typically do not have eosinophils as a prominent part of the inflammatory infiltrate and lack the vascular proliferation.

True epithelioid vascular tumors described later in this article are also in the differential diagnosis. Epithelioid hemangiomas with a paucity or lack of eosinophils and mixed spindled and epithelioid growth patterns, as well as intravascular epithelioid hemangiomas, can cause concern for epithelioid hemangioendothelioma. Additionally, distinction of osseous epithelioid hemangiomas from epithelioid hemangioendotheliomas may be particularly problematic, as multifocality can occur in both. Epithelioid hemangioendothelioma, with rare exceptions, lacks well-formed vascular channels. Instead, the neoplastic cells of epithelioid hemangioendothelioma are arranged in angiocentric cords and chains in a myxohyaline or chondroid stroma. Epithelioid hemangioendothelioma has a recurrent translocation, for which testing may be helpful in difficult cases (see later in this article).

When epithelioid hemangioma shows a more solid pattern with a dearth of inflammation, it can be almost impossible to histologically distinguish from cutaneous epithelioid angiomatous nodules. This distinction may be largely academic, as some consider these two entities to represent ends of a spectrum.[28,29]

Although epithelioid hemangiomas recur in approximately one-third to one-half of cases, virtually none have metastasized and none caused death. Indeed, the report of micrometastasis in the regional lymph node of one patient reported by Reed and Terazakis[30] appears to be an extraordinarily unique finding. Simple excision is adequate treatment.

Pathologic Key Features
EPITHELIOID HEMANGIOMA

- Usually presents on head and neck, most commonly around the ear

- Lobular proliferation of well-formed capillaries

- Capillaries lined by epithelioid endothelial cells

- Prominent inflammatory infiltrate with lymphoid aggregates and eosinophils

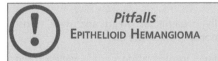

Differential Diagnosis
EPITHELIOID HEMANGIOMA

Epithelioid Hemangioma Versus	Helpful Distinguishing Features
Kimura disease	• Clinical differences: lymphadenopathy, peripheral eosinophilia, elevated serum IgE, variable renal abnormalities
	• Vascular component lacks epithelioid endothelial cells
IgG4-related skin disease	• Similar clinical presentation on the head and neck
	• Similar inflammatory infiltrate, but lacks vascular proliferation
Bacillary angiomatosis	• Lobular proliferation of capillaries lined by epithelioid endothelial cells admixed with neutrophils and histiocytes instead of lymphocytes and eosinophils
	• Amphophilic granular material representing collections of bacteria
	• Warthin-Starry stain will highlight bacteria
Cutaneous epithelioid angiomatous nodule	• Solid sheetlike proliferation of epithelioid endothelial cells
	• Vascular channel formation inapparent
	• Inflammatory infiltrate absent or mild
Epithelioid sarcomalike hemangioendothelioma	• Solid sheets and fascicles of epithelioid and spindled cells
	• Lacks vasoformative channels
	• Admixed neutrophils in 50% of cases
Epithelioid hemangioendothelioma	• Cordlike growth pattern
	• Myxohyaline matrix
	• No inflammatory infiltrate
Epithelioid angiosarcoma	• Infiltrative
	• Prominent nuclear atypia
	• High mitotic rate with atypical mitotic figures
	• Lacks conspicuous inflammatory infiltrate

Pitfalls
EPITHELIOID HEMANGIOMA

! Occasional cases can have solid areas

! Mitotic activity common, but atypical mitotic figures are not seen

! Inflammatory infiltrate can obscure underlying vascular proliferation

CUTANEOUS EPITHELIOID ANGIOMATOUS NODULE

Cutaneous epithelioid angiomatous nodule is a relatively new entity first described in 2004 by Brenn and Fletcher[31] in a series of 15 cases studied based on their unclassifiable nature at the time of investigation. These lesions were often submitted in consultation because of concern for epithelioid angiosarcoma. Clinically, cutaneous epithelioid angiomatous nodule typically presents as a small (<1.0 cm) violaceous superficial nodule or papule in middle-aged adults, although the age range at presentation is broad. Most cases are solitary lesions but occasional multiple or eruptive forms have been described.[32–34] Most lesions are described on the trunk or extremities, but presentation on the head and neck also occurs.

Microscopically, cutaneous epithelioid angiomatous nodule is a unilobular, dermal, circumscribed tumor (Fig. 5A). Recognizable vascular channel formation is usually present only focally. They are largely solid and composed of sheets of epithelioid endothelial cells with abundant eosinophilic cytoplasm. Intracytoplasmic vacuoles are usually apparent. The nuclei do not show significant pleomorphism, but they are somewhat enlarged with vesicular chromatin and conspicuous nucleoli, similar to the nuclei seen in the tumor

cells of epithelioid hemangioma (see Fig. 5B). Mitotic activity is typically conspicuous, with a mitotic rate up to 5 mitotic figures per 10 HPFs, however atypical forms are not seen. There is a variable inflammatory infiltrate that is usually sparse in nature consisting of admixed lymphocytes, histiocytes, and sometimes eosinophils.

The differential diagnosis of cutaneous epithelioid angiomatous nodule includes epithelial hemangioma. As previously noted, epithelioid hemangioma is more often multilobular, with relatively more well-formed capillaries lined by epithelioid endothelial cells. Interestingly, in a series of 10 cases of cutaneous epithelioid angiomatous nodules, reported by Sangüeza and colleagues,[28] most lesions were found to be clinically present on the head and neck. The investigators concluded that cutaneous epithelioid angiomatous nodule is best classified as a solid variant of

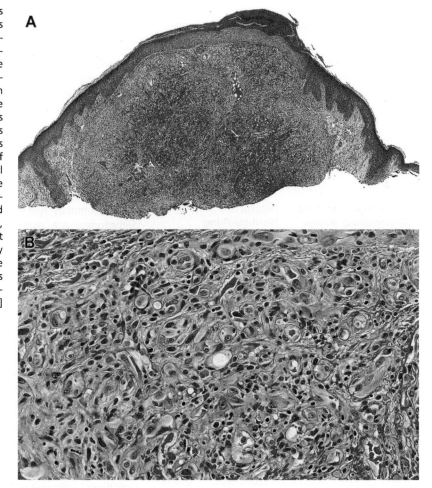

Fig. 5. (*A*) Cutaneous epithelioid angiomatous nodule. This lesion typically presents as a circumscribed nodule in the dermis. Intratumoral hemorrhage is a common finding and a clue to the diagnosis. (*B*) Cutaneous epithelioid angiomatous nodule. The tumor is composed of sheets of epithelioid endothelial cells. The tumor cells have abundant eosinophilic cytoplasm with enlarged nuclei, fine chromatin, and a single distinct nucleolus. Mitotic activity is commonly seen. Note the admixed erythrocytes (Hematoxylin-eosin, original magnification [*A*] ×40; [*B*] ×200).

epithelioid hemangioma, given the overlapping histologic and clinical features with epithelioid hemangioma.

Cutaneous epithelioid angiomatous nodule has been mistaken for angiosarcoma, especially when presenting in chronically sun-exposed skin.[35] The solid growth pattern of large, mitotically active, epithelioid endothelial cells is the source of confusion. In contrast to epithelioid angiosarcoma, cutaneous epithelioid angiomatous nodule has a circumscribed silhouette (see **Fig. 5**A) and lacks the pleomorphism of epithelioid angiosarcoma.

Like epithelioid hemangioma, cutaneous epithelioid angiomatous nodule is a benign tumor. Simple excision is curative.

Pathologic Key Features
CUTANEOUS EPITHELIOID ANGIOMATOUS NODULE

- Circumscribed
- Sheetlike proliferation of epithelioid endothelial cells
- Vascular channel formation absent or focal

Differential Diagnosis
CUTANEOUS EPITHELIOID ANGIOMATOUS NODULE

Cutaneous Epithelioid Angiomatous Nodule Versus	Helpful Distinguishing Features
Epithelioid hemangioma	• Lobular proliferation of well-formed capillaries • Prominent inflammatory infiltrate with lymphoid aggregates and eosinophils
Epithelioid angiosarcoma	• Infiltrative, not circumscribed • More nuclear atypia • May have complex vasoformative channels

Pitfalls
CUTANEOUS EPITHELIOID ANGIOMATOUS NODULE

! Mitotic activity common, but atypical mitotic figures not seen

! Tumor cells have conspicuous nucleoli, but not macro nucleoli

! Can express epithelial markers by immunohistochemistry

EPITHELIOID HEMANGIOENDOTHELIOMA

Epithelioid hemangioendothelioma was originally described by Weiss and Enzinger[36] in 1982 as an unusual vascular tumor of intermediate malignancy that was frequently misdiagnosed as carcinoma. Epithelioid hemangioendothelioma typically occurs in middle-aged adult patients as a solitary mass in the deep soft tissue, viscera, bone, or skin in a range of anatomic locations. The tumor is often angiocentric and can occasionally present with symptoms related to large vessel occlusion rather than as a mass lesion. Grossly, tumors associated with a vessel may resemble an organizing thrombus, whereas tumors not associated with a large vessel have a nondescript gross appearance, usually with a white-gray appearance. Cutaneous examples appear as a skin-colored nodule that clinically does not resemble a vascular neoplasm.

Approximately half of epithelioid hemangioendotheliomas are associated with a preexisting vessel and can histologically be seen growing within (**Fig. 6**A) or around and expanding the affected vessel. In these cases, the tumor cells radiate out from the associated vessel. Intravascular growth is less common in cutaneous epithelioid hemangioendothelioma. The most typical growth pattern of epithelioid hemangioendothelioma is infiltrative cords or nests of epithelioid endothelial cells embedded in a myxohyaline stroma (see **Fig. 6**B, C). The tumor cells may demonstrate rudimentary attempts at vasoformation in the way of individual intracytoplasmic lumens or vacuoles (so-called "blister cells") that may contain red blood cells (see **Fig. 6**D). The nuclear features are usually relatively bland but significant cytologic atypia may be seen in up to 25% of cases. Immunohistochemical evidence of endothelial differentiation is often needed to

Fig. 6. (*A*) Epithelioid hemangioendothelioma. This epithelioid hemangioendothelioma is arising in association with a vessel. The vessel is expanded, and the tumor extends into the adjacent soft tissue as cords of tumor cells. (*B*) Epithelioid hemangioendothelioma. The tumor cells are typically arranged as cords or small nests of epithelioid tumor cells embedded in a myxohyaline stroma.

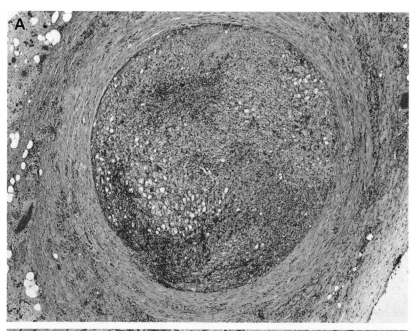

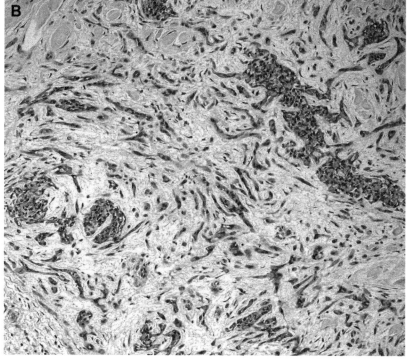

confirm the diagnosis. Epithelioid hemangioendotheliomas are immunoreactive for at least one vascular marker (CD31, CD34, or ERG).[35] Rare cases are negative for CD34 or CD31. Importantly,

approximately 25% of cases also will show immunoreactivity for cytokeratin.[35]

There has been recent insight into the pathogenesis of epithelioid hemangioendothelioma. It

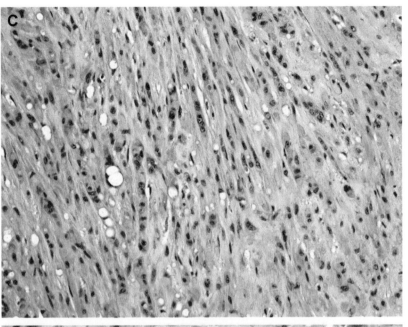

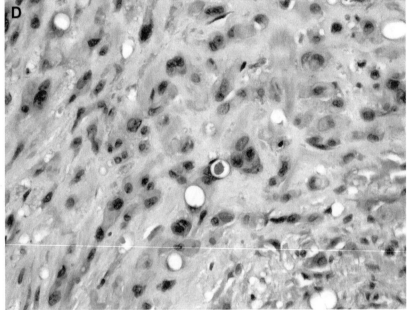

Fig. 6. (continued). (C) Epithelioid hemangioendothelioma. The cords of tumor cells often have individual cells with intracytoplasmic vacuoles. (D) Epithelioid hemangioendothelioma. The intracytoplasmic vacuoles are thought to represent primitive vascular lumens. Occasionally, erythrocytes are found inside the vacuoles (Hematoxylin-eosin, original magnification [A] ×40; [B] ×100; [C] ×200; [D] ×400).

is now known that this tumor has a consistently recurring t(1;3) involving *WWTR1* and *CAMTA1*. *WWTR1* (also called *TAZ*), on 3q25, is involved in 14-3-3T transcription factor activation and signaling in the Hippo pathway that is normally highly expressed in endothelial cells. *WWTR1* fuses to *CAMTA1*, on 1p36, which belongs to a family of calmodulin-binding transcription activators, normally found only in brain.[37,38] How this fusion protein mechanistically relates to the pathogenesis of epithelioid hemangioendothelioma is an area of active research. Fluorescence in situ hybridization to detect the t(1;3) can be a useful diagnostic tool in difficult cases.[39] A smaller subset of cases lacks the WWTR1-CAMTA1 fusion and has a YAP1-TFE3 fusion. The YAP1 transcriptional coactivator is a downstream effector of the Hippo pathway and shows homology to WWTR1. The tumors with this fusion tend to have more abundant eosinophilic cytoplasm, mild to moderate cytologic atypia, and relatively more well-formed vessels in addition to the cordlike arrangement more typical of this entity. TFE3 immunoreactivity is seen in these cases,[40] although nuclear TFE3 staining appears to not be specific for the YAP1-TFE3 fusion.[41]

The primary differential diagnosis of epithelioid hemangioendothelioma includes epithelioid sarcoma and epithelioid sarcomalike hemangioendothelioma. Epithelioid angiosarcoma also may come into the differential diagnosis in cases of epithelioid hemangioendothelioma with increased nuclear atypia, especially if sample size is limited. The cordlike growth pattern and myxohyaline stroma contrasts with these entities. Epithelioid sarcoma typically has a more solid nodular proliferation of epithelioid cells, often with central necrosis reminiscent of granulomas, although occasional cases can have a focal cordlike arrangement of tumor cells. Epithelioid sarcoma is sometimes considered in the differential diagnosis because of immunophenotypic overlap. In addition to strong keratin expression and EMA positivity, approximately 50% of epithelioid sarcomas are positive for CD34. Depending on which antibody is used, epithelioid sarcoma also may be positive for ERG.[42] Epithelioid sarcoma is negative for CD31 and shows loss of SMARCB1 (INI-1).[43]

Epithelioid sarcomalike hemangioendothelioma has a more solid growth pattern, and is composed of myoid-appearing spindled cells in loose fascicles. It is consistently negative for CD34. It also has a different cytogenetic abnormality, as discussed later in this article.

Epithelioid angiosarcoma in its pure form shows a diffuse, sheetlike growth pattern of epithelioid tumor cells with frequent coexpression of vascular and epithelial markers. The diffuse architecture, higher cellularity, higher mitotic activity, more prominent nucleoli, areas of necrosis, hemorrhagic background, multicellular vasoformative channels, and lack of angiocentric growth are used as distinguishing features from epithelioid hemangioendothelioma.[41]

Epithelioid hemangioendotheliomas can be confused with metastatic carcinoma, as described in the seminal description of the entity.[34] The cordlike growth pattern can be reminiscent of metastatic breast carcinoma; in particular, infiltrating lobular carcinoma. Immunoreactivity for vascular markers can readily distinguish epithelioid hemangioendothelioma from metastatic carcinoma.

Due to the myxohyaline matrix, cutaneous epithelioid hemangioendothelioma can have some morphologic overlap with a cutaneous mixed tumor or other myoepithelial tumors. Evidence of true epithelial differentiation, including ducts, cysts, squamous metaplasia, and apocrine differentiation allows distinction in more differentiated tumors. In tumors lacking more overt histologic evidence of an epithelial component, immunoreactivity for myoepithelial markers allows distinction.

Epithelial hemangioendothelioma recurs in approximately 10% to 15% of cases and metastasizes to regional lymph nodes or the lungs in 20% to 30% of cases. The overall mortality is approximately 10% to 20%.[12,35] Striking nuclear atypia, an increasing number of spindled cells, solid angiosarcomalike foci, and greater than 2 mitoses per 10 HPFs tended to be related to poor clinical outcome in the study by Mentzel and colleagues,[35] but only nuclear atypia and high proliferative activity showed a significant influence in bivariate statistical analysis. However, in multivariate analysis, only a mitotic rate greater than 6 mitoses per 10 HPFs correlated with bad prognosis. In a more recent multivariate analysis of 51 cases of epithelioid hemangioendothelioma, size greater than 3 cm and greater than 3 mitotic figures per 50 HPFs predicted an adverse outcome; atypia was not an independent adverse factor.[44]

Key Pathologic Features
EPITHELIOID HEMANGIOENDOTHELIOMA

- Vasculocentric in 50%
- Cordlike to nested growth pattern
- Vacuolated tumor cells ("blister cells")
- Myxohyaline stroma
- t(1;3)WWTR1-CAMTA1

Differential Diagnosis
EPITHELIOID
HEMANGIOENDOTHELIOMA

EHE Versus	Helpful Distinguishing Features
ESH/PH	• Solid sheets and fascicles of epithelioid and spindled cells
	• Negative for CD34
	• Lacks myxohyaline matrix
	• t(7;19)*Serpine1-FOSB*
Epithelioid sarcoma	• Nodular growth pattern, often with central necrosis
	• Negative for CD31
	• Lacks myxohyaline matrix
	• Lacks vacuolated tumor cells
Metastatic carcinoma	• Negative for vascular markers
Myoepithelioma/ mixed tumor	• Growth pattern more nested
	• Lacks vacuolated tumor cells
	• May have true ductal differentiation
	• Positive for myoepithelial markers

Abbreviations: EHE, epithelioid hemangioendothelioma; ESH/PH, epithelioid sarcomalike hemangioendothelioma/ pseudomyogenic hemangioendothelioma.

Pitfalls
EPITHELIOID
HEMANGIOENDOTHELIOMA

! Keratin immunoreactivity common and causes confusion with metastatic carcinoma, epithelioid sarcoma, or epithelioid sarcomalike hemangioendothelioma

! Myxohyaline matrix similar to matrix of myoepithelial tumors

! Usually has bland nuclear features

EPITHELIOID SARCOMALIKE HEMANGIOENDOTHELIOMA (PSEUDOMYOGENIC HEMANGIOENDOTHELIOMA)

Epithelioid sarcomalike hemangioendothelioma is a rare vascular tumor of intermediate malignancy. It was originally described in 2003 in a series of 7 identical cases that were submitted in consultation with the presumptive diagnosis of epithelioid sarcoma.[45] The same tumor was described in 2011 under the name pseudomyogenic hemangioendothelioma.[46] It is now recognized that epithelioid sarcomalike hemangioendothelioma and pseudomyogenic hemangioendothelioma are the same entity. This tumor typically occurs on the extremities of younger to middle-aged adults, with the lower extremities of men being more common. Superficial lesions may present as an ulcerated nodule, similar to epithelioid sarcoma. Cases clinically resembling dermatofibromas also have been reported.[47] Most are multifocal on presentation, often involving multiple different tissue planes (**Fig. 7**). Not surprisingly, given their microscopic features, they do not resemble a vascular neoplasm grossly. They typically have a nondescript tan-gray appearance on gross examination.

Microscopically, tumors are composed of sheets and nodules of eosinophilic epithelioid to spindled endothelial cells with dense eosinophilic cytoplasm (**Fig. 8**). Vascular differentiation is essentially inapparent. There are no well-formed vessels and only rare intracytoplasmic lumens. Cytologic atypia is usually mild to moderate, and mitotic activity is low (<5/50 HPFs). Admixed neutrophils are seen in approximately 50% of cases, and this can be a clue to the diagnosis (see **Fig.** 8C, D). The tumor has a rather unique immunophenotype. It is consistently and strongly keratin positive, positive for Fli-1 and ERG, frequently positive for CD31 (50%–83%), but negative for CD34.[45,46] Nuclear expression of SMARCB1 (INI-1) is retained.[46]

A balanced t(7;19) (q22;q13) has been identified as the sole abnormality in many of these tumors, resulting in a *SERPINE1-FOSB* fusion. SERPINE1, which is highly expressed in vascular cells, is likely to promote FOSB. The FOSB transcription factor belongs to the FOS family of proteins, which acts with JUN family transcription factors as major components of the activating protein 1 (AP-1) complex involved in cell growth and survival.[48,49] As described previously, rearrangement of *FOSB* also is present in a subset of epithelioid hemangiomas. The *FOSB* fusions are likely to result in the upregulation of FOSB protein and AP-1 activation.

Fig. 7. Epithelioid sarcomalike hemangioendothelioma/pseudomyogenic hemangioendothelioma. This tumor frequently presents as multifocal lesions. The lesions often involve multiple tissue planes in a given area, and involvement of the skin is relatively common.

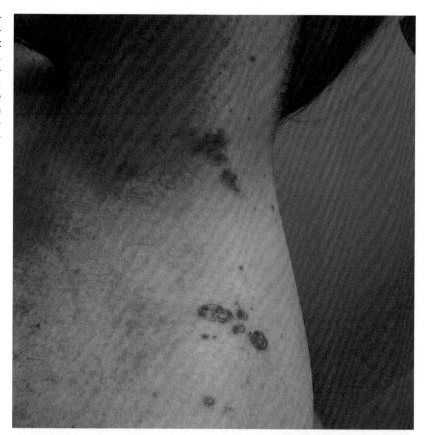

Similarly, these findings reinforce the view that epithelioid sarcomalike/pseudomyogenic hemangioendothelioma is distinct from both epithelioid sarcoma and epithelioid hemangioendothelioma.

The primary differential diagnosis is epithelioid sarcoma. This differential is quite difficult. Epithelioid sarcomas tend to be composed of smaller, well-defined nodules rather than sheetlike growth and show greater nuclear atypia. Although there is immunophenotypic overlap, absence of immunoreactivity for CD31, Fli-1, and SMARCB1 (INI-1) helps distinguish epithelioid sarcoma.[50] Absence or weak immunoreactivity for ERG in epithelioid sarcoma also can be helpful if antibody to C-terminus is used; epithelioid sarcomas are frequently ERG positive with antibodies against the N-terminus.[42,43]

In predominantly spindled cases, leiomyosarcoma may be considered. Epithelioid sarcomalike hemangioendothelioma lacks the intersecting fascicular pattern of a true smooth muscle tumor and is negative for smooth muscle markers by immunohistochemistry.

Other epithelioid vascular tumors, such as cutaneous epithelioid angiomatous nodule and epithelioid hemangioendothelioma, could, as discussed previously, be considered. Both have different growth patterns, however. Cutaneous epithelioid angiomatous nodule is circumscribed and epithelioid hemangioendothelioma has a distinct cordlike to nested growth pattern.

The behavior of epithelioid sarcomalike hemangioendothelioma appears to be that of a vascular tumor of intermediate malignancy. There is

A

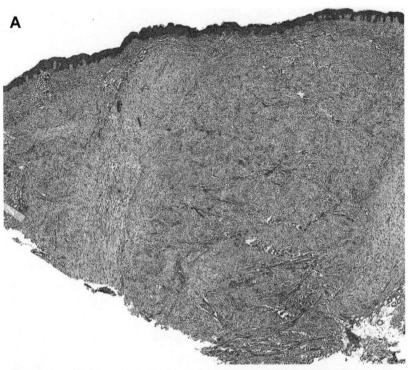

Fig. 8. (A) Epithelioid sarcomalike hemangioendothelioma/pseudomyogenic hemangioendothelioma. The tumor has an infiltrative growth pattern and is composed of sheets and fascicles of neoplastic cells. Its vascular nature is inapparent with routine microscopy. (B) Epithelioid sarcomalike hemangioendothelioma/ pseudomyogenic hemangioendothelioma. The tumor is frequently composed of a combination of epithelioid and spindled tumor cells with relatively abundant eosinophilic cytoplasm.

B

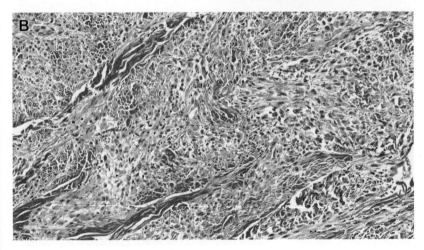

significant risk of local recurrence, but low risk of distant metastasis.[51–53] Surgical resection is the treatment of choice. However, in some cases, the multifocal nature of the tumor may be quite widespread.[46] In such cases, surgery may not be a practical approach unless a radical procedure is attempted. Some patients have been treated with adjuvant radiation therapy and chemotherapy, but a clearly defined role for these modalities has not been established.[46] Now that a tumor-defining cytogenetic abnormality has been described, future targeted therapies may be developed as more is learned about this rare neoplasm.[48,49]

Fig. 8. (continued). (*C*) Epithelioid sarcomalike hemangioendothelioma/ pseudomyogenic hemangioendothelioma. This example was composed predominantly of polygonal epithelioid tumor cells. Scattered admixed neutrophils were present. (*D*) Epithelioid sarcomalike hemangioendothelioma/ pseudomyogenic hemangioendothelioma. This tumor was predominantly composed of spindled cells with dense eosinophilic cytoplasm, imparting a myoid appearance to the lesion. Again, note the admixed neutrophils (Hematoxylin-eosin, original magnification [*A*] ×20; [*B*] ×100; [*C*] ×200; [*D*] ×200).

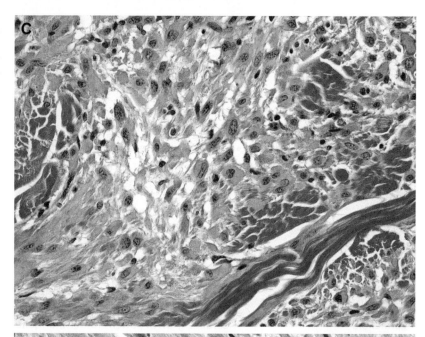

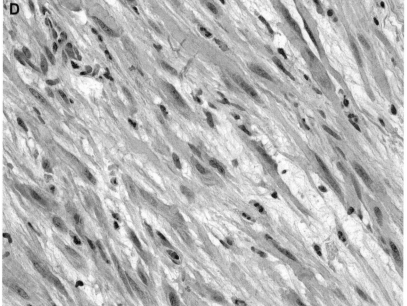

Pathologic Key Features
EPITHELIOID SARCOMALIKE HEMANGIOENDOTHELIOMA/PSEUDOMYOGENIC HEMANGIOENDOTHELIOMA

- Frequently multifocal

- Solid sheets and fascicles of epithelioid to spindled cells

- Dense eosinophilic cytoplasm

- Admixed neutrophils common

- Unique immunophenotype: Cytokeratin AE1/3+, ERG+, Fli1+, CD31+/−, CD34−, SMARCB1 (INI-1) retained

- t(7;19)*SERPINE1-FOSB*

Differential Diagnosis
ESH/PH

ESH/PH Versus	Helpful Distinguishing Features
Epithelioid sarcoma	• Often grows as smaller nodules of tumor cells with central necrosis
	• Negative for CD31, Fli-1
	• Positive for CD34 in 50%–60%
	• Loss of nuclear immunoreactivity for SMARCB1 (INI-1)
Leiomyosarcoma	• Intersecting fascicular pattern
	• Elongated cigar-shaped nuclei
	• Immunoreactivity for SMA, desmin
Cutaneous epithelioid angiomatous nodule	• Circumscribed
	• Positive for CD34
Epithelioid hemangioendothelioma	• Cordlike growth pattern rather than solid
	• Myxohyaline matrix
	• Positive for CD34
	• t(1;3)*WWTR1-CAMTA1*

Abbreviations: ESH/PH, epithelioid sarcomalike hemangioendothelioma/pseudomyogenic hemangioendothelioma; SMA, smooth muscle actin.

Pitfalls
EPITHELIOID SARCOMALIKE HEMANGIOENDOTHELIOMA/ PSEUDOMYOGENIC HEMANGIOENDOTHELIOMA

! Keratin immunoreactivity and histologic features cause confusion with epithelioid sarcoma

! CD34 consistently negative

! CD31 negative in 20% to 50% of cases

EPITHELIOID ANGIOSARCOMA

Epithelioid angiosarcomas most often present in deep soft tissue,[54,55] but can arise in any location. In contrast to conventional cutaneous angiosarcoma that arises on sun-damaged skin of the head and neck in elderly patients, epithelioid angiosarcoma of the skin appears to have a broader age range of involvement with very rare cases affecting pediatric patients, where the involvement of extremities is more common.[56,57] Epithelioid angiosarcomas also can be seen as an iatrogenic phenomenon in lymphedema-associated angiosarcoma (Stewart-Treves syndrome) and postradiation angiosarcoma.[58,59] Like other angiosarcomas, epithelioid angiosarcomas present as erythematous to violaceous lesions. Grossly, they are usually ill-defined, infiltrative hemorrhagic tumors. Occasional cases with a more solid growth pattern may have a less hemorrhagic appearance grossly.

Epithelioid variants of angiosarcoma may show a range of features with complex interanastomosing vessels lined by epithelioid endothelial cells to solid sheets of atypical epithelioid endothelial cells in which it is difficult to recognize its true vascular nature. The presence of erythrocytes within the solid sheets and cells with intracytoplasmic vacuoles can be a clue to the diagnosis in cases with a predominantly solid growth pattern (Fig. 9A). Areas with more obvious vascular channel formation may be present at the periphery of tumors with a solid growth pattern, although these areas may not be evident in small biopsies (see Fig. 9B). The tumor cells are polygonal in nature with abundant amphophilic, grayish cytoplasm and prominent nuclear atypia. Mitotic activity is typically brisk with frequent atypical forms. Apoptotic cells

Fig. 9. (*A*) Epithelioid angiosarcoma. This tumor was predominantly composed of solid sheets of epithelioid tumor cells. The presence of intracytoplasmic vacuoles and extravasation of erythrocytes are a clue to the diagnosis. (*B*) Epithelioid angiosarcoma. There may be a variety of growth patterns in epithelioid angiosarcoma. At the periphery of tumors with a largely solid growth pattern, more obvious vasoformative channels may be present. (*C*) Epithelioid angiosarcoma. The cytoplasm of the tumor cells of epithelioid angiosarcoma often has a characteristic purple-gray hue. This feature in combination with hemorrhage is a useful clue to the diagnosis (Hematoxylin-eosin, original magnification [*A*] ×100; [*B*] ×100; [*C*] ×200).

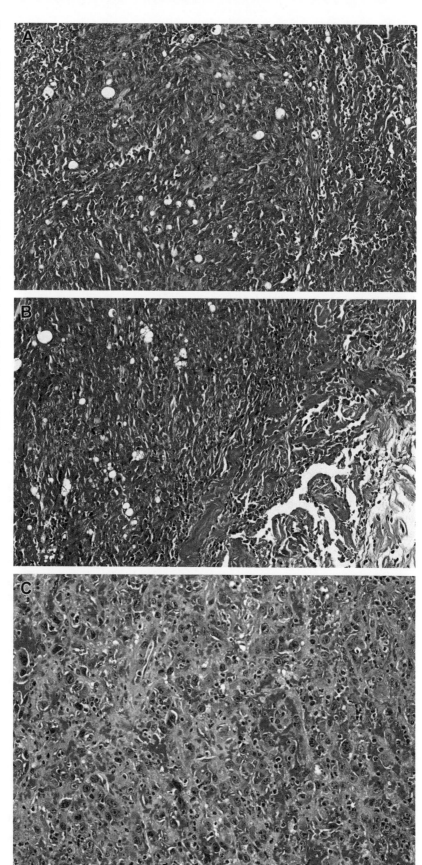

and tumor necrosis are often seen (see **Fig. 9C**). Epithelioid angiosarcomas are positive for vascular markers, including CD31, CD34, and ERG.[59,60] Immunoreactivity for cytokeratin, neuro-endocrine markers, and CD30 also has been described and represents diagnostic pitfalls.[61]

Immunoreactivity for epithelial markers and the morphology can cause confusion with poorly differentiated carcinomas. The amphophilic cyto-plasm and associated erythrocytes can be a clue to consider the diagnosis of epithelioid angiosar-coma based on histologic findings. Immunoreac-tivity for vascular markers allows distinction, although it should be mentioned that a small sub-set (10%) of angiosarcomas can be negative for CD31, and that other entities, such as atypical fi-broxanthoma, can be positive for this marker.[62,63] Immunostains for ERG are more specific than CD31 and CD34.[64] Similarly, in cases with immu-noreactivity for CD30, anaplastic large-cell lymphoma is a differential consideration, but addi-tional immunostains for vascular markers will allow recognition of epithelioid angiosarcoma.[65] Other epithelioid vascular tumors can be considered (see previously). As a rule, none of the other epithelioid vascular tumors have the degree of aty-pia seen in epithelioid angiosarcoma.

All angiosarcomas are aggressive neoplasms with a high rate of local recurrence and metastatic potential; there is no inherent difference in the behavior of epithelioid angiosarcoma. Surgery is the ideal therapeutic intervention, but even with aggressive surgery, recurrence is common, as is metastasis. The overall 5-year survival is approxi-mately 30% to 40%.[2]

Key Pathologic Features
Epithelioid Angiosarcoma

- Often has vasoformative channels
- Prominent nuclear atypia
- Abundant amphophilic cytoplasm
- Intracytoplasmic vacuoles
- Intratumoral hemorrhage
- Positive for vascular markers

Differential Diagnosis
Epithelioid Angiosarcoma

Epithelioid Angiosarcoma Versus	Helpful Distinguishing Feature
Epithelioid hemangioma	• Well-formed, not complex vessels
	• Less nuclear atypia
	• Eosinophilic cytoplasm
	• Admixed lymphoid ag-gregates and eosinophils
CEAN	• Circumscribed and small
	• Less nuclear atypia
	• Eosinophilic cytoplasm
ESH/PH	• Tumor cells often spindled
	• Dense eosinophilic cytoplasm
	• Less nuclear atypia and low mitotic rate
	• Negative for CD34
Poorly differentiated carcinoma	• Usually lacks intratumoral hemorrhage
	• Cytoplasm often more eosinophilic
	• Negative for vascular markers
Anaplastic large-cell lymphoma	• Lacks intratumoral hemorrhage
	• Lacks vacuolated tumor cells
	• Admixed lymphoid cells
	• Negative for vascular markers

Abbreviations: CEAN, cutaneous epithelioid angiomatous nodule; ESH/PH, epithelioid sarcomalike hemangioendo-thelioma/pseudomyogenic hemangioendothelioma.

Pitfalls
Epithelioid Angiosarcoma

! Often has solid sheetlike growth pattern

! Immunoreactivity for epithelial markers common

! Rare cases with immunoreactivity for CD30

Table 1
Summary table of epithelioid vascular tumors

	EH	CEAN	EHE	ESH/PH	EAS
Growth pattern	Lobular, well-formed vessels	Solid, circumscribed	Cords and nests	Sheets and fascicles	Sheets and complex vessels
Inflammation	Lymphoid aggregates and eosinophils	Variable: occasional eosinophils	Not prominent	Neutrophils (50%)	Not prominent
Nuclei	Uniform, open chromatin; small nucleolus	Uniform, open chromatin; small nucleolus	Hyperchromatic, mild to moderate atypia	Mild to moderate atypia	Moderate to severe atypia
Immunophenotype	CD31+, CD34+, ERG+, CK−/+	CD31+, CD34+, ERG+, CK−/+	CD31+, CD34+, ERG+, CK−/+	CD31+/−, CD34−, ERG+, Fli-1+, SMARCB1 retained	CD31+, CD34+, ERG+, CK−/+, CD30−/+

Abbreviations: CEAN, cutaneous epithelioid angiomatous nodule; CK, cytokeratin; EAS, epithelioid angiosarcoma; EH, epithelioid hemangioma; EHE, epithelioid hemangioendothelioma; ESH/PH, epithelioid sarcomalike hemangioendothelioma/pseudomyogenic hemangioendothelioma.

SUMMARY

Epithelioid vascular tumors pose diagnostic difficulty. Careful attention to histologic features with judicious use of immunohistochemical stains allows recognition of these challenging tumors. Key histologic features of this group of epithelioid vascular tumors are presented in **Table 1**.

REFERENCES

1. Wells GC, Whimster IW. Subcutaneous angiolymphoid hyperplasia with eosinophilia. Br J Dermatol 1969;81(1):1–14.
2. Enzinger and Weiss's soft tissue tumors. In: Goldblum JR, Folpe AL, Weiss SW, editors. Malignant vascular tumors. 6th edition. Philadelphia: Mosby; 2014. p. 703–32.
3. Buder K, Ruppert S, Trautmann A, et al. Angiolymphoid hyperplasia with eosinophilia and Kimura's disease—a clinical and histopathological comparison. J Dtsch Dermatol Ges 2014;12(3):224–8.
4. Azari AA, Kanavi MR, Lucarelli M, et al. Angiolymphoid hyperplasia with eosinophilia of the orbit and ocular adnexa: report of 5 cases. JAMA Ophthalmol 2014;132(5):633–6.
5. San Nicoló M, Mayr D, Berghaus A. Angiolymphoid hyperplasia with eosinophilia of the external ear: case report and review of the literature. Eur Arch Otorhinolaryngol 2013;270(10):2775–7.
6. Ohmori S, Sugita K, Sawada Y, et al. Angiolymphoid hyperplasia with eosinophilia occurring on the penis. Eur J Dermatol 2010;20(4):545–6.
7. Fetsch JF, Sesterhenn IA, Miettinen M, et al. Epithelioid hemangioma of the penis: a clinicopathologic and immunohistochemical analysis of 19 cases, with special reference to exuberant examples often confused with epithelioid hemangioendothelioma and epithelioid angiosarcoma. Am J Surg Pathol 2004;28(4):523–33.
8. Haas AF, La Perriere R, King EJ. Angiolymphoid hyperplasia with eosinophilia of the hand. A case report. J Dermatol Surg Oncol 1991;17(9):731–4.
9. Sharp JF, Rodgers MJ, MacGregor FB, et al. Angiolymphoid hyperplasia with eosinophilia. J Laryngol Otol 1990;104(12):977–9.
10. Rosai J, Akerman LR. Intravenous atypical vascular proliferation. A cutaneous lesion simulating a malignant blood vessel tumor. Arch Dermatol 1974; 109(5):714–7.
11. Requena L, Sangueza OP. Cutaneous vascular proliferation. Part II. Hyperplasias and benign neoplasms. J Am Acad Dermatol 1997;37(6):887–919 [quiz: 920–2].
12. Weiss SW, Ishak KG, Dail DH, et al. Epithelioid hemangioendothelioma and related lesions. Semin Diagn Pathol 1986;3(4):259–87.
13. Cooper PH. Is histiocytoid hemangioma a specific pathologic entity? Am J Surg Pathol 1988;12(11): 815–7.

14. Tsang WY, Chan JK. The family of epithelioid vascular tumors. Histol Histopathol 1993;8(1): 187–212.

15. Olsen TG, Helwig EB. Angiolymphoid hyperplasia with eosinophilia. A clinicopathologic study of 116 patients. J Am Acad Dermatol 1985;12(5 Pt 1):781–96.

16. Macarenco RS, do Canto AL, Gonzalez S. Angiolymphoid hyperplasia with eosinophilia showing prominent granulomatous and fibrotic reaction: a morphological and immunohistochemical study. Am J Dermatopathol 2006;28(6):514–7.

17. Nielsen GP, Srivastava A, Kattapuram S, et al. Epithelioid hemangioma of bone revisited: a study of 50 cases. Am J Surg Pathol 2009;33(2):270–7.

18. Miteva M, Galimberti ML, Ricotti C, et al. D2-40 highlights lymphatic vessel proliferation of angiolymphoid hyperplasia with eosinophilia. J Cutan Pathol 2009;36(12):1316–22.

19. Fetsch JF, Weiss SW. Observations concerning the pathogenesis of epithelioid hemangioma (angiolymphoid hyperplasia). Mod Pathol 1991;4:449.

20. Antonescu CR, Chen HW, Zhang L, et al. ZFP36-FOSB fusion defines a subset of epithelioid hemangioma with atypical features. Genes Chromosomes Cancer 2014;53(11):951–9.

21. Kung IT, Gibson JB, Bannatyne PM. Kimura's disease: a clinicopathological study of 21 cases and its distinction from angiolymphoid hyperplasia with eosinophilia. Pathology 1984;16:39.

22. Urabe A, Tsuneyoshi M, Enjoji M. Epithelioid hemangioma versus Kimura's disease. A comparative clinicopathologic study. Am J Surg Pathol 1987;11(10): 758–66.

23. Googe PB, Harris NL, Mihm MC Jr. Kimura's disease and angiolymphoid hyperplasia with eosinophilia: two distinct histopathological entities. J Cutan Pathol 1987;14(5):263–71.

24. Helander SD, Peters MS, Kuo TT, et al. Kimura's disease and angiolymphoid hyperplasia with eosinophilia: new observations from immunohistochemical studies of lymphocyte markers, endothelial antigens, and granulocyte proteins. J Cutan Pathol 1995;22(4): 319–26.

25. Hamaguchi Y, Fujimoto M, Matsushita Y, et al. IgG4-related skin disease, a mimic of angiolymphoid hyperplasia with eosinophilia. Dermatology 2011; 223(4):301–5.

26. Hattori T, Miyanaga T, Tago O, et al. Isolated cutaneous manifestation of IgG4-related disease. J Clin Pathol 2012;65(9):815–8.

27. Sato Y, Takeuchi M, Takata K, et al. Clinicopathologic analysis of IgG4-related skin disease. Mod Pathol 2013;26(4):523–32.

28. Sangüeza OP, Walsh SN, Sheehan DJ, et al. Cutaneous epithelioid angiomatous nodule: a case series and proposed classification. Am J Dermatopathol 2008;30:16–20.

29. Al-Daraji WI, Prescott RJ, Abdellaoui A, et al. Cutaneous epithelioid angiomatous nodule: different views or interpretations in the analysis of ten new cases. Dermatol Online J 2009;15(3):2. 29.

30. Reed RJ, Terazakis N. Subcutaneous angioblastic lymphoid hyperplasia with eosinophilia (Kimura's disease). Cancer 1972;29:489.

31. Brenn T, Fletcher CD. Cutaneous epithelioid angiomatous nodule: a distinct lesion in the morphologic spectrum of epithelioid vascular tumors. Am J Dermatopathol 2004;26:14–21.

32. Lo CS, Lee MC. Case of a cutaneous epithelioid angiomatous nodule on the foot. J Dermatol 2013; 40(6):480–1.

33. Dastgheib L, Aslani FS, Sepaskhah M, et al. A young woman with multiple cutaneous epithelioid angiomatous nodules (CEAN) on her forearm: a case report and follow-up of therapeutic intervention. Dermatol Online J 2013;19(3):1.

34. Pavlidakey PG, Burroughs C, Karrs T, et al. Cutaneous epithelioid angiomatous nodule: a case with metachronous lesions. Am J Dermatopathol 2011; 33(8):831–4.

35. Mentzel T, Beham A, Calonje E, et al. Epithelioid hemangioendothelioma of skin and soft tissues: clinicopathologic and immunohistochemical study of 30 cases. Am J Surg Pathol 1997;21(4):363–74.

36. Weiss SW, Enzinger FM. Epithelioid hemangioendothelioma: a vascular tumor often mistaken for a carcinoma. Cancer 1982;50(5):970–81.

37. Tanas MR, Sboner A, Oliveira AM, et al. Identification of a disease-defining gene fusion in epithelioid hemangioendothelioma. Sci Transl Med 2011;3: 98ra82.

38. Errani C, Zhang L, Sung YS, et al. A novel WWTR1-CAMTA1 gene fusion is a consistent abnormality in epithelioid hemangioendothelioma of different anatomic sites. Genes Chromosomes Cancer 2011;50:644–53.

39. Anderson T, Zhang L, Hameed M, et al. Thoracic epithelioid malignant vascular tumors: a clinicopathologic study of 52 cases with emphasis on pathologic grading and molecular studies of WWTR1-CAMTA1 fusions. Am J Surg Pathol 2015; 39(1):132–9.

40. Antonescu CR, Le Loarer F, Mosquera JM, et al. Novel YAP1-TFE3 fusion defines a distinct subset of epithelioid hemangioendothelioma. Genes Chromosomes Cancer 2013;52(8):775–84.

41. Flucke U, Vogels RJ, de Saint Aubain Somerhausen N, et al. Epithelioid hemangioendothelioma: clinicopathologic, immunohistochemical, and molecular genetic analysis of 39 cases. Diagn Pathol 2014;9:131.

42. Miettinen M, Wang Z, Sarlomo-Rikala M, et al. ERG expression in epithelioid sarcoma: a diagnostic pitfall. Am J Surg Pathol 2013;37(10):1580–5.

43. Stockman DL, Hornick JL, Deavers MT, et al. ERG and FLI1 protein expression in epithelioid sarcoma. Mod Pathol 2014;27(4):496–501.

44. Deyrup AT, Tighiouart M, Montag AG, et al. Epithelioid hemangioendothelioma of soft tissue: a proposal for risk stratification based on 49 cases. Am J Surg Pathol 2008;32(6):924–7.

45. Billings SD, Folpe AL, Weiss SW. Epithelioid sarcoma-like hemangioendothelioma. Am J Surg Pathol 2003;27:4857.

46. Hornick JL, Fletcher CD. Pseudomyogenic hemangioendothelioma: a distinctive often multicentric tumor with indolent behavior. Am J Surg Pathol 2011;35:190.

47. Stuart LN, Gardner JM, Lauer SR, et al. Epithelioid sarcoma-like (pseudomyogenic) hemangioendothelioma, clinically mimicking dermatofibroma, diagnosed by skin biopsy in a 30-year-old man. J Cutan Pathol 2013;40(10):909–13.

48. Trombetta D, Magnusson L, von Steyern FV, et al. Translocation t(7;19)(q22;q13)—a recurrent chromosome aberration in pseudomyogenic hemangioendothelioma? Cancer Genet 2011;204(4):211–5.

49. Walther C, Tayebwa J, Lilljebjörn H, et al. A novel SERPINE1-FOSB fusion gene results in transcriptional up-regulation of FOSB in pseudomyogenic haemangioendothelioma. J Pathol 2014;232(5):534–40.

50. Patel RM, Billings SD. Cutaneous soft tissue tumors that make you say, "Oh $*&%!". Adv Anat Pathol 2012;19(5):320–30.

51. Mangham DC, Kindblom LG. Rarely metastasizing soft tissue tumours. Histopathology 2014;64(1):88–100.

52. Requena L, Santonja C, Martinez-Amo JL, et al. Cutaneous epithelioid sarcomalike (pseudomyogenic) hemangioendothelioma: a little-known low-grade cutaneous vascular neoplasm. JAMA Dermatol 2013;149(4):459–65.

53. Billings SD, Folpe AL, Weiss SW. Epithelioid sarcoma-like hemangioendothelioma (pseudomyogenic hemangioendothelioma). Am J Surg Pathol 2011;35(7):1088 [author reply: 1088–9].

54. Fletcher CD. 3rd edition. Diagnostic histopathology of tumors, vol. 1. Philadelphia: Elsevier Limited; 2007. p. 66–7.

55. Fletcher CDM, Beham A, Bekir S, et al. Epithelioid angiosarcoma of deep soft tissue: a distinctive tumor readily mistaken for an epithelial neoplasm. Am J Surg Pathol 1991;15(10):915–24.

56. Suchak R, Thway K, Zelger B, et al. Primary cutaneous epithelioid angiosarcoma: a clinicopathologic study of 13 cases of a rare neoplasm occurring outside the setting of conventional angiosarcomas and with predilection for the limbs. Am J Surg Pathol 2011;35:60–9.

57. Bacchi CE, Silva TR, Zambrano E, et al. Epithelioid angiosarcoma of the skin: a study of 18 cases with emphasis on its clinicopathologic spectrum and unusual morphologic features. Am J Surg Pathol 2010;34:1334–43.

58. Billings SD, McKenney JK, Folpe AL, et al. Cutaneous angiosarcoma following breast-conserving surgery and radiation: an analysis of 27 cases. Am J Surg Pathol 2004;28(6):781–8.

59. Alessi E, Sala F, Berti E. Angiosarcomas in lymphedematous limbs. Am J Dermatopathol 1986;8(5):371–8.

60. Mobini N. Cutaneous epithelioid angiosarcoma: a neoplasm with potential pitfalls in diagnosis. J Cutan Pathol 2009;36:362–9.

61. Tessier Cloutier B, Costa FD, Tazelaar HD, et al. Aberrant expression of neuroendocrine markers in angiosarcoma: a potential diagnostic pitfall. Hum Pathol 2014;45(8):1618–24.

62. Tatsas AD, Keedy VL, Florell SR, et al. Foamy cell angiosarcoma: a rare and deceptively bland variant of cutaneous angiosarcoma. J Cutan Pathol 2010;37(8):901–6.

63. Luzar B, Calonje E. Morphological and immunohistochemical characteristics of atypical fibroxanthoma with a special emphasis on potential diagnostic pitfalls: a review. J Cutan Pathol 2010;37:301–9.

64. Thum C, Husain EA, Mulholland K, et al. Atypical fibroxanthoma with pseudoangiomatous features: a histological and immunohistochemical mimic of cutaneous angiosarcoma. Ann Diagn Pathol 2013;17(6):502–7.

65. Alimchandani M, Wang ZF, Miettinen M. CD30 expression in malignant vascular tumors and its diagnostic and clinical implications: a study of 146 cases. Appl Immunohistochem Mol Morphol 2014;22(5):358–62.

Diagnostically Challenging Spindle Cell Neoplasms of the Retroperitoneum

Inga-Marie Schaefer, MD,
Christopher D.M. Fletcher, MD, FRCPath*

KEYWORDS

• Retroperitoneum • Spindle cell • Liposarcoma • Nerve sheath tumor • Smooth muscle tumor

ABSTRACT

The diagnostic spectrum of spindle cell neoplasms arising in the retroperitoneum is wide and, in the presence of commonly shared morphologic features, it may be challenging to establish a correct diagnosis in certain cases. Beyond seemingly undifferentiated spindle cell morphology, most neoplasms may reveal distinctive adipocytic, smooth muscle or myofibroblastic or nerve sheath differentiation and show additional diagnostic clues or characteristic molecular abnormalities. Obtaining sufficient and representative biopsy material, a thorough work-up, and extensive sampling of gross specimens followed by a combined histopathologic, immunohistochemical, and, if necessary, molecular work-up of these cases is advisable so as not to miss important diagnostic and/or prognostic indicators.

amounts of material are obtained by CT-guided biopsy for histopathologic and molecular analyses.

Retroperitoneal sarcomas in general account for approximately 15% of all soft tissue sarcomas. They are usually slow growing and present at advanced disease stages with local infiltration of adjacent structures, rendering their management particularly challenging. Local disease progression is the most common cause of death. Surgical resection remains the mainstay of therapy, but local recurrence eventually develops in a majority of patients despite aggressive surgery.

OVERVIEW

A wide spectrum of tumors with spindle cell morphology arises in the retroperitoneum, including tumors showing adipocytic, smooth muscle, and myofibroblastic differentiation as well as tumors of peripheral nerves. The differential diagnosis of these entities may sometimes be straightforward. In certain situations, however, it can be particularly challenging to establish a correct diagnosis, for instance, if only limited

DEDIFFERENTIATED LIPOSARCOMA

INTRODUCTION

Dedifferentiated liposarcoma represents 10% of liposarcomas and accounts for the vast majority of retroperitoneal malignant spindle cell neoplasms. Most cases of dedifferentiated liposarcoma arise in this location, followed by deep soft tissue of the extremities, trunk, mediastinum, spermatic cord, and the head and neck region. Patients are most often 40 to 60 years of age. Dedifferentiated liposarcoma develops from well-differentiated liposarcoma, with approximately 90% of cases occurring de novo in a primary liposarcoma and the remaining 10% arising in recurrences.

Department of Pathology, Brigham and Women's Hospital, Harvard Medical School, 75 Francis Street, Boston, MA 02115, USA
* Corresponding author.
E-mail address: cfletcher@partners.org

Surgical Pathology 8 (2015) 353–374
http://dx.doi.org/10.1016/j.path.2015.05.007

GROSS FEATURES

Dedifferentiated liposarcoma most often presents as a large mass and usually shows transition from well-differentiated areas, grossly resembling mature adipose tissue, to nonlipogenic sarcoma with a firm, whitish to tan appearance. This transition is usually sharply demarcated (**Fig. 1**) but may occasionally be subtle, with both components intimately intermingled. Multiple discontiguous masses are common. Thorough sampling is important for correctly diagnosing these cases and areas of well-differentiated liposarcoma may be mistaken for normal adipose tissue by surgeons and pathologists. Regions with a different appearance on gross examination should be sampled carefully because clues to establish the correct diagnosis may be present only focally.

MICROSCOPIC FEATURES

Dedifferentiated liposarcoma (**Fig. 2**) shows a wide range of histologic appearances (**Fig. 3**): an unclassified storiform or pleomorphic morphology is most common, followed by myxofibrosarcoma-like or not otherwise specified spindle cell morphology, sometimes with a neutrophilic infiltrate.[1] Dedifferentiated liposarcoma accounts for the majority of tumors diagnosed as so-called inflammatory malignant fibrous histiocytoma (MFH) in the past.[1] Areas of well-differentiated liposarcoma resemble mature adipose tissue, at least in the lipoma-like variant, with marked variation in adipocyte size and focal nuclear atypia in adipocytes and/or stromal cells. The sclerosing variant of well-differentiated liposarcoma consists mostly of collagenous fibrous tissue, often with bizarre multinucleate cells, which predominates over areas with fatty morphology.

In dedifferentiated liposarcoma, the higher-grade, nonlipogenic component usually lacks any specific differentiation but may often express smooth muscle actin (SMA) and/or desmin,

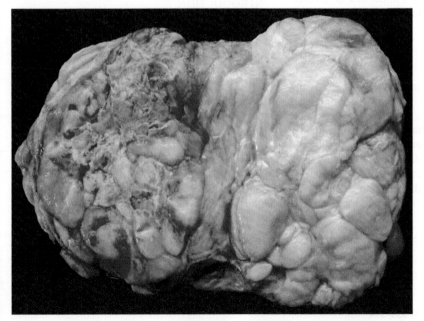

Fig. 1. Grossly, transition from (*right*) well-differentiated liposarcoma resembling mature adipose tissue to (*left*) areas of dedifferentiated liposarcoma, appearing as firm tan-gray areas with focal necrosis, may be appreciated.

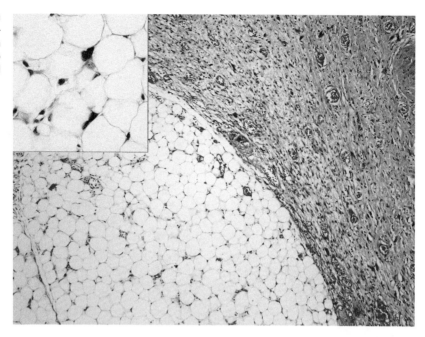

Fig. 2. Abrupt transition from (*left*) well-differentiated liposarcoma (×100; *inset*, ×400) to (*right*) dedifferentiated liposarcoma (×100).

suggesting myofibroblastic differentiation. Lipoblasts may not always be readily identifiable and, on the other hand, may be found in benign adipocytic tumors (eg, chondroid lipoma and lipoblastoma). Lipoblasts are characterized by 2 or more large cytoplasmic vacuoles, scalloping hyperchromatic, atypical nuclei. Lipoblasts are not regarded as a requirement for diagnosis of liposarcoma.

Up to 10% of tumors exhibit heterologous rhabdomyosarcomatous or leiomyosarcomatous, and more rarely osteosarcomatous or angiosarcomatous, differentiation.[2–4] Some cases may show micronodular meningioma-like whorls, which are often associated with ossification and a plasmacytic infiltrate,[5] whereas others may exhibit homologous lipoblastic differentiation resembling pleomorphic liposarcoma (**Fig. 4**).[6] The nonlipogenic component may be morphologically low grade, a phenomenon described as low-grade dedifferentiation,[7] although Evans[8] disputes this categorization.

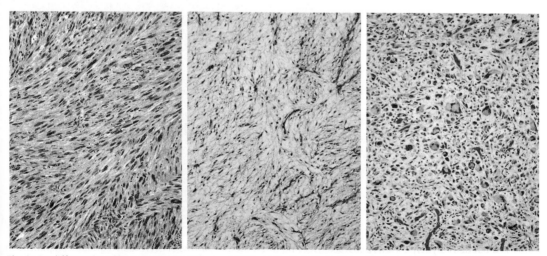

Fig. 3. Dedifferentiated liposarcoma may show varied morphology, including a fascicular/storiform spindle cell appearance (*left*), myxoid change resembling myxofibrosarcoma (*middle*), or pleomorphic morphology (*right*) (×200).

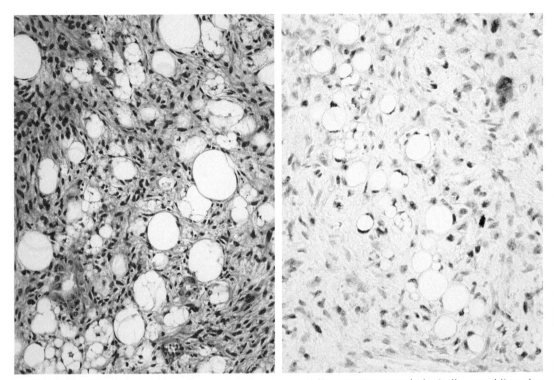

Fig. 4. (*Left*) Dedifferentiated liposarcoma with homologous differentiation, morphologically resembling pleomorphic liposarcoma, shows (*right*) overexpression of MDM-2 by tumor cells (×200).

DIAGNOSIS AND DIFFERENTIAL DIAGNOSIS

The combination of tumor site, presence of an adjacent well-differentiated component, and immunohistochemical and molecular findings establishes the diagnosis of dedifferentiated liposarcoma in a majority of cases. These liposarcomas frequently show ring or giant marker chromosomes with amplification of the 12q13–15 locus, which includes *MDM2*, *CDK4*, and *HMGA2* genes; and molecular analyses, such as fluorescence in situ hybridization (FISH), consistently reveal high-level amplification of *MDM2* (**Fig. 5**).[9–11] Additional complex genomic aberrations are common. Both the lipogenic and nonlipogenic components show diffuse nuclear

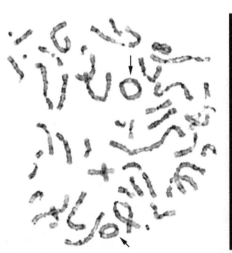
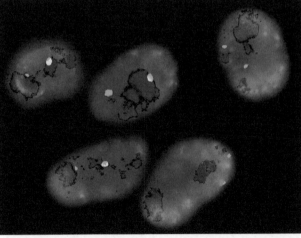

Fig. 5. A G-banded karyotype shows 2 characteristic ring chromosomes (*arrows*). FISH reveals high-level amplification of the 12q13–15 region (*red probe*), including *MDM2* and *CDK4*. The green probe is directed to the centromere of chromosome 12. (*Courtesy of* Dr Jonathan Fletcher, Department of Pathology, Brigham & Women's Hospital, Boston, USA.)

expression of MDM-2 as well as CDK-4 by immunohistochemistry, the latter more diffuse and often stronger in the dedifferentiated component.[11,12]

Other liposarcoma subtypes, pleomorphic sarcomas arising in the retroperitoneum, and sarcomatoid carcinoma might be considered in the differential diagnosis of dedifferentiated liposarcoma. In particular, if well-differentiated areas are absent, the correct diagnosis may be difficult when made only on morphologic grounds.

Pleomorphic liposarcoma, accounting for 5% of liposarcomas, is usually deep seated and more frequently arises in the limbs than in the trunk and retroperitoneum. Pleomorphic liposarcomas histologically demonstrate lipogenic areas to a variable extent and show marked cytologic pleomorphism. Multivacuolated lipoblasts are a characteristic feature and intracytoplasmic eosinophilic globules or droplets are often present. High-grade pleomorphic/spindle cell sarcoma, myxofibrosarcoma-like or epithelioid morphology may be observed. Pleomorphic liposarcoma expresses SMA in approximately half of cases and focally keratin and/or desmin in a subset of cases.[13] In contrast to dedifferentiated liposarcoma, pleomorphic liposarcoma lacks *MDM2* amplification and MDM-2/CDK-4 overexpression and instead may show complex chromosomal aberrations.

Myxofibrosarcoma is the most common type of soft tissue sarcoma in elderly patients, usually develops in the limbs, and is vanishingly rare in the retroperitoneum. There is no well-differentiated fatty component. Even though MDM-2/CDK-4 overexpression may be present, myxofibrosarcoma lacks high-level *MDM2* amplification.

Leiomyosarcoma can be distinguished from dedifferentiated liposarcoma by tumor cells exhibiting brightly eosinophilic cytoplasm, cigar-shaped nuclei, a more consistently fascicular architecture, and usually strong expression of SMA, desmin, and/or caldesmon. More restricted expression of these markers may be detected in a subset of dedifferentiated liposarcomas. Leiomyosarcomas usually lack *MDM2* amplification and nuclear MDM-2/CDK-4 overexpression.

Malignant peripheral nerve sheath tumor (MPNST) most often consists of a relatively uniform spindle cell population with tapering or wavy, elongated nuclei, pale cytoplasm, alternating cellularity, and perivascular condensation. In no more than 40% to 50% of cases, S-100 protein and, to a lesser extent, glial fibrillary acidic protein (GFAP), SOX-10, and MDM-2 may be expressed at least focally by a subset of tumor cells, but CDK-4 positivity and *MDM2* amplification are generally absent in MPNST.

By definition, undifferentiated pleomorphic sarcoma is a diagnosis of exclusion and the presence of MDM-2/CDK-4 overexpression and *MDM2* amplification favors dedifferentiated liposarcoma.

Finally, sarcomatoid carcinomas that exhibit pleomorphic spindle cell morphology can be distinguished from dedifferentiated liposarcoma by their expression of epithelial markers in the absence of *MDM2* amplification. In many patients, a primary visceral carcinoma may be identified clinically.

PROGNOSIS

Dedifferentiated liposarcoma has a 5-year survival rate of 60% to 70%, with a recurrence rate of approximately 40% and a metastatic risk of approximately 20% in this time frame. With 10 to 20 years' follow-up, virtually all retroperitoneal tumors of this type ultimately recur. Dedifferentiated liposarcoma classified as low-grade harbors the same prognosis as tumors of high-grade categories.[7] Retroperitoneal dedifferentiated liposarcomas are often large tumors, presenting at an advanced stage with local infiltration of adjacent structures and may not be amenable to complete or margin-negative surgical resection. In these cases, death often results from local progression and compromise of vital structures rather than from metastases.

CELLULAR SCHWANNOMA

INTRODUCTION

Schwannomas are benign tumors of peripheral nerves and may arise at various locations. They usually affect adult patients of both genders equally and either are sporadic or, more rarely, occur in the setting of neurofibromatosis type 2,[14] Carney complex,[15] or schwannomatosis.[16] Variants include ancient schwannoma with prominent degenerative changes, plexiform schwannoma mostly arising in younger patients as painful mass on the trunk, melanotic schwannoma (sometimes in association with Carney complex), epithelioid schwannoma, microcystic/reticular schwannoma, and cellular schwannoma.[17–19]

Cellular schwannomas occur in deep soft tissue, most often in the retroperitoneum, paravertebral region, pelvis, or mediastinum, where they may arise from a major nerve.[17–19] Middle-aged patients with a slight female predominance are most frequently affected, and a subset of patients has a diagnosis of NF-2.[19] In these patients, biallelic inactivation of the *NF2* gene located at 22q12.2 leads to loss of expression of the tumor suppressor merlin. Approximately 15% to 30% of cellular schwannomas were misdiagnosed as sarcoma in the past.[17,19]

> ### *Key Features*
> #### CELLULAR SCHWANNOMA
>
> - Adult patients, women more than men
> - Sporadic or occasionally in patients with neurofibromatosis type 2
> - Large soft tissue mass, encapsulated
> - Histology: cellular fascicles, often lacks Antoni B pattern, contains hyalinized blood vessels, mitoses, sometimes infiltrative
> - Tumor cells express S-100 strongly and diffusely, keratin often positive in mediastinum/retroperitoneum; epithelial membrane antigen (EMA) highlights perineurial capsule
> - Molecular features: *NF2* inactivation
> - Prognosis: recurrence in less than 5%; very rare transformation to epithelioid MPNST/epithelioid angiosarcoma

GROSS FEATURES

Cellular schwannomas are solitary, encapsulated tumors but sometimes show a focally infiltrative growth and even erode bone – a feature that may be worrisome for malignancy.[17] Origin from a major nerve can be observed in a subset of cases. Cellular schwannomas show a firm, white to tan cut surface.

MICROSCOPIC FEATURES

Histologically, cellular schwannomas are well circumscribed (Fig. 6) and show a uniformly hypercellular fascicular or whorled growth. They can be distinguished from conventional schwannoma by the absence or only focal presence of Antoni B areas, which are less cellular and more myxoid. The spindled tumor cells with tapering nuclei and palely eosinophilic cytoplasm grow in dense fascicles (Fig. 7). Verocay bodies consisting of palisaded Schwann cells with intervening eosinophilic cytoplasm are rare in cellular schwannoma. Scattered xanthoma cells (Fig. 8), a peritumoral lymphoid cuff, and hyalinized blood vessels, typical of schwannomas, may serve as diagnostic clues. Despite its benign nature, degenerative nuclear pleomorphism, mitoses (usually <10/10 high-power fields [HPFs]), focal necrosis, and infiltrative growth may be observed.

DIAGNOSIS AND DIFFERENTIAL DIAGNOSIS

Cellular schwannomas express nuclear and cytoplasmic S-100 protein strongly and diffusely (Fig. 9). A perineurial capsule is often highlighted by EMA expression. In addition, GFAP is expressed in a subset of tumors.[20] Particularly when located in the mediastinum or retroperitoneum, keratin expression can be observed in cellular schwannomas, possibly as a result of cross-reaction with GFAP.[20] Scattered axons may be revealed by staining with neurofilament protein. Molecular studies show either monosomy

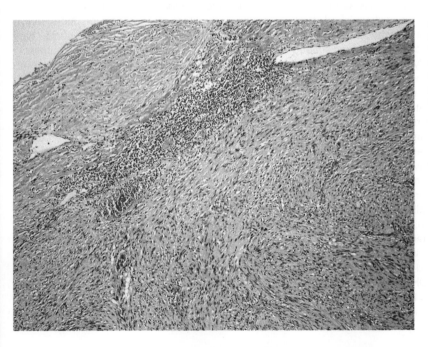

Fig. 6. Cellular schwannomas are typically well-circumscribed and encapsulated tumors, often with a peritumoral lymphoid cuff (×100).

Fig. 7. Uniform hypercellularity, representing Antoni A areas, with tumor cells arranged in fascicles or whorls is characteristic of cellular schwannoma (×200).

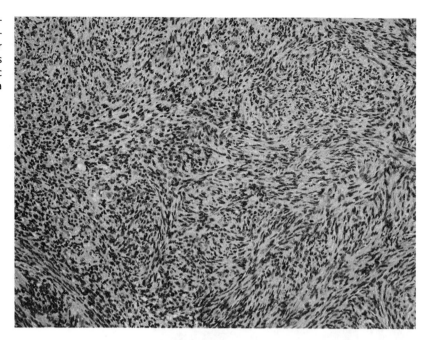

22q or deletion of the *NF2* locus in the majority of schwannomas.[21]

The diagnosis of cellular schwannoma can be difficult in limited biopsy material, and hypercellularity, nuclear atypia, focal necrosis, and mitotic figures may raise concern for malignancy. Principal differential diagnoses include deep-seated sarcomas with spindle cell morphology, such as MPNST, leiomyosarcoma, and monophasic synovial sarcoma.

As opposed to cellular schwannoma, MPNST frequently shows zonation of alternating hyper- and hypocellularity. Cytologic atypia, nuclear pleomorphism, and mitoses are more prominent in MPNST than in cellular schwannoma. Furthermore, MPNST characteristically shows perivascular accentuation of tumor cells, lacks hyalinized blood vessels, and expresses weak and/or focal S-100 protein in only a subset of cases.

Fig. 8. Accumulations of xanthoma cells as well as blood vessels with hyaline walls are common in cellular schwannoma (×200).

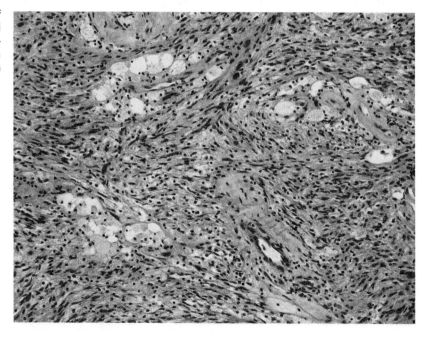

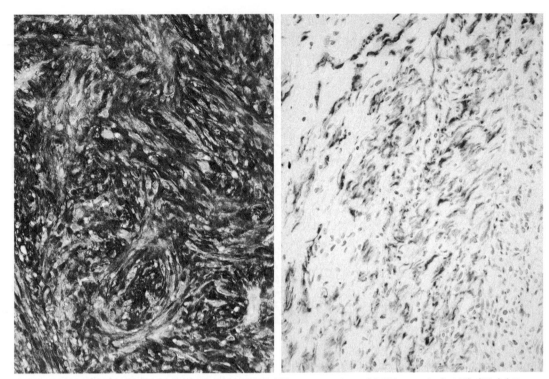

Fig. 9. (*Left*) Cellular schwannomas show strong and diffuse expression of S-100 protein (×400). (*Right*) Expression of keratins, in this case AE1/AE3, may be observed in a subset of cellular schwannomas, particularly when arising in the retroperitoneum or mediastinum (×400).

Leiomyosarcomas may be distinguished from cellular schwannoma by the presence of spindle cells with brightly eosinophilic cytoplasm and cigar-shaped nuclei. Furthermore, they diffusely express SMA, desmin, and/or caldesmon as markers of myogenic differentiation but generally lack S-100 positivity.

Monophasic synovial sarcoma is rare in the retroperitoneum but consists of fascicles of monomorphic spindle cells with tapering, often overlapping nuclei and pale, ill-defined cytoplasm. The tumor cells are surrounded by a variably collagenous matrix with hemangiopericytoma-like vessels. They usually express epithelial markers at least focally (EMA more than keratin). In contrast to cellular schwannoma, nuclear TLE-1 is expressed in a majority of cases.[22] Up to 30% of synovial sarcomas show limited S-100 positivity. Synovial sarcoma harbors the pathognomonic t(X;18) resulting in *SS18-SSX* fusion, which is detectable by molecular testing.[22]

PROGNOSIS

Cellular schwannomas only extremely rarely show malignant transformation to either epithelioid MPNST or epithelioid angiosarcoma. Local recurrence is rare unless excision is incomplete.[19]

MALIGNANT PERIPHERAL NERVE SHEATH TUMOR

INTRODUCTION

MPNST accounts for approximately 5% of soft tissue sarcomas and mostly arise in the limbs, followed by the trunk/retroperitoneum and head and neck region. They occur sporadically (30%–50%), in the setting of neurofibromatosis type 1 (NF-1) (30%–50%),[23] or after radiation therapy (10%), usually with a latency of at least 10 years.[24] Sporadic MPNSTs affect both genders equally and are more common in adults than children. Patients with NF-1 have a lifetime risk of developing MPNST of approximately 5% to 10%.[25] In this setting, men are affected more frequently than women and are 10 to 15 years younger than reported for sporadic MPNST.

Diagnostic criteria for MPNSTs include identifiable origin from a peripheral nerve or benign nerve sheath tumor, evidence of Schwann cell differentiation, or the development of a spindle cell sarcoma in a patient with NF-1. Approximately 50% of MPNSTs develop from a preexisting neurofibroma (with the plexiform subtype harboring the highest risk of malignant transformation), although a few reported cases originate from schwannoma[26] or ganglioneuroma,[27] and approximately 40% arise de novo. NF-1–associated MPNSTs more often show origin from either a peripheral nerve or neurofibroma. Most MPNSTs are high-grade tumors with aggressive behavior.

Key Features
MALIGNANT PERIPHERAL NERVE SHEATH TUMOR

- Sporadic, associated with NF-1, or postradiation

- Sporadic MPNST: patients aged 40 to 50 years, women the same as men

- NF-1–associated MPNST: patients aged approximately 30 years, men more than women

- Trunk/retroperitoneum is second most common site, tumors often large at diagnosis

- Histology: alternating cellularity, perivascular accentuation; frequent mitoses; heterologous differentiation in 10% to 15%

- Tumor cells express weak or focal S-100 (<50%), GFAP (30%), SOX-10 (30%)

- Molecular features: *NF1* inactivation (17q11), PRC2 inactivation, additional complex aberrations

- Prognosis: 5-year survival rate 30% to 60%

GROSS FEATURES

Deep MPNSTs are often large (>10 cm) at initial diagnosis and may present as a fusiform swelling if arising from a peripheral nerve. Most MPNSTs are pseudoencapsulated but may be infiltrative. If arising from a preexistent neurofibroma, transition to MPNST may be discernible. MPNSTs usually show a firm white to tan fleshy, occasionally gelatinous cut surface with focal hemorrhage and necrosis. Some MPNSTs show a thin pseudocapsule.

MICROSCOPIC FEATURES

MPNST most often shows a spindled, fascicular growth pattern with alternation of more cellular and looser, myxoid areas with perivascular condensation or whorling (Fig. 10). Relatively monomorphic tumor cells exhibit elongated tapering, wavy, hyperchromatic nuclei, and scant eosinophilic cytoplasm with ill-defined borders (Fig. 11). Mitoses can be numerous. Up to 10% of cases show predominantly myxoid morphology. Besides Schwannian differentiation, MPNST rarely shows perineurial features with a whorled growth resembling perineurioma.[28] Heterologous differentiation occurs in 10% to 15% of MPNSTs, more frequently in the setting of NF-1, and includes rhabdomyosarcomatous differentiation (so-called malignant Triton tumor) (Fig. 12)[29] followed by osteosarcomatous, chondrosarcomatous, and rarely

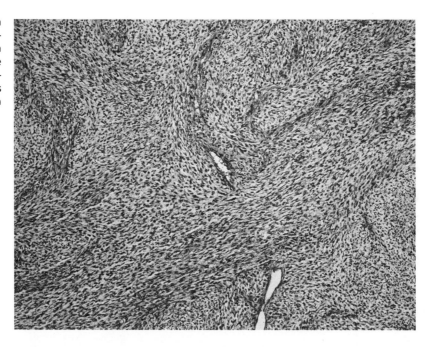

Fig. 10. MPNST often shows a spindled, fascicular growth pattern with alternation of more cellular and looser, myxoid areas as well as perivascular condensation (×100).

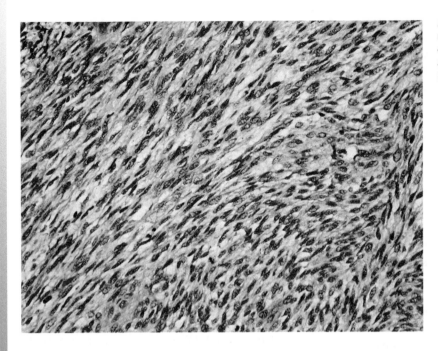

Fig. 11. Relatively mono-morphic tumor cells with elongated tapering nuclei are a common feature of MPNST (×200).

angiosarcomatous or epithelial (mostly glandular) differentiation. Variants of MPNST include epithelioid MPNST, which is more commonly superficial and accounts for less than 5% of cases arising in deep soft tissue, usually unassociated with NF-1.

DIAGNOSIS AND DIFFERENTIAL DIAGNOSIS

MPNST expresses S-100 protein in less than 50% of cases, and often less than 10% of tumor cells stain positively (**Fig. 13**). GFAP and SOX-10 are expressed in approximately 30% of cases and may serve as second-line markers.

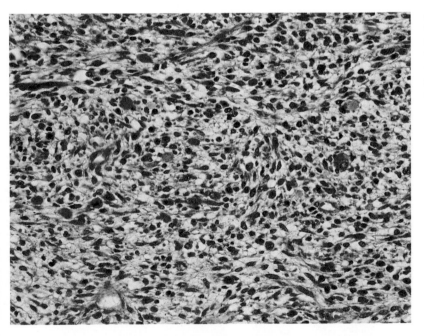

Fig. 12. A case of MPNST with heterologous rhab-domyosarcomatous differentiation (so-called malignant Triton tumor) showing numerous plump eosinophilic rhabdomyo-blasts (×400).

Fig. 13. Expression of S-100 protein in a minor subset of tumor cells in MPNST (×400).

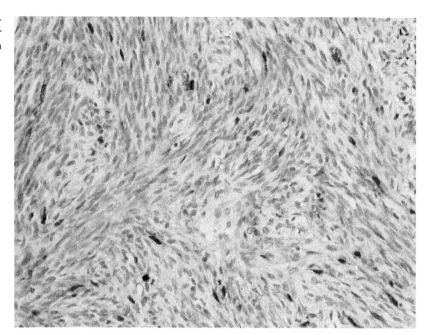

Both sporadic and NF-1–associated MPNSTs show 17q loss or *NF1* mutations as well as complex karyotypes with high numbers of chromosomal aberrations, including numerous structural and numerical changes.[21,30] A stepwise progression from neurofibroma to atypical neurofibroma and finally to MPNST has been proposed, and evidence suggests that genomic inactivation of *CDKN2A* encoding for p16 represents an early event in progression to MPNST.[31] Furthermore, dysregulation of the Polycomb repressive complex 2 (PRC2), which plays a role in Ras-driven transcriptional activation, has recently been demonstrated in MPNST.[32]

Differential diagnoses are cellular schwannoma, leiomyosarcoma, and monophasic synovial sarcoma.

Leiomyosarcoma has more eosinophilic cytoplasm and lacks the typical zonation and perivascular accentuation observed in MPNST. Furthermore, leiomyosarcomas generally do not express S-100 protein but instead show diffuse positivity for myogenic markers, such as SMA, desmin, and/or caldesmon.

Monophasic synovial sarcoma expresses TLE-1 in a majority of cases, in contrast to MPNST, which shows focal TLE-1 positivity in approximately 15%

of cases.[22] A subset of synovial sarcomas express S-100 protein, but SOX-10 expression is less frequent in synovial sarcoma (7% vs 67% in MPNST).[33] In cases in which a clear distinction between both entities is difficult based on histomorphology and immunohistochemical profile, FISH or RT-PCR may confirm the *SS18-SSX* fusion in synovial sarcoma.

Dedifferentiated liposarcoma can be distinguished from MPNST by the presence of fatty differentiation and more consistent nuclear MDM-2/CDK-4 overexpression. Although a subset of MPNST is reported to show *MDM2* amplification,[34] CDK-4 positivity favors the diagnosis of dedifferentiated liposarcoma.

PROGNOSIS

The prognosis of MPNST is generally unfavorable, with a 5-year survival rate of 30% to 60%, and local recurrences and distant metastases (mostly hematogeneous spread to the lung) are described to occur in 40% to 68% of patients.[35] Whether MPNSTs arising in NF-1 patients have a worse prognosis than sporadic MPNST is still controversial. MPNST with heterologous differentiation often behaves particularly aggressively and frequently metastasizes.

Differential Diagnosis

Cellular schwannoma

- Sporadic or in NF-2 or in schwannomatosis
- Hypercellular without Antoni B pattern
- Sometimes degenerative nuclear atypia
- Hyalinized blood vessels
- Mitoses generally <10/10 HPFs
- Tumor cells express S-100 strongly and diffusely, sometimes keratin
- Molecular feature: *NF2* inactivation (22q12)

MPNST

- Sporadic, in NF-1, or postradiation
- Alternating cellularity, zonation
- Hyperchromatic nuclei, at least focal nuclear atypia
- Perivascular accentuation of tumor cells
- Mitoses and necrosis frequent
- In <50% of cases, tumor cells express S-100 weak and focal, sometimes GFAP and SOX-10
- Molecular feature: *NF1* inactivation (17q11), PRC2 inactivation, additional complex aberrations

DEEP LEIOMYOMA

INTRODUCTION

Leiomyomas occur in various anatomic locations and the following compartments are distinguished for diagnostic and prognostic purposes: deep soft tissue, including retroperitoneum/abdominal cavity, skin, subcutis, and external genitalia.[36] Leiomyomas of deep soft tissue are rare and affect middle-aged adults with a predilection for women.[37,38] They mostly arise in the retroperitoneum, followed by the limbs and trunk. Criteria for malignancy in leiomyoma differ in both genders and depend on tumor site.[36]

Key Features
RETROPERITONEAL LEIOMYOMA

- Adult patients, peak approximately 40 years, women more than men
- Rare, slowly growing, well-circumscribed, lobulated, greater than 5 cm in size
- Histology: cigar-shaped nuclei, brightly eosinophilic cytoplasm
- Mitotic rate: female patients less than 10 mitoses/50 HPFs, male patients less than 1 mitosis/50 HPFs
- No necrosis, no/minimal nuclear atypia
- Tumor cells express SMA, desmin, caldesmon, ER/PR (male patients lack ER)
- Prognosis: almost no recurrence, no metastases

GROSS FEATURES

Deep leiomyomas are slowly growing tumors and are often large at initial diagnosis, with a mean size of approximately 16 cm.[37] They are well circumscribed and lobulated, with a firm gray-white, whorled, rubbery cut surface.

MICROSCOPIC FEATURES

Deep leiomyomas consist of usually long intersecting fascicles of mature smooth muscle cells (ie, spindle cells with brightly eosinophilic cytoplasm and elongated, blunt-ended, cigar-shaped nuclei [**Figs. 14** and **15**], sometimes with nuclear palisading). Deep leiomyomas of the retroperitoneum may resemble their uterine counterparts by exhibiting trabecular architecture and degenerative changes, such as fibrosis, myxoid change, scattered osteoclastic giant cells, stromal hyalinization, focal calcification, ossification, hemorrhage, and cystic change. In deep leiomyomas, degenerative nuclear atypia does not necessarily indicate malignancy.[39]

DIAGNOSIS AND DIFFERENTIAL DIAGNOSIS

Leiomyomas consistently show diffuse expression of SMA, desmin (**Fig. 16**), and/or caldesmon. Up to 40% of cases additionally express epithelial markers, such as EMA or keratin, whereas S-100 and CD34 positivity are less common. Similar to uterine leiomyomas, a majority of retroperitoneal leiomyomas in women show ER (see **Fig. 16**) and PR positivity, whereas only the latter is expressed in male patients.[37] Rarely, retroperitoneal leiomyomas show DOG-1 positivity (approximately 10%).[40]

Fig. 14. Deep leiomyomas usually consist of long intersecting fascicles of well-differentiated smooth muscle cells (×100).

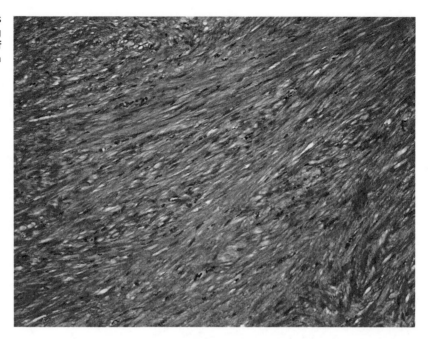

Criteria for malignancy differ depending on anatomic location: for instance, in deep smooth muscle tumors arising in the extremities, tumors with greater than 1 mitosis/50 HPFs are regarded as malignant.[36] In contrast, a higher mitotic rate is permitted in retroperitoneal leiomyomas (most of which arise in women), where tumors with less than 10 mitoses/50 HPFs seem to be benign, as long as there is no atypia or necrosis. In men, in whom such lesions are exceedingly rare, the threshold in retroperitoneal leiomyomas is less than 1 mitosis/50 HPFs. *MED12* mutations have also been described in extrauterine leiomyoma, in which they seem to occur less frequently than in uterine leiomyoma (15% vs 75%).[41,42] Leiomyomas usually show normal or noncomplex karyotypes in the diploid range.[41]

Fig. 15. The spindled tumor cells of leiomyoma have brightly eosinophilic cytoplasm and elongated, cigar-shaped, or more tapering nuclei (×200).

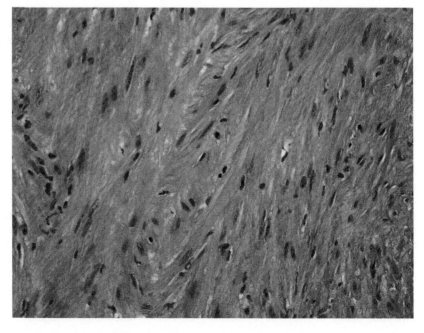

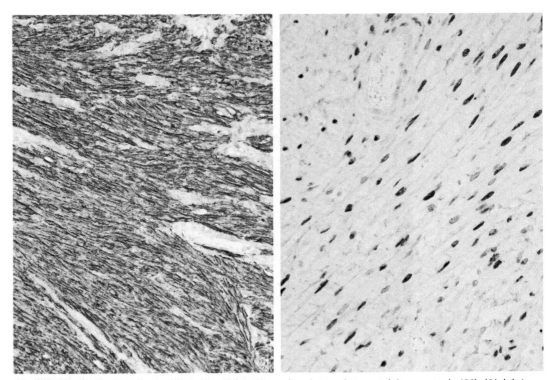

Fig. 16. (*Left*) Strong and diffuse expression of desmin can be observed in most leiomyomas (×400). (*Right*) A majority of retroperitoneal leiomyomas show expression of estrogen receptor (×400).

The differential diagnosis of retroperitoneal leiomyoma includes leiomyosarcoma, cellular schwannoma, perivascular epithelioid cell tumor (PEComa), and gastrointestinal stromal tumor (GIST).

Leiomyosarcoma is diagnosed in cases with more than minimal nuclear atypia, necrosis, or a higher mitotic rate than acceptable for deep leiomyoma.[36]

Cellular schwannoma presents as an encapsulated, uniformly cellular spindle cell neoplasm but, unlike leiomyoma, lacks the typical cytologic features of smooth muscle differentiation and instead consists of tumor cells with wavy, elongated, and tapering nuclei. Cellular schwannomas show strong and diffuse S-100 expression but lack SMA, desmin, and caldesmon positivity.

PEComas show evidence of myomelanocytic differentiation.[43] Similar to retroperitoneal leiomyomas, they predominantly occur in women and histologically show eosinophilic tumor cells, often having rather granular cytoplasm, which are mostly epithelioid or polygonal but sometimes spindled. In addition to myogenic markers (SMA and desmin), PEComas characteristically coexpress HMB-45 or melan-A.[43,44]

If located in the abdominal cavity, GIST may enter the differential diagnosis. The tumor cells exhibit syncytial, palely eosinophilic cytoplasm, do not show the typical cigar-shaped nuclei of leiomyoma, and lack degenerative changes. GIST shows diffuse positivity for DOG-1 in 98% and KIT in 95% of cases. Desmin expression is observed in only approximately 5% of GISTs.[45] Furthermore, oncogenic mutations in either one of the receptor tyrosine kinases *KIT* or *PDGFRA* are detectable by genomic sequencing in 85% of GISTs and may be diagnostically useful in cases with unusual morphology or immunohistochemical profile.

PROGNOSIS

Local recurrence in leiomyomas occurs in less than 10% of cases, sometimes after a long latency. Soft tissue leiomyomas do not metastasize.[37]

LEIOMYOSARCOMA

INTRODUCTION

Intra-abdominal leiomyosarcoma accounts for 40% to 45% of leiomyosarcomas and includes tumors arising in the retroperitoneum, mesentery, or omentum and major blood vessels, such as the inferior vena cava.[46] They mostly affect women aged 40 to 60 years. Retroperitoneal leiomyosarcomas are often large at presentation, and surgical resection with negative margins can be challenging.

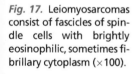

Key Features
RETROPERITONEAL LEIOMYOSARCOMA

- Patients aged approximately 40 to 60 years, women more than men

- Well-circumscribed, thin pseudocapsule, usually greater than 5 cm in size

- Mitotic rate: female patients greater than or equal to 10 mitoses/50 HPFs, male patients greater than or equal to 1 mitosis/50 HPFs

- Necrosis, more than minimal nuclear atypia

- Tumor cells express SMA, desmin, caldesmon, also in 30% to 40% keratin/EMA

- Prognosis: 5-year survival rate 20% to 30%

GROSS FEATURES

Deep leiomyosarcomas are large, well-circumscribed and occasionally infiltrative tumors with a thin pseudocapsule. They exhibit a fleshy gray-white to tan, whorled cut surface that may show a heterogeneous appearance in higher-grade tumors with areas of necrosis, hemorrhage, myxoid change, and cystic degeneration.

MICROSCOPIC FEATURES

Leiomyosarcomas consist of fascicles of spindle cells with brightly eosinophilic, sometimes fibrillary cytoplasm (Fig. 17) and vesicular, elongated to cigar-shaped nuclei (Fig. 18). Necrosis, hyalinization, or cystic change is frequent. Morphologic variants include tumors with marked pleomorphism (Fig. 19), a prominent inflammatory infiltrate, myxoid morphology, granular cell change,[47] and rarely dedifferentiation to undifferentiated sarcoma without evidence of smooth muscle differentiation (Fig. 20).[48]

DIAGNOSIS AND DIFFERENTIAL DIAGNOSIS

Immunohistochemically, leiomyosarcomas express SMA in a majority of cases, desmin in 70% to 80%,[49] and caldesmon in approximately 60% of cases. Of note, 30% to 40% of leiomyosarcomas may show positivity for epithelial markers, such as keratin or EMA.[49] Molecular studies reveal that extrauterine leiomyosarcomas, in contrast to their uterine counterpart, lack *MED12* mutations.[41] They usually have complex karyotypes with extensive intra- and intertumoral heterogeneity.[50]

The differential diagnosis of retroperitoneal leiomyosarcomas includes mainly deep leiomyoma and dedifferentiated liposarcoma.

Deep leiomyomas may exhibit degenerative changes but the presence of necrosis, more than minimal nuclear atypia, and a mitotic rate greater than or equal to 10/50 HPFs in women or greater than or equal to 1/50 HPFs in men indicates leiomyosarcoma.

Dedifferentiated liposarcoma, in most cases, lacks convincing smooth muscle differentiation. In dedifferentiated liposarcoma with heterogeneous

Fig. 17. Leiomyosarcomas consist of fascicles of spindle cells with brightly eosinophilic, sometimes fibrillary cytoplasm (×100).

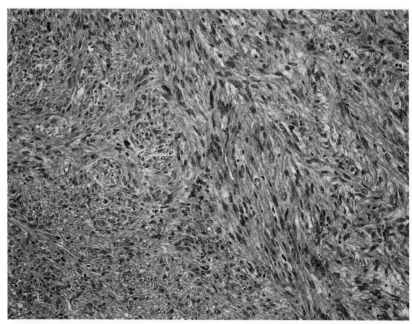

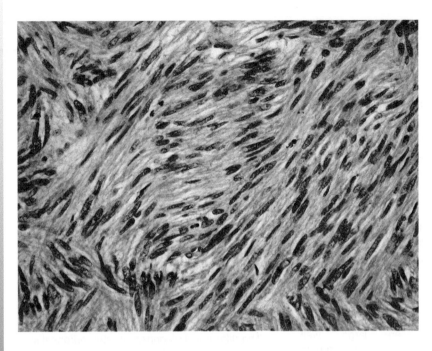

Fig. 18. Tumor cells of leiomyosarcoma with somewhat hyperchromatic, elongated to cigar-shaped nuclei and scattered mitoses (×200).

leiomyosarcomatous differentiation, however, the distinction from primary leimyosarcoma can be challenging – in particular, when only limited biopsy material is available. In this setting, overexpression of MDM-2/CDK-4 and *MDM2* amplification may prove helpful because they are consistently present in dedifferentiated liposarcoma with myosarcomatous differentiation, similar to conventional dedifferentiated liposarcoma.[4] In contrast, leiomyosarcomas are negative for MDM-2/CDK-4 and only a subset of cases show low-level *MDM2* amplification. It is important to differentiate between leiomyosarcoma and dedifferentiated liposarcoma with myosarcomatous differentiation because the latter has a significantly lower metastatic potential.[4]

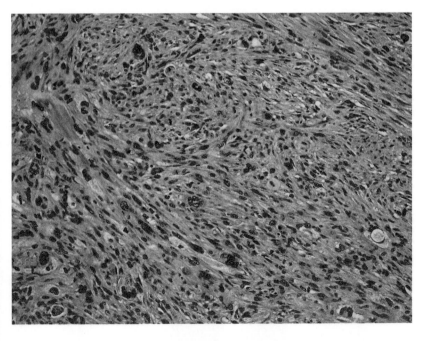

Fig. 19. Pleomorphic leiomyosarcoma showing highly pleomorphic and atypical tumor cells with only a partially fascicular architecture (×200).

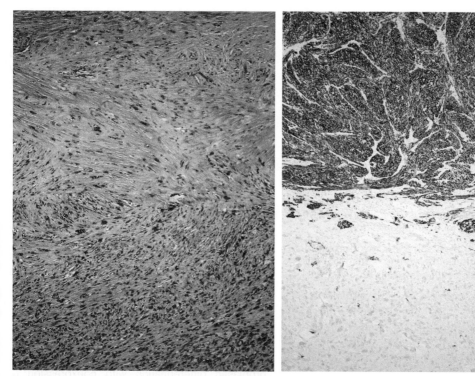

Fig. 20. Rarely, abrupt transition from (*top*) well-differentiated leiomyosarcoma to (*bottom*) dedifferentiated leiomyosarcoma with loss of desmin expression may be observed (×100).

PROGNOSIS

Due to their size and deep location, complete surgical resection of retroperitoneal leiomyosarcomas may be difficult. A majority of patients develop local recurrence and distant metastases (mostly pulmonary and hepatic). The 5-year survival rate ranges approximately from 20% to 30%.

MAMMARY-TYPE MYOFIBROBLASTOMA

INTRODUCTION

Mammary-type myofibroblastoma histologically is identical to myofibroblastoma of the breast but arises in soft tissue at extramammary sites, most commonly in the inguinal/groin region, followed by the trunk, lower limb and retroperitoneum,

Differential Diagnosis

Retroperitoneal leiomyoma	Retroperitoneal leiomyosarcoma
• Female patients peak around 40 years of age	• Female patients peak around 40 to 60 years of age
• Mitoses—women: less than 10/50 HPFs, men: less than 1/50 HPFs	• Mitoses—women: greater than or equal to 10/50 HPFs, men: greater than or equal to 1/50 HPFs
• No necrosis, no/minimal atypia	• Necrosis, more than minimal atypia
• Molecular features: normal or noncomplex karyotype, *MED12* mutations in 15%	• Molecular features: complex karyotype, no *MED12* mutations
• Prognosis: almost no recurrence, no metastases	• Prognosis: recurrence and metastases common

and in the past years increasingly recognized at various other locations.[51,52] The mean age of patients is approximately 55 years but a wide age distribution can be observed, and approximately two-thirds of cases occur in male patients.[52]

Key Features
MAMMARY-TYPE MYOFIBROBLASTOMA

- Adult patients, wide age range but mainly adults, men more than women

- Most common in the groin/inguinal region, well-circumscribed, unencapsulated

- Histology: tumor cells with myofibroblastic differentiation, intervening collagen, variable adipose tissue, mast cells

- Tumor cells express CD34 and desmin, occasionally SMA; loss of Rb expression

- Molecular features: del13q14 (*RB1, FOXO1*)

GROSS FEATURES

Mammary-type myofibroblastoma presents as a slow-growing or incidentally detected mass with a median size of approximately 6 cm. The tumors are well circumscribed but unencapsulated, showing a firm tan, pink, white, or brown cut surface with a whorled or nodular, rarely mucoid appearance lacking necrosis or hemorrhage.

MICROSCOPIC FEATURES

Mammary-type myofibroblastoma consists of spindle to oval tumor cells with stubby or pointed nuclei and inconspicuous nucleoli, indistinct palely eosinophilic to amphophilic cytoplasm with ill-defined borders and variable cellularity (**Figs. 21** and **22**). The cells are arranged haphazardly in fascicles of variable size with intervening hyalinized collagenous stroma. A variable amount (10%–60%) of adipose tissue is usually part of the tumor, often showing variation in adipocyte size.[51] Few mitoses and focal atypia with nuclear pleomorphism may be present, and mast cells are typically scattered throughout the tumor. Some cases (at least in the breast) may show smooth muscle or cartilaginous differentiation. Epithelioid morphology, rare atypical or multinucleate cells, and focal myxoid stromal change have also been described.

DIAGNOSIS AND DIFFERENTIAL DIAGNOSIS

Mammary-type myofibroblastoma shows myofibroblastic differentiation with coexpression of both CD34 and desmin (**Fig. 23**). Approximately 30% of tumors additionally express SMA. Mammary-type myofibroblastomas harbor partial monosomy 13q14, which includes *RB1* and *FOXO1*, which assigns it to the spectrum of tumors with 13q abnormalities and loss of Rb1 expression (see **Fig. 23**), such as cellular angiofibroma and spindle-cell/pleomorphic lipoma.

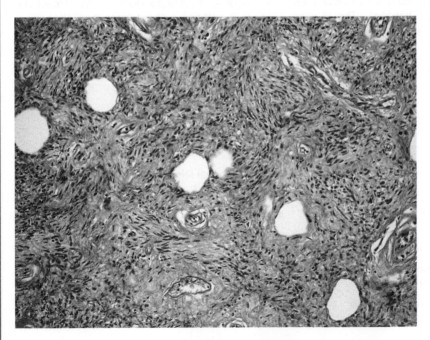

Fig. 21. Mammary-type myofibroblastoma contains spindle cells arranged haphazardly in fascicles with intervening collagenous stroma (×100).

Fig. 22. Tumor cells with stubby or pointed nuclei distributed in a collagenous stroma with variable numbers of mature adipocytes (×200).

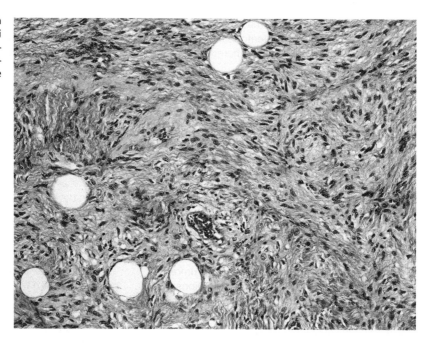

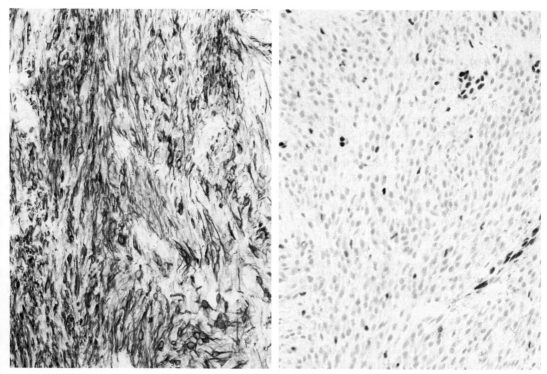

Fig. 23. (*Left*) Expression of desmin is characteristic of mammary-type myofibroblastoma (×400). (*Right*) Abnormalities of the 13q14 locus lead to loss of Rb1 expression in a majority of cases; endothelial cells serve as a positive internal control (×400).

The differential diagnosis of mammary-type my-ofibroblastoma in the retroperitoneum includes smooth muscle tumors and well-differentiated liposarcoma with spindle cell features.

Well-differentiated liposarcoma, which may have a spindle cell component, is usually larger than mammary-type myofibroblastoma and often multi-lobulated. Well-differentiated liposarcoma with spindle cell areas comprises tumor cells with more clearly evident nuclear atypia and hyperchromasia than mammary-type myofibroblastoma, scattered in a myxoid or collagenous stroma. Furthermore, lipoblasts may be observed. Similar to mammary-type myofibroblastoma, CD34 may be expressed but desmin is usually more limited. MDM-2/CDK-4 overexpression and *MDM2* amplification is variable in well-differentiated liposarcoma with spindle cell features and instead some tumors, which have been referred to as spindle cell liposarcoma or well-differentiated adipocytic neoplasm with spindle cell features, show monosomy 7 and 13q14 deletions (including *RB1*).[53]

PROGNOSIS

Mammary-type myofibroblastoma is a benign tumor and usually does not recur, even if excision is marginal.

SUMMARY

The diagnostic spectrum of spindle cell neoplasms arising in the retroperitoneum is wide and, in the presence of commonly shared morphologic features, it may be challenging to establish a correct diagnosis in certain cases. Beyond seemingly un-differentiated spindle cell morphology, however, most neoplasms may reveal distinctive adipocytic, smooth muscle or myofibroblastic or nerve sheath differentiation and show additional diagnostic clues or characteristic molecular abnormalities. Obtaining sufficient and representative biopsy material, a thorough work-up, and extensive sampling of gross specimens followed by a combined histopathologic, immunohistochemical, and – if necessary – molecular work-up of these cases is advisable so as not to miss important diagnostic and/or prognostic indicators.

REFERENCES

1. Coindre JM, Hostein I, Maire G, et al. Inflammatory malignant fibrous histiocytomas and dedifferentiated liposarcomas: histological review, genomic profile, and MDM2 and CDK4 status favour a single entity. J Pathol 2004;203:822–30.

2. McCormick D, Mentzel T, Beham A, et al. Dedifferentiated liposarcoma. Clinicopathologic analysis of 32 cases suggesting a better prognostic subgroup among pleomorphic sarcomas. Am J Surg Pathol 1994;18:1213–23.

3. Henricks WH, Chu YC, Goldblum JR, et al. Dedifferentiated liposarcoma: a clinicopathological analysis of 155 cases with a proposal for an expanded definition of dedifferentiation. Am J Surg Pathol 1997; 21:271–81.

4. Binh MB, Guillou L, Hostein I, et al. Dedifferentiated liposarcomas with divergent myosarcomatous differentiation developed in the internal trunk: a study of 27 cases and comparison to conventional dedifferentiated liposarcomas and leiomyosarcomas. Am J Surg Pathol 2007;31:1557–66.

5. Nascimento AG, Kurtin PJ, Guillou L, et al. Dedifferentiated liposarcoma: a report of nine cases with a peculiar neurallike whorling pattern associated with metaplastic bone formation. Am J Surg Pathol 1998;22:945–55.

6. Marino-Enriquez A, Fletcher CD, Dal CP, et al. Dedifferentiated liposarcoma with "homologous" lipoblastic (pleomorphic liposarcoma-like) differentiation: clinicopathologic and molecular analysis of a series suggesting revised diagnostic criteria. Am J Surg Pathol 2010;34:1122–31.

7. Elgar F, Goldblum JR. Well-differentiated liposarcoma of the retroperitoneum: a clinicopathologic analysis of 20 cases, with particular attention to the extent of low-grade dedifferentiation. Mod Pathol 1997;10:113–20.

8. Evans HL. Atypical lipomatous tumor, its variants, and its combined forms: a study of 61 cases, with a minimum follow-up of 10 years. Am J Surg Pathol 2007;31:1–14.

9. Coindre JM, Pedeutour F, Aurias A. Well-differentiated and dedifferentiated liposarcomas. Virchows Arch 2010;456:167–79.

10. Rosai J, Akerman M, Dal CP, et al. Combined morphologic and karyotypic study of 59 atypical lipomatous tumors. Evaluation of their relationship and differential diagnosis with other adipose tissue tumors (a report of the CHAMP Study Group). Am J Surg Pathol 1996;20:1182–9.

11. Sirvent N, Coindre JM, Maire G, et al. Detection of MDM2-CDK4 amplification by fluorescence in situ hybridization in 200 paraffin-embedded tumor samples: utility in diagnosing adipocytic lesions and comparison with immunohistochemistry and real-time PCR. Am J Surg Pathol 2007;31:1476–89.

12. Binh MB, Sastre-Garau X, Guillou L, et al. MDM2 and CDK4 immunostainings are useful adjuncts in diagnosing well-differentiated and dedifferentiated liposarcoma subtypes: a comparative analysis of 559 soft tissue neoplasms with genetic data. Am J Surg Pathol 2005;29:1340–7.

13. Hornick JL, Bosenberg MW, Mentzel T, et al. Pleomorphic liposarcoma: clinicopathologic analysis of 57 cases. Am J Surg Pathol 2004;28:1257–67.

14. Martuza RL, Eldridge R. Neurofibromatosis 2 (bilateral acoustic neurofibromatosis). N Engl J Med 1988;318:684–8.

15. Carney JA. Psammomatous melanotic schwannoma. A distinctive, heritable tumor with special associations, including cardiac myxoma and the Cushing syndrome. Am J Surg Pathol 1990;14:206–22.

16. Hadfield KD, Newman WG, Bowers NL, et al. Molecular characterisation of SMARCB1 and NF2 in familial and sporadic schwannomatosis. J Med Genet 2008;45:332–9.

17. Woodruff JM, Godwin TA, Erlandson RA, et al. Cellular schwannoma: a variety of schwannoma sometimes mistaken for a malignant tumor. Am J Surg Pathol 1981;5:733–44.

18. Fletcher CD, Davies SE, McKee PH. Cellular schwannoma: a distinct pseudosarcomatous entity. Histopathology 1987;11:21–35.

19. Casadei GP, Scheithauer BW, Hirose T, et al. Cellular schwannoma. A clinicopathologic, DNA flow cytometric, and proliferation marker study of 70 patients. Cancer 1995;75:1109–19.

20. Fanburg-Smith JC, Majidi M, Miettinen M. Keratin expression in schwannoma; a study of 115 retroperitoneal and 22 peripheral schwannomas. Mod Pathol 2006;19:115–21.

21. Mertens F, Dal CP, De Wever I, et al. Cytogenetic characterization of peripheral nerve sheath tumours: a report of the CHAMP study group. J Pathol 2000; 190:31–8.

22. Foo WC, Cruise MW, Wick MR, et al. Immunohistochemical staining for TLE1 distinguishes synovial sarcoma from histologic mimics. Am J Clin Pathol 2011;135:839–44.

23. Ghosh BC, Ghosh L, Huvos AG, et al. Malignant schwannoma. A clinicopathologic study. Cancer 1973;31:184–90.

24. Foley KM, Woodruff JM, Ellis FT, et al. Radiation-induced malignant and atypical peripheral nerve sheath tumors. Ann Neurol 1980;7:311–8.

25. Widemann BC. Current status of sporadic and neurofibromatosis type 1-associated malignant peripheral nerve sheath tumors. Curr Oncol Rep 2009;11:322–8.

26. Woodruff JM, Selig AM, Crowley K, et al. Schwannoma (neurilemoma) with malignant transformation. A rare, distinctive peripheral nerve tumor. Am J Surg Pathol 1994;18:882–95.

27. Fletcher CD, Fernando IN, Braimbridge MV, et al. Malignant nerve sheath tumour arising in a ganglioneuroma. Histopathology 1988;12:445–8.

28. Hirose T, Scheithauer BW, Sano T. Perineurial malignant peripheral nerve sheath tumor (MPNST): a clinicopathologic, immunohistochemical, and ultrastructural study of seven cases. Am J Surg Pathol 1998;22:1368–78.

29. Daimaru Y, Hashimoto H, Enjoji M. Malignant "triton" tumors: a clinicopathologic and immunohistochemical study of nine cases. Hum Pathol 1984;15: 768–78.

30. Bottillo I, Ahlquist T, Brekke H, et al. Germline and somatic NF1 mutations in sporadic and NF1-associated malignant peripheral nerve sheath tumours. J Pathol 2009;217:693–701.

31. Beert E, Brems H, Daniels B, et al. Atypical neurofibromas in neurofibromatosis type 1 are premalignant tumors. Genes Chromosomes Cancer 2011; 50:1021–32.

32. Lee W, Teckie S, Wiesner T, et al. PRC2 is recurrently inactivated through EED or SUZ12 loss in malignant peripheral nerve sheath tumors. Nat Genet 2014;46: 1227–32.

33. Kang Y, Pekmezci M, Folpe AL, et al. Diagnostic utility of SOX10 to distinguish malignant peripheral nerve sheath tumor from synovial sarcoma, including intraneural synovial sarcoma. Mod Pathol 2014;27:55–61.

34. Wallander ML, Tripp S, Layfield LJ. MDM2 amplification in malignant peripheral nerve sheath tumors correlates with p53 protein expression. Arch Pathol Lab Med 2012;136:95–9.

35. Zou C, Smith KD, Liu J, et al. Clinical, pathological, and molecular variables predictive of malignant peripheral nerve sheath tumor outcome. Ann Surg 2009;249:1014–22.

36. Hornick JL, Fletcher CD. Criteria for malignancy in nonvisceral smooth muscle tumors. Ann Diagn Pathol 2003;7:60–6.

37. Paal E, Miettinen M. Retroperitoneal leiomyomas: a clinicopathologic and immunohistochemical study of 56 cases with a comparison to retroperitoneal leiomyosarcomas. Am J Surg Pathol 2001;25:1355–63.

38. Billings SD, Folpe AL, Weiss SW. Do leiomyomas of deep soft tissue exist? An analysis of highly differentiated smooth muscle tumors of deep soft tissue supporting two distinct subtypes. Am J Surg Pathol 2001;25:1134–42.

39. Fletcher CD, Kilpatrick SE, Mentzel T. The difficulty in predicting behavior of smooth-muscle tumors in deep soft tissue. Am J Surg Pathol 1995;19:116–7.

40. Miettinen M, Wang ZF, Lasota J. DOG1 antibody in the differential diagnosis of gastrointestinal stromal tumors: a study of 1840 cases. Am J Surg Pathol 2009;33:1401–8.

41. Ravegnini G, Marino-Enriquez A, Slater J, et al. MED12 mutations in leiomyosarcoma and extra-uterine leiomyoma. Mod Pathol 2013;26:743–9.

42. Bertsch E, Qiang W, Zhang Q, et al. MED12 and HMGA2 mutations: two independent genetic events in uterine leiomyoma and leiomyosarcoma. Mod Pathol 2014;27:1144–53.

43. Hornick JL, Fletcher CD. PEComa: what do we know so far? Histopathology 2006;48:75–82.

44. Folpe AL, Mentzel T, Lehr HA, et al. Perivascular epithelioid cell neoplasms of soft tissue and gynecologic origin: a clinicopathologic study of 26 cases and review of the literature. Am J Surg Pathol 2005;29:1558–75.

45. Corless CL, Fletcher JA, Heinrich MC. Biology of gastrointestinal stromal tumors. J Clin Oncol 2004; 22:3813–25.

46. Wile AG, Evans HL, Romsdahl MM. Leiomyosarcoma of soft tissue: a clinicopathologic study. Cancer 1981;48:1022–32.

47. Mentzel T, Wadden C, Fletcher CD. Granular cell change in smooth muscle tumours of skin and soft tissue. Histopathology 1994;24:223–31.

48. Chen E, O'Connell F, Fletcher CD. Dedifferentiated leiomyosarcoma: clinicopathological analysis of 18 cases. Histopathology 2011;59:1135–43.

49. Iwata J, Fletcher CD. Immunohistochemical detection of cytokeratin and epithelial membrane antigen in leiomyosarcoma: a systematic study of 100 cases. Pathol Int 2000;50:7–14.

50. Mandahl N, Fletcher CD, Dal CP, et al. Comparative cytogenetic study of spindle cell and pleomorphic leiomyosarcomas of soft tissues: a report from the CHAMP Study Group. Cancer Genet Cytogenet 2000;116:66–73.

51. McMenamin ME, Fletcher CD. Mammary-type myofibroblastoma of soft tissue: a tumor closely related to spindle cell lipoma. Am J Surg Pathol 2001;25: 1022–9.

52. Howitt BE, Fletcher CD. Mammary-type myofibroblastoma: clinicopathologic characterization in a series of 143 cases. Am J Surg Pathol 2015, in press.

53. Mentzel T, Palmedo G, Kuhnen C. Well-differentiated spindle cell liposarcoma ('atypical spindle cell lipomatous tumor') does not belong to the spectrum of atypical lipomatous tumor but has a close relationship to spindle cell lipoma: clinicopathologic, immunohistochemical, and molecular analysis of six cases. Mod Pathol 2010;23:729–36.

Diagnostically Challenging "Fatty" Retroperitoneal Tumors

Karen J. Fritchie, MD*

KEYWORDS

- Adipocytic • Fatty • Retroperitoneal • Sarcoma • Liposarcoma

ABSTRACT

A variety of benign and malignant retroperitoneal mesenchymal lesions may have a component of adipose tissue, including entities such as lipoma, myolipoma, angiomyolipoma, solitary fibrous tumor, genital stromal tumors, and well-differentiated/dedifferentiated liposarcoma. Although definitive diagnosis is usually straightforward on the complete resection specimen, it is often more difficult to workup these lesions on small biopsy samples. This review focuses on challenging diagnostic scenarios of retroperitoneal lesions with a "fatty" component and provides major differential diagnoses for commonly encountered morphologic patterns, clinicopathologic features of the various entities, and strategy for use of ancillary techniques, such as immunohistochemistry and cytogenetic studies.

OVERVIEW

One of the most commonly encountered specimens in soft tissue consultation practice is the biopsy or resection of a retroperitoneal mass. Oftentimes these specimens harbor a component of fat. Although the differential diagnosis of a "fatty" retroperitoneal tumor includes well-differentiated liposarcoma and dedifferentiated liposarcoma, it is also important to consider benign entities, such as lipoma, myolipoma, angiomyolipoma, the lipomatous variant of solitary fibrous tumor, and genital stromal tumors.

There are 4 main rules that pertain to this topic (Key Points). The first 3 are critical in the workup of any adipocytic tumor, and the fourth applies to retroperitoneal sarcomas. Not only do these rules provide a starting point in the evaluation of these cases, but they also keep the pathologist out of trouble. The first rule is location, location, location. Although not absolute, superficial fatty tumors are often benign, whereas those occurring in deep soft tissue (intramuscular, retroperitoneal, groin, mediastinum) are more likely to be malignant. This rule is especially true in the retroperitoneum, as well-differentiated/dedifferentiated liposarcoma should be on the differential diagnosis of virtually every lipomatous mass at this site.

Key Points

1. Location: Superficial (above the fascia) fatty tumors are typically benign, whereas those occurring in deep soft tissue (intramuscular, retroperitoneum, groin, mediastinum) are more worrisome for malignancy.

2. Do not look for lipoblasts. The diagnostic cell of well-differentiated liposarcoma is the atypical hyperchromatic stromal cell.

3. Most fatty tumors have recurrent cytogenetic aberrations.

4. The main differential diagnosis of a retroperitoneal sarcoma is well-differentiated liposarcoma, dedifferentiated liposarcoma, and leiomyosarcoma.

Disclosure/conflict of interest: The author declares no conflict of interest.
Department of Laboratory Medicine and Pathology, Mayo Clinic, 200 First Street, Southwest, Rochester, MN 55905, USA
* Department of Anatomic Pathology, Mayo Clinic, Hilton 11, 200 First Street, Southwest, Rochester, MN 55905.
E-mail address: fritchie.karen@mayo.edu

The second rule of fatty tumors is, do not look for lipoblasts. Searching for lipoblasts is a time sink that does more harm than good. Lipoblasts are neoplastic cells that recapitulate the development of normal fat (Fig. 1A). It is important to realize that lipoblasts may be found in both benign and malignant fatty tumors. Except for the diagnosis of pleomorphic liposarcoma, lipoblasts are not requisite for the diagnosis of liposarcoma. Furthermore, many cell types, including atrophic adipocytes (see Fig. 1B), vacuolated histiocytes (see Fig. 1C), and signet-ring cell carcinomas (see Fig. 1D), can mimic lipoblasts, leading to diagnostic chaos. The key cell of atypical lipomatous tumor/well-differentiated liposarcoma and dedifferentiated liposarcoma is the atypical hyperchromatic stromal cell (see Fig. 1E).

Most lipomatous tumors harbor chromosomal aberrations, and the third rule is that we can often exploit these cytogenetic findings, especially on small biopsy specimens. Atypical lipomatous tumors/well-differentiated liposarcoma and dedifferentiated liposarcoma have giant and ring chromosomes with 12q13–15 amplicons containing genes such as MDM2 and CDK4, whereas lipomas do not.[1] Consequently, the identification of MDM2 amplification by fluorescence in situ hybridization (FISH) is a sensitive and specific tool in the evaluation of well-differentiated fatty tumors (lipoma vs atypical lipomatous tumor/well-differentiated liposarcoma), and this technique is especially helpful with limited tissue (Fig. 2).[2,3] Although MDM2/CDK4 amplification also may be detected by immunohistochemistry, FISH studies may be preferable due to occasional nonspecific staining and lower sensitivity and specificity encountered with CDK4 and MDM2 immunostains.[3] Approximately 75% of lipomas have abnormal karyotypes, with translocations involving the region of 12q13–15 (HMGA2 locus) being the most common finding; other benign lipomatous tumors that are occasionally found in the retroperitoneum, such as hibernoma, lipoblastoma, and myelolipoma, also have chromosomal aberrations.[4–7] Because it often is not possible to look for these abnormalities because of lack of readily available FISH probes, sending fresh tissue for cytogenetic analysis from the resection of any lipomatous neoplasm may yield helpful information.

The last important rule to consider is the differential diagnosis of a retroperitoneal sarcoma, and by far the most common entities include well-differentiated liposarcoma/dedifferentiated liposarcoma and leiomyosarcoma. Although other sarcomas may occur at this location, the pathologist should consider the former diagnoses before entertaining other ideas.

The remainder of this review emphasizes these key principles while discussing frequent morphologic patterns of retroperitoneal masses with an adipocytic component.

PATTERN 1: MATURE ADIPOSE TISSUE AND ATYPICAL HYPERCHROMATIC STROMAL CELLS

This scenario is commonly seen on biopsy and resection specimens of adipocytic lesions in the retroperitoneum. Morphologic review shows mature adipocytes admixed with variable amounts of atypical spindled cells with hyperchromatic and smudgy nuclei (Fig. 3A). Some of the atypical cells may have a floretlike multinucleated appearance (see Fig. 3B).

When one encounters a retroperitoneal mass harboring these features, it is helpful to recall the rules mentioned earlier. First, the fatty mass is at a deep site (retroperitoneum), which should trigger the pathologist to think about well-differentiated liposarcoma. Second, the diagnostic cell type (atypical hyperchromatic stromal cell) has been identified, confirming the diagnosis of well-differentiated liposarcoma. Note that in this situation we do not need lipoblasts or ancillary testing for diagnosis. Be aware that fat necrosis is common in lipomatous lesions and may raise concern for malignancy (Pitfall: Fat necrosis). Although foci of fat necrosis can be quite cellular, the components include histiocytes, fibroblasts, and inflammatory cells without cytologic atypia (Fig. 4).

Pitfalls

Fat necrosis

! Fat necrosis is common in adipocytic tumors

! Fat necrosis shows a mixed population of fibroblasts, histiocytes, and inflammatory cells without atypia

! Be careful not to misinterpret cells in fat necrosis as atypical hyperchromatic stromal cells

! Histiocytes are often positive for MDM2 by immunohistochemistry; therefore, it is advised that both MDM2 and CDK4 immunostains are used in conjunction, as histiocytes are negative for CDK4

Fig. 1. Lipoblasts (*A*) exhibit hyperchromatic nuclei that are scalloped by one or multiple fat vacuoles. Histologic mimics of lipoblasts include fat atrophy (*B*), vacuolated histiocytes (*C*), and signet-ring carcinomas (*D*). The diagnostic cell of welldifferentiated liposarcoma is the atypical hyperchromatic stromal cell, which contains an enlarged, hyperchromatic, and smudgy nucleus (*E*). (Hematoxylin-eosin, original magnification [*A*] ×100; [*B*] ×100; [*C*] ×100; [*D*] ×100; [*E*] ×100)

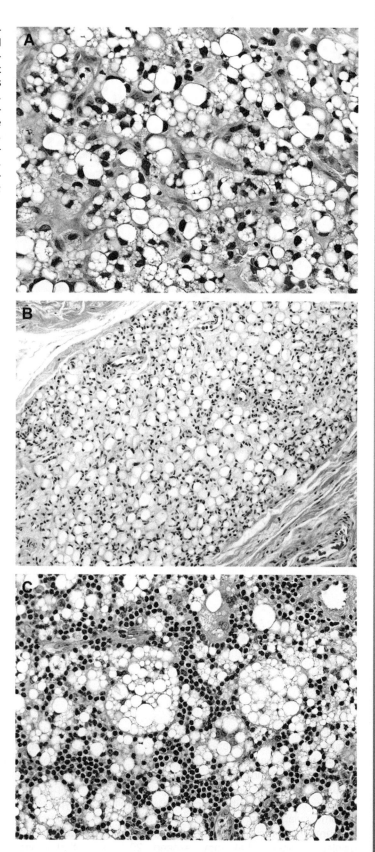

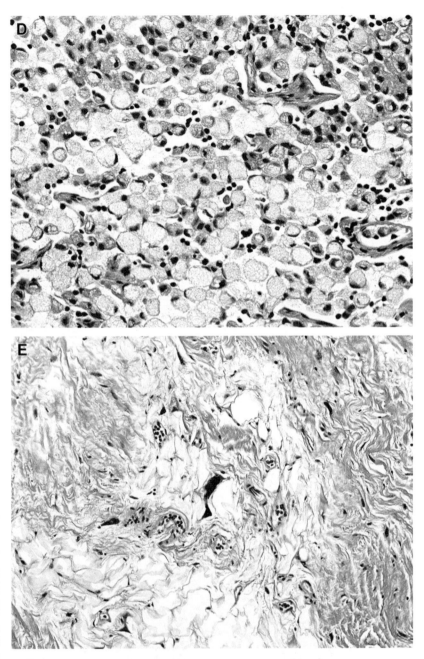

Fig. 1. (*continued*).

Well-differentiated liposarcoma is a locally aggressive but nonmetastasizing adipocytic neoplasm that peaks in incidence in the sixth decade of life. Although rare examples do occur in superficial soft tissue, this entity typically arises at deep soft tissue sites, including extremities (intramuscular), groin, retroperitoneum, and mediastinum. These tumors present as slowly growing painless masses that may exceed 20 cm.

Well-differentiated liposarcoma shows more heterogeneity than lipoma on gross examination with indurated firm areas and fibrous bands, which should be sampled. Histologic examination shows adipocytes and variable numbers of atypical hyperchromatic stromal cells. The atypical hyperchromatic stromal cells are the diagnostic cell type and exhibit enlarged dark smudgy nuclei that are visible from low magnification. These cells

Fig. 2. Well-differentiated liposarcoma shows amplification of *MDM2* by FISH studies (*A*), whereas lipomas do not (*B*).

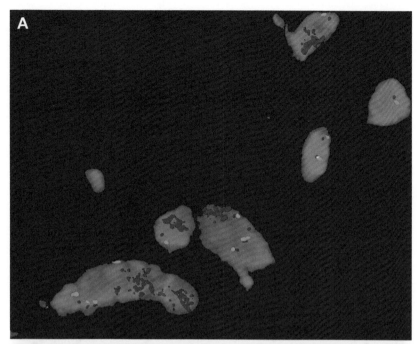

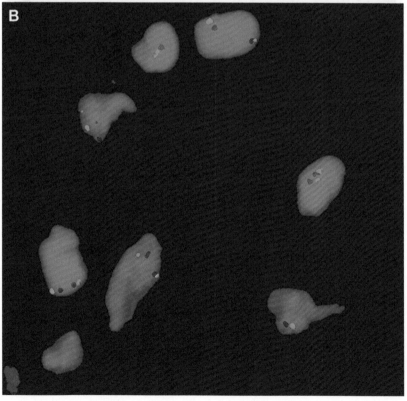

are best appreciated in fibrous septa (**Fig. 5**A) and within the walls of blood vessels (see **Fig. 5**B). When this tumor occurs in the extremities, it is more amenable to complete resection; however, it is often difficult to completely excise this tumor when it arises in the retroperitoneum, leading to high recurrence and mortality rates (>90% and >80%, respectively).[4,8] Consequently, even

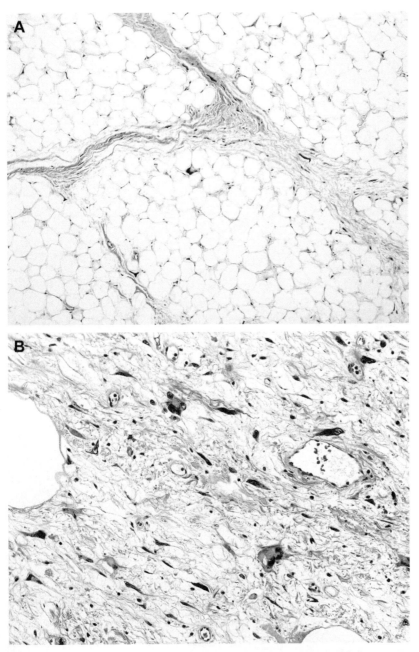

Fig. *3.* This specimen shows a well-differentiated lipomatous neoplasm with easily identifiable atypical hyperchromatic stromal cells (*A*), some of which exhibit a floretlike multinucleated appearance (*B*) (Hematoxylin-eosin, original magnification [*A*] ×40; [*B*] ×100).

though the terms "atypical lipomatous tumor" and "well-differentiated liposarcoma" are synonymous in the current World Health Organization Classification of Bone and Soft Tissue Tumors, "well-differentiated liposarcoma" is the preferred term when this entity occurs in the retroperitoneum.[8]

PATTERN 2: MATURE ADIPOSE TISSUE WITHOUT CYTOLOGIC ATYPIA

Although well-differentiated lipomatous neoplasms without atypia in superficial soft tissue

Fig. 4. A focus of fat necrosis in a lipomatous tumor. Although there are histiocytes and inflammatory cells, no cytologic atypia is appreciated (Hematoxylin-eosin, original magnification ×200).

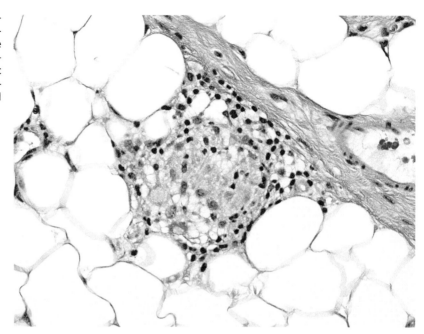

are readily labeled as lipomas, the story is more complicated in the retroperitoneum. When one encounters material from a retroperitoneal mass that shows only mature adipose tissue (Fig. 6), again remember the rules discussed earlier. First, based on the location, we should be concerned about well-differentiated liposarcoma. Even though lipomas can occur in the retroperitoneum, they are greatly outnumbered by well-differentiated liposarcoma.[9] It also is important to realize that the morphology of well-differentiated liposarcoma can be deceptively bland, with large areas resembling mature adipose tissue and only rare atypical hyperchromatic stromal cells. Consequently, atypical hyperchromatic stromal cells may be missed due to sampling error, especially on core biopsy. Fortunately, in this situation we are able to take advantage of the cytogenetic features of well-differentiated liposarcoma (third rule). In well-differentiated liposarcoma, all the cells in the lesion, even those resembling benign fat, will harbor amplification of *MDM2* by FISH. Cells of lipoma will be negative for *MDM2* amplification. For these reasons, FISH studies for *MDM2* amplification (or immunohistochemistry for MDM and CDK4) should be performed on every well-differentiated lipomatous proliferation of the retroperitoneum without unequivocal cytologic atypia.[10] If FISH testing is positive for *MDM2*

amplification, the diagnosis of well-differentiated liposarcoma can be made (biopsy or resection). If FISH testing on a biopsy specimen fails to show *MDM2* amplification, the case is best signed out as "mature adipose tissue," with a main differential diagnosis including retroperitoneal lipoma and nonneoplastic fat. If FISH testing is negative on a well-sampled resection specimen, I would advocate labeling the tumor as lipoma with a comment stating that our experience with primary retroperitoneal lipomas is limited and clinical follow-up is recommended. Fresh tissue sent for cytogenetic analysis and showing translocations of 12q13–15, rearrangements of 6p21 to 23, or 13q deletions but not ring or giant marker chromosomes would be helpful in supporting the diagnosis of lipoma.[7]

PATTERN 3: MATURE ADIPOSE TISSUE WITH ATYPICAL HYPERCHROMATIC STROMAL CELLS ADMIXED WITH UNDIFFERENTIATED PLEOMORPHIC SARCOMA

If the pathologist encounters a high-grade malignancy in the retroperitoneum, the differential diagnosis is exceedingly broad, and entities such as sarcomatoid carcinoma, melanoma, and lymphoma should be excluded. However, the key to

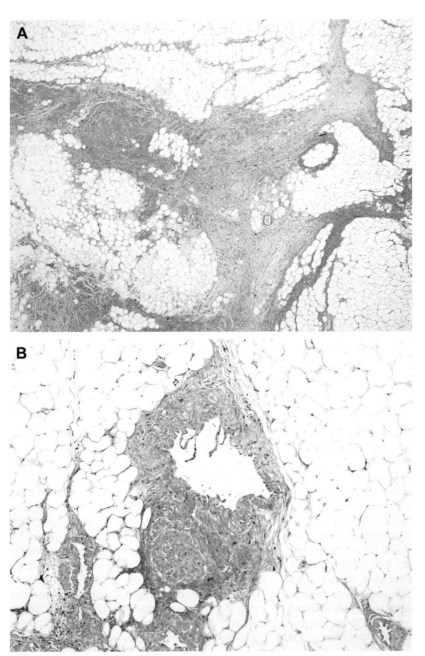

Fig. 5. Atypical hyperchromatic stromal cells of well-differentiated liposarcoma are best appreciated in fibrous septa (*A*) and the walls of blood vessels (*B*). These cells can be appreciated at low power (Hematoxylin-eosin, original magnification [*A*] ×20; [*B*] ×100).

this diagnostic scenario is to remember that dedifferentiated liposarcoma is one of the most common sarcoma in this location. Convincing evidence of a biphasic pattern of well-differentiated liposarcoma and nonlipogenic sarcoma is diagnostic of dedifferentiated liposarcoma.

Dedifferentiated liposarcoma is a high-grade malignancy that reaches peak incidence in the seventh decade, with equal distribution between men and women.[4] Although dedifferentiated liposarcoma can occur in deep soft tissues of the extremities, it is much more likely to occur in the

Fig. 6. Histologic review of this retroperitoneal mass shows a well-differentiated fatty tumor without cytologic atypia. This tumor was positive for *MDM2* amplification by FISH, supporting the diagnosis of well-differentiated liposarcoma (Hematoxylin-eosin, original magnification ×100).

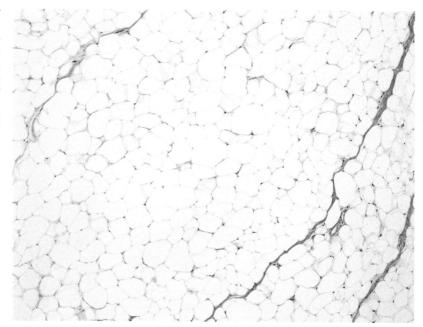

retroperitoneum and groin. Dedifferentiation is a time-dependent phenomenon, and almost 20% of well-differentiated liposarcomas of the retroperitoneum will eventually undergo dedifferentiation.[11] Gross examination typically reveals a large multinodular mass with fatty and solid components corresponding to well-differentiated and dedifferentiated areas, respectively (Fig. 7A). Histologically, these tumors are biphasic, with areas of mature adipose tissue with atypical hyperchromatic stromal cells admixed with areas of nonlipogenic sarcoma (see Fig. 7B–D). Although, in most cases the nonlipogenic component resembles high-grade undifferentiated pleomorphic sarcoma, the dedifferentiated areas can have a wide spectrum of morphologic patterns, including meningothelial-like whorls (Fig. 8A), metaplastic bone (see Fig. 8B), myxoid change, or divergent rhabdomyosarcomatous (see Fig. 8C) or osteosarcomatous (see Fig. 8D) elements.[12–17] Cases of dedifferentiated liposarcoma with homologous pleomorphic liposarcomatous differentiation also have been reported.[18,19] Dedifferentiated liposarcomas share cytogenetic aberrations with well-differentiated liposarcoma, specifically

12q13–15 amplification. Up to 20% of these tumors metastasize, with 5-year overall mortality rates of approximately 30%.[11,12]

The most straightforward manifestation of this scenario is the resection of a retroperitoneal mass with areas resembling high-grade undifferentiated pleomorphic sarcoma. Although it is tempting to focus on solid areas when grossing such a specimen, it is critical to sample regions resembling mature fat or fat with fibrous septa. Most of the time, morphologic review of these areas will yield atypical hyperchromatic stromal cells, and the diagnosis of dedifferentiated liposarcoma can be made without a large immunohistochemical workup or FISH analysis.

Occasionally the pathologist will be lucky enough to see both well-differentiated and differentiated components on a core biopsy (Fig. 9); however, it is important to distinguish dedifferentiated liposarcoma from other pleomorphic sarcomas or nonmesenchymal pleomorphic neoplasms infiltrating fat. Unless there is unequivocal evidence of a well-differentiated liposarcomatous component in the sample, the pathologist should consider other sarcomatoid

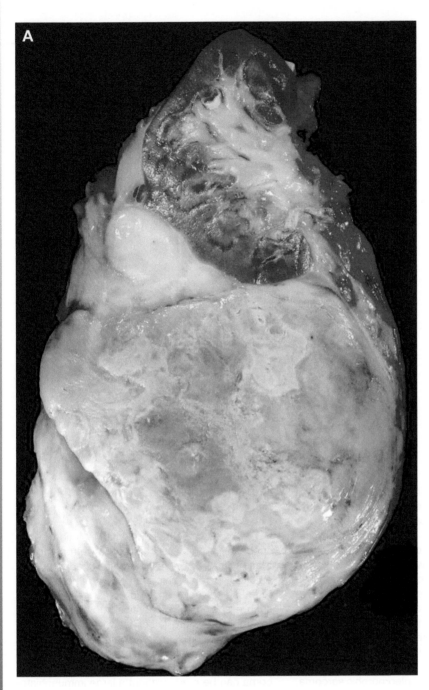

Fig. 7. Gross image of a large retroperitoneal dedifferentiated liposarcoma showing a multinodular heterogeneous cut surface (*A*).

malignancies, such as sarcomatoid carcinoma, pleomorphic lymphomas, and melanoma, as well as specific sarcomas, such as angiosarcoma, rhabdomyosarcoma, and pleomorphic leiomyosarcoma. Once these other entities have been excluded, the presence of *MDM2* amplification by FISH helps support the diagnosis of dedifferentiated liposarcoma.

Fig. 7. (continued). Histologic review demonstrates an abrupt transition between the well-differentiated (*left*) and dedifferentiated (*right*) components (*B*).

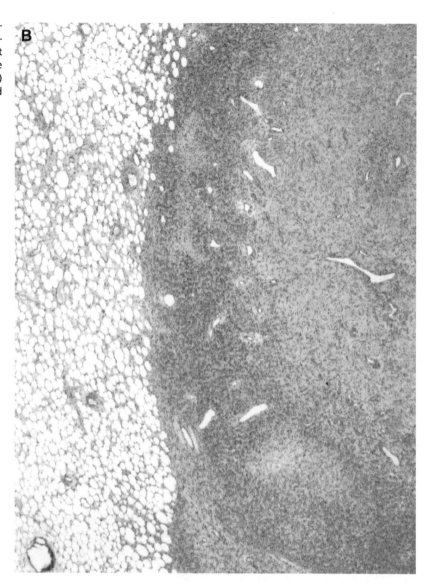

PATTERN 4: MATURE ADIPOSE TISSUE WITH LOW-GRADE SPINDLE-CELL PROLIFERATION

One of the most difficult diagnostic scenarios is the evaluation of a lesion composed of adipose tissue and bland spindled cells, because the differential diagnosis includes tumors that are variably associated with adipocytic differentiation. Again, the first step is to take location into consideration and rule out dedifferentiated liposarcoma. Occasionally the dedifferentiated areas of dedifferentiated liposarcoma may be deceptively bland and

mimic fibromatosis or a low-grade spindle-cell sarcoma (**Fig. 10**). If convincing atypical hyperchromatic stromal cells are not identified, immunohistochemistry for MDM2 and CDK4 or FISH studies for *MDM2* amplification can be performed. Once dedifferentiated liposarcoma has been ruled out, focus should shift to less common soft tissue neoplasms, including myolipoma, angiomyolipoma, the lipomatous variant of solitary fibrous tumors, and genital stromal tumors (**Table 1**).

Myolipoma is an uncommon benign lipomatous tumor composed of mature fat and mature smooth

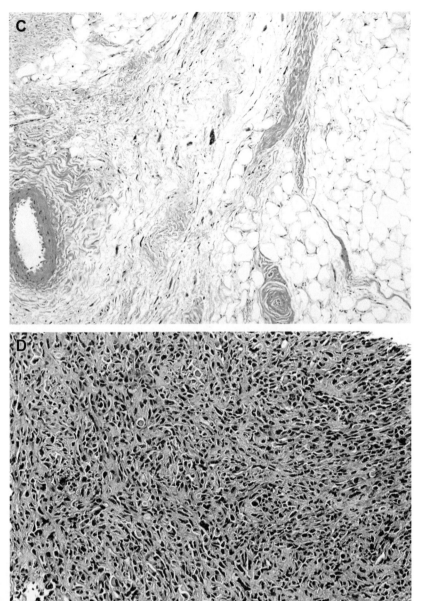

Fig.   7. (continued).
Higher magnification of the well-differentiated areas (*C*) shows mature adipose with atypical hyperchromatic stromal cells, whereas the dedifferentiated foci (*D*) resemble a high-grade undifferentiated pleomorphic sarcoma (Hematoxylin-eosin, original magnification [*B*] ×40; [*C*] ×100; [*D*] ×200).

muscle that typically occurs in women in the fifth and sixth decades of life. This tumor has a predilection for the retroperitoneum, abdomen, and pelvis. Sectioning of myolipoma reveals a smooth

yellow-white cut surface. Histologic examination shows a mixture of mature adipocytes and smooth muscle without cytologic atypia (Fig. 11A, B). The smooth muscle component will mark with smooth

Fig. 8. The spectrum of morphology that can be seen in dedifferentiated liposarcoma is diverse and includes meningothelial-like whorls (*A*), metaplastic bone (*B*), and heterologous rhabdomyosarcomatous (*C*) or osteosarcomatous (*D*) differentiation (Hematoxylin-eosin, original magnification [*A*] ×100; [*B*] ×100; [*C*] ×200; [*D*] ×200).

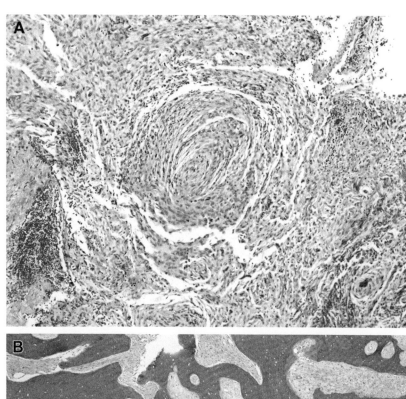

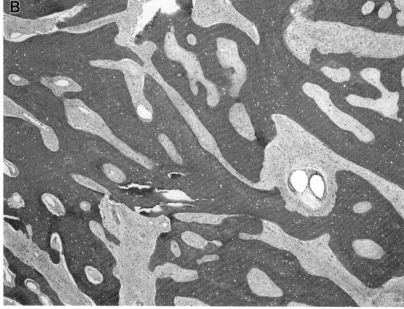

muscle actin (see **Fig. 11C**) and desmin (see **Fig. 11D**).

Angiomyolipoma belongs to a family of tumors termed PEComas (perivascular epithelioid cell tumors), which are composed of cells with reactivity for smooth muscle and melanocytic markers and are usually associated with the walls of blood vessels. Although angiomyolipomas typically arise in the kidney, they also may occur in the retroperitoneum and other sites such as liver and colon. They

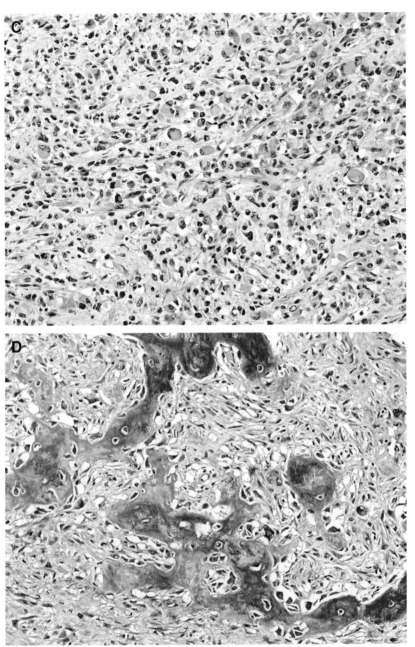

Fig. 8. (continued).

are more common in women than men, and most present in middle adulthood. Although the average size is approximately 9 cm, they may reach sizes larger than 20 cm. Microscopic examination reveals a triphasic morphology: mature adipose tissue, thick-walled blood vessels, and spindle cells in a perivascular arrangement (Fig. 12A). The spindle-cell component will show immunoreactivity for smooth muscle actin (see Fig. 12B), as well as melanocytic markers (see Fig. 12C).

Solitary fibrous tumors are mesenchymal neoplasms that primarily occur in adults, with an equal sex distribution. They mainly occur in deep soft tissue sites, including the pelvis and retroperitoneum. Histologically, solitary fibrous tumors show a

Fig. 9. Rare example of a core biopsy that contains both well-differentiated (*right*) and dedifferentiated components (*left*) of dedifferentiated liposarcoma (Hematoxylin-eosin, original magnification ×20).

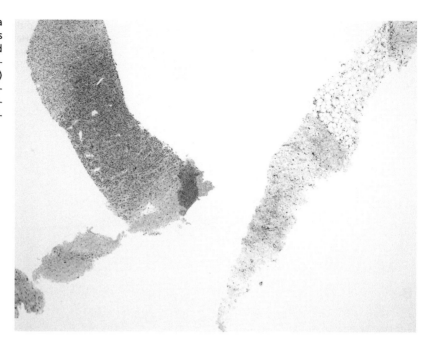

variably cellular proliferation of relatively uniform spindled to ovoid cells arranged around staghorn-shaped thick-walled blood vessels. The lipomatous variant of solitary fibrous tumor has been well described, and some tumors may harbor up to 75% of a fatty component (**Fig. 13**).[20–23] Immunohistochemical analysis usually shows the lesional cells to be positive for CD34. Recent work has shown most solitary fibrous tumors to harbor *NAB2-STAT6* fusions, and STAT6 immunostain is a relatively sensitive and specific marker for this tumor.[24–27] However, rare cases of dedifferentiated liposarcoma have exhibited STAT6 expression, so a combination of FISH for *MDM2* amplification and STAT6 immunohistochemistry may be necessary with a limited sample (Pitfall: STAT6).[25,28]

Pitfalls

STAT6

! Rare cases of dedifferentiated liposarcoma may show STAT6 immunoexpression

Genital stromal tumors, such as cellular angiofibroma (also known as angiomyofibroblastoma-like tumor of the male genital tract) and mammary-type myofibroblastoma, occasionally may present as pelvic or retroperitoneal masses. Cellular angiofibroma is characterized by a well-marginated proliferation of bland spindled cells, wispy collagen, and small to medium-sized blood vessels. Mammary-type myofibroblastomas are well-circumscribed masses composed of short fascicles of slender cells admixed with thick collagen bundles. Not only do these 2 entities share immunophenotypic findings, including variable reactivity for desmin, actin, CD34, and estrogen receptor, they also are linked genetically by loss of *RB1*.[4,29–33] Furthermore, both cellular angiofibroma (**Fig. 14**A) and mammary-type myofibroblastoma (see **Fig. 14**B) may contain a component of mature adipose tissue.[4,34]

On complete resection specimen, definitive diagnosis may be possible on morphology alone, but immunohistochemistry is often needed when dealing with a small biopsy. If a battery of immunostains, including smooth muscle actin, desmin, CD34, melanocytic markers, and STAT6 yields inconclusive results, these specimens can be signed out descriptively such as "fat-containing spindle-cell neoplasm," with definitive diagnosis deferred to complete resection.

PATTERN 5: MYXOID SARCOMA WITH A FATTY COMPONENT

It is often tempting for pathologists to suggest the diagnosis of myxoid liposarcoma when faced with a myxoid sarcoma in the retroperitoneum. However, myxoid liposarcoma virtually never arises in the retroperitoneum, and examination of these specimens typically reveals the

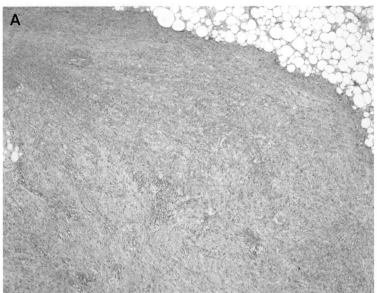

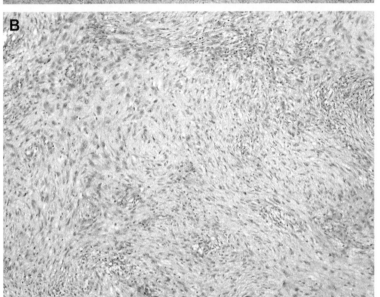

Fig. 10. Low-power (*A*) and high-power (*B*) views of dedifferentiated liposarcoma with only mild cytologic atypia (Hematoxylin-eosin, original magnification [*A*] ×40; [*B*] ×100).

Table 1
Mature adipose tissue with low-grade spindle-cell proliferation

Diagnosis	Key Morphologic Features	Helpful Immunostains	FISH for *MDM2* Amplification
Dedifferentiated liposarcoma	Atypical hyperchromatic stromal cells	—	Positive
Myolipoma	Bundles of smooth muscle	Positive for actin and desmin	Negative
Angiomyolipoma	Spindle cells appear to spin-off blood vessels	Positive for actin, HMB45, and MelanA	Negative
Lipomatous solitary fibrous tumor	Hyalinized staghorn-shaped blood vessels	Positive for CD34 and STAT6	Negative
Cellular angiofibroma	Uniform spindle cells, wispy collagen, highly vascular	Variable CD34, actin, desmin, estrogen receptor	Negative
Extra-mammary myofibroblastoma	Uniform spindle cells, thick collagen bundles	Positive for desmin, CD34, variable actin	Negative

Abbreviation: FISH, fluorescence in situ hybridization.

Fig. 11. Low-power (*A*) and high-power (*B*) views of myolipoma showing a mixture of bland smooth muscle and mature fat. Immunohistochemical studies show the spindle cell population to express smooth muscle actin (*C*) and desmin (*D*) (Hematoxylin-eosin, original magnification [*A*] ×40; [*B*] ×200; [*C*] ×200, smooth muscle actin; [*D*] ×200, desmin).

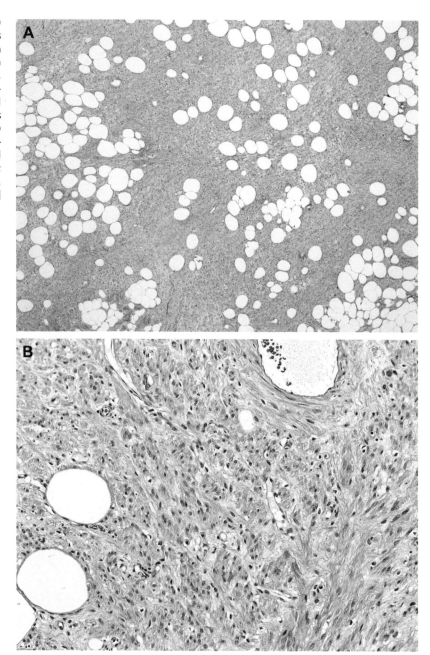

presence of markedly atypical spindled cells or floretlike giant cells (**Fig. 15**), which are characteristic of well-differentiated/dedifferentiated liposarcoma and not present in myxoid liposarcoma. The lesional cells in myxoid liposarcoma are uniform with round to ovoid morphology. Even though well-differentiated/dedifferentiated liposarcoma can have myxoid change and a plexiform vasculature mimicking myxoid liposarcoma, studies have confirmed that virtually all tumors with such morphology are well-differentiated/dedifferentiated liposarcoma.[16,17]

Again, when encountering such a specimen, remember that the main differential diagnosis of a retroperitoneal sarcoma includes well-differentiated/dedifferentiated liposarcoma and leiomyosarcoma but not myxoid liposarcoma. If the entire mass has been resected, thorough

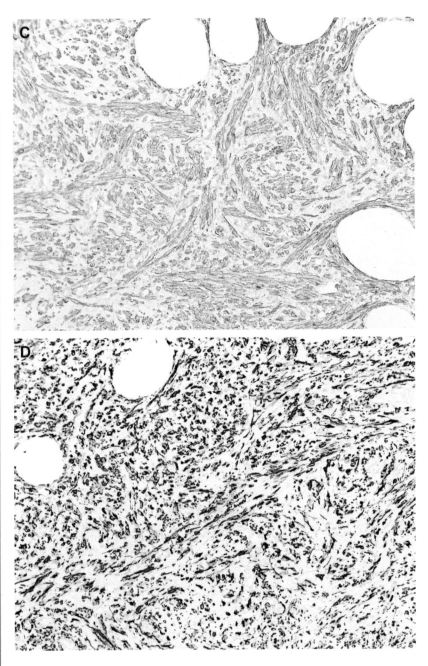

Fig. 11. (continued).

sampling will likely yield foci of mature adipose tissue and atypical hyperchromatic stromal cells diagnostic of well-differentiated/dedifferentiated liposarcoma. However, if the pathologist has limited material, the presence of *MDM2* amplification by FISH will help support the diagnosis of well-differentiated/dedifferentiated liposarcoma.

Fig. 12. Angiomyolipomas show a tri-phasic appearance, including mature adipose tissue, spindled cells, and blood vessels (*A*). Note that the spindle cells appear to "spin-off" the vessels. These tumors are positive for smooth muscle actin (*B*) and melanocytic markers such as Melan A (*C*) (Hematoxylin-eosin, original magnification [*A*] ×100; [*B*] ×100, smooth muscle actin; [*C*] ×100, Melan A).

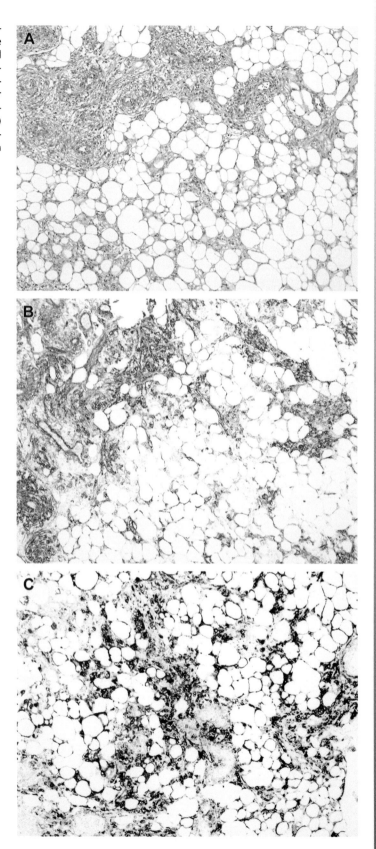

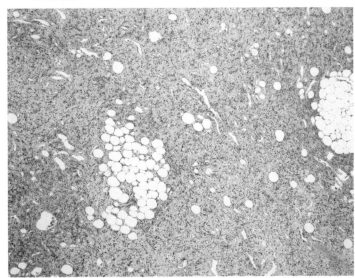

Fig. 13. Example of a solitary fibrous tumor composed of scattered staghorn-shaped blood vessels with hyalinized walls and a component of mature adipose tissue (Hematoxylin-eosin, original magnification ×40).

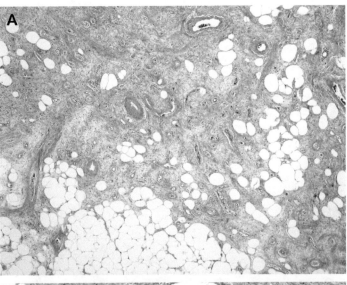

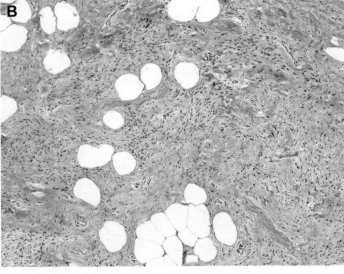

Fig. 14. Examples of cellular angiofibroma (*A*) and mammary-type myofibroblastoma (*B*) with adipocytic components (Hematoxylin-eosin, original magnification [*A*] ×100; [*B*] ×100).

Fig. 15. Well-differentiated liposarcoma with myxoid stroma and a plexiform vascular network mimicking myxoid liposarcoma (*A*). However, careful examination reveals atypical hyperchromatic stromal cells (*B*) and floretlike multinucleated cells (*C*), which are not present in myxoid liposarcoma but, instead, diagnostic of well-differentiated liposarcoma (Hematoxylin-eosin, original magnification [*A*] ×100; [*B*] ×200; [*C*] ×200).

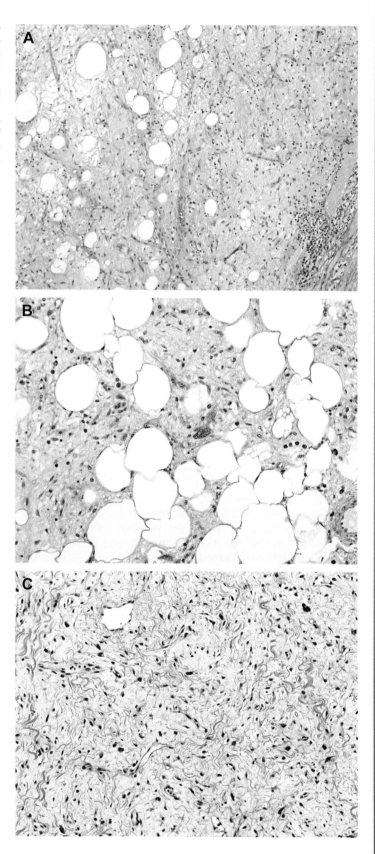

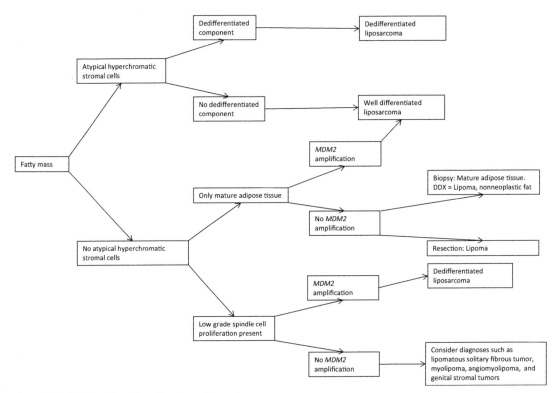

Fig. 16. Evaluation of a "fatty" retroperitoneal mass.

SUMMARY

Although mesenchymal neoplasms can be intimidating, the 4 rules discussed in the article provide pathologists with a framework for working up fatty lesions in the retroperitoneum (**Fig. 16**). Although well-differentiated and dedifferentiated liposarcoma should be the primary considerations of a "fatty" retroperitoneal neoplasm, pathologists should be aware that benign adipocytic and nonadipocytic tumors with a fatty component also may occur at this site.

REFERENCES

1. Rosai J, Akerman M, Dal Cin P, et al. Combined morphologic and karyotypic study of 59 atypical lipomatous tumors. Evaluation of their relationship and differential diagnosis with other adipose tissue tumors (a report of the CHAMP Study Group). Am J Surg Pathol 1996;20:1182–9.
2. Weaver J, Downs-Kelly E, Goldblum JR, et al. Fluorescence in situ hybridization for MDM2 gene amplification as a diagnostic tool in lipomatous neoplasms. Mod Pathol 2008;21:943–9.
3. Weaver J, Rao P, Goldblum JR, et al. Can MDM2 analytical tests performed on core needle biopsy be relied upon to diagnose well-differentiated liposarcoma? Mod Pathol 2010;23:1301–6.
4. Goldblum JR, Folpe AL, Weiss SW. Enzinger and Weiss's soft tissue tumors. Philadelphia: Elsevier Saunders; 2014.
5. Mandahl N, Hoglund M, Mertens F, et al. Cytogenetic aberrations in 188 benign and borderline adipose tissue tumors. Genes Chromosomes Cancer 1994;9:207–15.
6. Sreekantaiah C, Leong SP, Karakousis CP, et al. Cytogenetic profile of 109 lipomas. Cancer Res 1991; 51:422–33.
7. Willen H, Akerman M, Dal Cin P, et al. Comparison of chromosomal patterns with clinical features in 165 lipomas: a report of the CHAMP study group. Cancer Genet Cytogenet 1998;102:46–9.
8. Fletcher CD, Bridge JA, Hogendoorn PC, et al, editors. World Health Organization classification of tumours. Lyon (France): International Agency for Research on Cancer; 2013.
9. Ida CM, Wang X, Erickson-Johnson MR, et al. Primary retroperitoneal lipoma: a soft tissue pathology heresy? Report of a case with classic histologic, cytogenetics, and molecular genetic features. Am J Surg Pathol 2008;32:951–4.
10. Zhang H, Erickson-Johnson M, Wang X, et al. Molecular testing for lipomatous tumors: critical analysis

and test recommendations based on the analysis of 405 extremity-based tumors. Am J Surg Pathol 2010;34:1304–11.

11. Weiss SW, Rao VK. Well-differentiated liposarcoma (atypical lipoma) of deep soft tissue of the extremities, retroperitoneum, and miscellaneous sites. A follow-up study of 92 cases with analysis of the incidence of "dedifferentiation". Am J Surg Pathol 1992; 16:1051–8.

12. Henricks WH, Chu YC, Goldblum JR, et al. Dedifferentiated liposarcoma: a clinicopathological analysis of 155 cases with a proposal for an expanded definition of dedifferentiation. Am J Surg Pathol 1997;21:271–81.

13. Salzano RP Jr, Tomkiewicz Z, Africano WA. Dedifferentiated liposarcoma with features of rhabdomyosarcoma. Conn Med 1991;55:200–2.

14. Song JS, Gardner JM, Tarrant WP, et al. Dedifferentiated liposarcoma with peculiar meningothelial-like whorling and metaplastic bone formation. Ann Diagn Pathol 2009;13:278–84.

15. Nascimento AG, Kurtin PJ, Guillou L, et al. Dedifferentiated liposarcoma: a report of nine cases with a peculiar neurallike whorling pattern associated with metaplastic bone formation. Am J Surg Pathol 1998;22:945–55.

16. de Vreeze RS, de Jong D, Tielen IH, et al. Primary retroperitoneal myxoid/round cell liposarcoma is a nonexisting disease: an immunohistochemical and molecular biological analysis. Mod Pathol 2009;22:223–31.

17. Sioletic S, Dal Cin P, Fletcher CD, et al. Well-differentiated and dedifferentiated liposarcomas with prominent myxoid stroma: analysis of 56 cases. Histopathology 2013;62:287–93.

18. Boland JM, Weiss SW, Oliveira AM, et al. Liposarcomas with mixed well-differentiated and pleomorphic features: a clinicopathologic study of 12 cases. Am J Surg Pathol 2010;34:837–43.

19. Marino-Enriquez A, Fletcher CD, Dal Cin P, et al. Dedifferentiated liposarcoma with "homologous" lipoblastic (pleomorphic liposarcoma-like) differentiation: clinicopathologic and molecular analysis of a series suggesting revised diagnostic criteria. Am J Surg Pathol 2010;34:1122–31.

20. Ceballos KM, Munk PL, Masri BA, et al. Lipomatous hemangiopericytoma: a morphologically distinct soft tissue tumor. Arch Pathol Lab Med 1999;123:941–5.

21. Folpe AL, Devaney K, Weiss SW. Lipomatous hemangiopericytoma: a rare variant of hemangiopericytoma that may be confused with liposarcoma. Am J Surg Pathol 1999;23:1201–7.

22. Guillou L, Gebhard S, Coindre JM. Lipomatous hemangiopericytoma: a fat-containing variant of solitary fibrous tumor? Clinicopathologic, immunohistochemical, and ultrastructural analysis of a series in favor of a unifying concept. Hum Pathol 2000;31:1108–15.

23. Nielsen GP, Dickersin GR, Provenzal JM, et al. Lipomatous hemangiopericytoma. A histologic, ultrastructural and immunohistochemical study of a unique variant of hemangiopericytoma. Am J Surg Pathol 1995;19:748–56.

24. Chmielecki J, Crago AM, Rosenberg M, et al. Whole-exome sequencing identifies a recurrent NAB2-STAT6 fusion in solitary fibrous tumors. Nat Genet 2013;45:131–2.

25. Doyle LA, Vivero M, Fletcher CD, et al. Nuclear expression of STAT6 distinguishes solitary fibrous tumor from histologic mimics. Mod Pathol 2014;27: 390–5.

26. Mohajeri A, Tayebwa J, Collin A, et al. Comprehensive genetic analysis identifies a pathognomonic NAB2/STAT6 fusion gene, nonrandom secondary genomic imbalances, and a characteristic gene expression profile in solitary fibrous tumor. Genes Chromosomes Cancer 2013;52:873–86.

27. Robinson DR, Wu YM, Kalyana-Sundaram S, et al. Identification of recurrent NAB2-STAT6 gene fusions in solitary fibrous tumor by integrative sequencing. Nat Genet 2013;45:180–5.

28. Doyle LA, Tao D, Marino-Enriquez A. STAT6 is amplified in a subset of dedifferentiated liposarcoma. Mod Pathol 2014;27:1231–7.

29. Flucke U, van Krieken JH, Mentzel T. Cellular angiofibroma: analysis of 25 cases emphasizing its relationship to spindle cell lipoma and mammary-type myofibroblastoma. Mod Pathol 2011;24:82–9.

30. Hameed M, Clarke K, Amer HZ, et al. Cellular angiofibroma is genetically similar to spindle cell lipoma: a case report. Cancer Genet Cytogenet 2007;177: 131–4.

31. Maggiani F, Debiec-Rychter M, Vanbockrijck M, et al. Cellular angiofibroma: another mesenchymal tumour with 13q14 involvement, suggesting a link with spindle cell lipoma and (extra)-mammary myofibroblastoma. Histopathology 2007;51: 410–2.

32. Maggiani F, Debiec-Rychter M, Verbeeck G, et al. Extramammary myofibroblastoma is genetically related to spindle cell lipoma. Virchows Arch 2006; 449:244–7.

33. Pauwels P, Sciot R, Croiset F, et al. Myofibroblastoma of the breast: genetic link with spindle cell lipoma. J Pathol 2000;191:282–5.

34. Iwasa Y, Fletcher CD. Cellular angiofibroma: clinicopathologic and immunohistochemical analysis of 51 cases. Am J Surg Pathol 2004;28:1426–35.

Selected Diagnostically Challenging Pediatric Soft Tissue Tumors

Alyaa Al-Ibraheemi, MD, Harry Kozakewich, MD,
Antonio R. Perez-Atayde, MD*

KEYWORDS

- Superficial Ewing sarcoma • Anaplastic chordoma
- DICER-associated nasal chondromesenchymal hamartoma

ABSTRACT

Many benign and malignant soft tissue tumors in children are challenging and their diagnosis requires knowledge of their vast diversity, histopathological complexity, and immunohistochemical, cytogenetic, and molecular characteristics. The importance of clinical and imaging features cannot be overstated. Soft tissue sarcomas account for 15% of all pediatric malignancies after leukemia/lymphoma, central nervous system tumors, neuroblastoma and Wilms tumor. This article discusses selected challenging pediatric soft tissue tumors with an update on recently described entities.

SUPERFICIAL EWING SARCOMA: OVERVIEW

The Ewing sarcoma (ES) family of tumors is a distinctive group of malignant small round cell sarcomas that occurs in bone and soft tissue and includes classic ES, malignant peripheral neuroectodermal tumor, so-called atypical ES, and the adamantinoma-like ES.[1-4]

Superficial ES (SES), defined by its occurrence in skin and subcutaneous tissue without involvement of the fascia, is rare.[5-23] SES affects children and young adults with a slight white female predominance.[9] It has a predilection for the extremities followed by the trunk. SES usually presents as a soft superficial and freely mobile mass that is occasionally painful or ulcerated.[9,15] A majority of tumors are small and single but are sometimes multiple.[5]

GROSS FEATURES

Typically, SES is well-demarcated, unencapsulated, and located in the mid-dermis, deep dermis, or subcutaneous tissue (Fig. 1). Involvement of the superficial dermis may produce pedunculation (Fig. 2).

On cut surface, SES has a fleshy white appearance and may have necrosis, cystification, and hemorrhage. Occasionally, it has a pigmented appearance from hemosiderin deposition. It is generally small with a median size of 2 cm (range 0.5–7 cm).

MICROSCOPIC FEATURES

At scanning examination, SES is centered in the dermis and may extend into the subcutis (see Fig. 2). Tumor satellites may be present (see Fig. 2B). The histopathology is similar to that of ES of bone and deep soft tissue. SES is densely cellular and composed of small cells with uniform round nuclei, fine chromatin, inconspicuous nucleoli, and scant clear-to-eosinophilic cytoplasm with indistinct borders (Fig. 3). Cytoplasmic clumps of PAS-positive glycogen are often present. Tumor cells are typically arranged in nests or sheets that are more clearly delineated by a reticulin stain. Mitoses, necrosis, and apoptotic bodies are frequently seen. SES can also have a fascicular pattern with spindled cell morphology or may be composed of moderately pleomorphic cells as in the atypical Ewing sarcoma.[23] Multinucleated giant tumor cells may be present (see Fig. 3B). Hemorrhage may result in pseudoendotheliomatous spaces with hemosiderin deposition.[12,18] Typically, tumor cells have diffuse and strong membranous

Department of Pathology, Boston Children's Hospital, 300 Longwood Ave, Boston, MA 02115, USA
* Corresponding author.
E-mail address: antonio.perez-atayde@childrens.harvard.edu

Surgical Pathology 8 (2015) 399–418
http://dx.doi.org/10.1016/j.path.2015.05.009

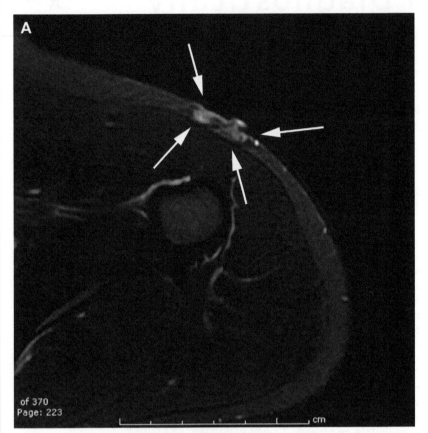

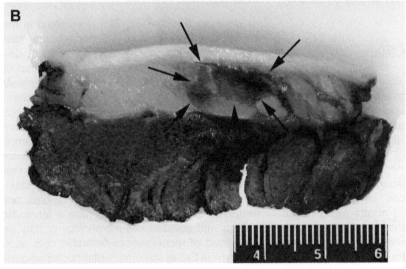

Fig. 1. SES. Imaging and gross. (*A*) MRI showing heterogeneously T2-enhancing lobulated, well-defined subcutaneous mass anterior to the left humeral head (*arrows*). (*B*) Subcutaneous mass (depicted in [*A*]) is lobulated and brown (*arrows*). The dark brown tissue at the bottom is skeletal muscle.

expression for CD99 (**Fig. 4**A). Additional immunopositivity is observed with FLI-1 as well as cytokeratins (20%) and occasionally desmin, synaptophysin, S-100 protein, and epithelial membrane antigen (EMA) (see **Fig. 4**; **Fig. 5**).[23]

DIFFERENTIAL DIAGNOSIS

The differential diagnosis of SES includes neuroendocrine (Merkel cell) carcinoma, cellular blue nevus, malignant melanoma, clear cell

Fig. 2. SES. Light microscopy. (*A*) Expansile densely cellular dermal nodule. (*B*) Satellite lesions in deep dermis and subcutaneous fat (hematoxylin-eosin).

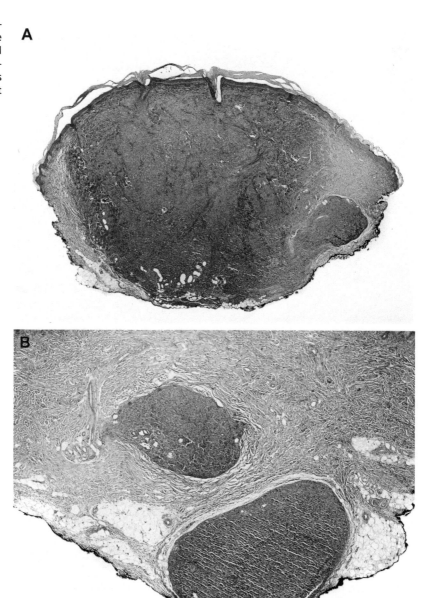

sarcoma, myoepithelial tumors, angiomatoid fibrous histiocytoma (AFH), neuroblastoma, rhabdomyosarcoma, and lymphoma. This wide differential diagnosis includes tumors that, like Ewing sarcoma, have rearrangement of the *EWSR1* gene, such as clear cell sarcoma, myoepithelial tumors, and AFH.[24] Therefore, rearrangement of the *EWSR1* gene by fluorescence in situ hybridization (FISH) does not exclude these tumors if the fusion partner is unknown.

Merkel cell carcinoma is rare in the pediatric age group and morphologically overlaps with SES. CK20 is a helpful marker to differentiate SES from Merkel cell carcinoma, because it is negative in SES. Cellular blue cell nevus, malignant

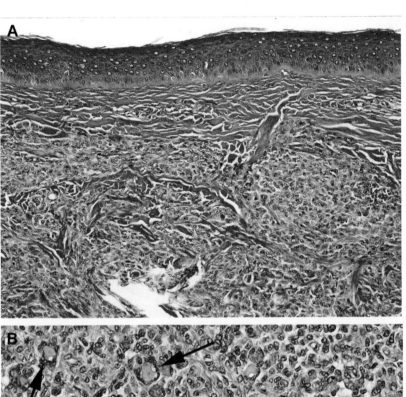

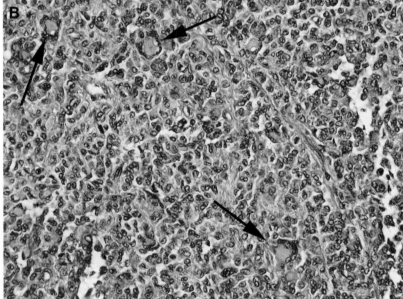

Fig. 3. SES. Light microscopy. (A) Dermal tumor in Fig. 2 composed of irregular nests of undifferentiated small round cells. (B) Irregular nuclei with variably sized nucleoli and poorly defined cell borders. Occasional giant multinucleated tumor cells (arrows) (hematoxylin-eosin).

melanoma, clear cell sarcoma, and myoepithelial tumors are important diagnostic considerations when SES expresses S-100 protein. Cellular blue nevus, malignant melanoma, and clear cell sarcoma typically express HMB-45 and Melan-A. Myoepithelial tumors can be exceptionally difficult to differentiate from SES because the latter may conspicuously express EMA and S-100 protein as well. Absence of membranous CD99 and loss of nuclear INI1 expression are helpful features, and documentation of the characteristic *ESWR1-POU5F1* translocation is diagnostic. AFH with pseudovascular spaces and hemosiderin deposition may mimic SES but, in the former, the biphasic pattern with both a small cell and a myofibroblastic component, a characteristic peripheral

Fig. 4. SES. Immunohisto-chemistry. (*A*) Intense and diffuse membranous immunoreactivity for CD99. (*B*) Focal immunopositivity for synaptophysin.

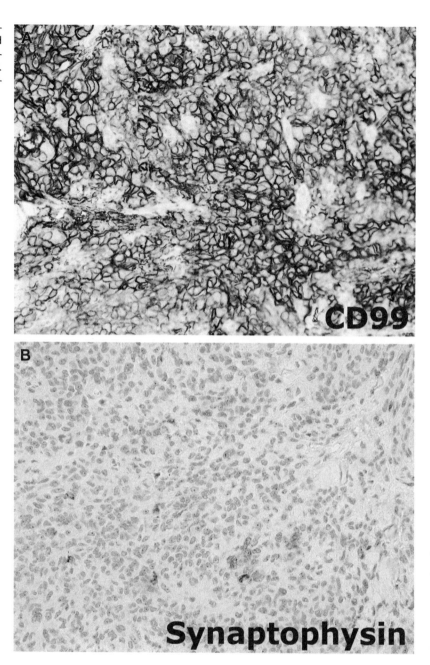

lymphoid infiltrate, and focal immunoreactivity for desmin, EMA, and CD99 are helpful in distinguishing the 2 lesions. Lingering uncertainty may require documentation of a specific translocation in AFH, namely *EWSR1-ATF1* or *EWSR1-CREB1*. Metastatic cutaneous neuroblastoma enters the differential diagnosis. It typically occurs, however, in children younger than 5 years. Neuropil, ganglionic differentiation; diffuse expression of synaptophysin, chromogranin, and protein gene product (PGP) 9.5; and lack of CD99 immunoreactivity are characteristic of neuroblastoma. Lymphoblastic lymphoma usually has diffuse CD99 expression, but other lymphoid markers

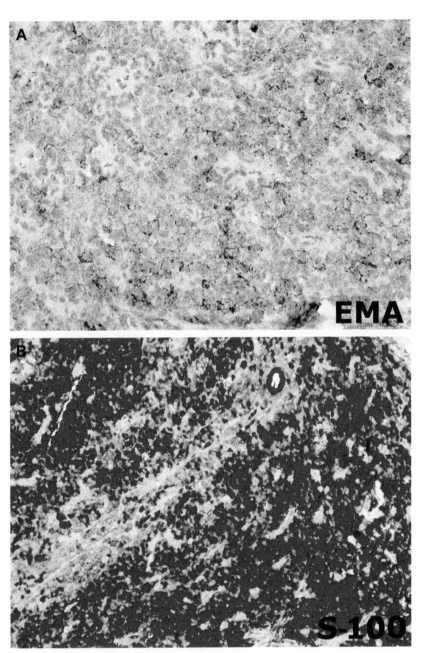

Fig. 5. SES. Immunohisto-chemistry. (*A*) Diffuse im-munoreactivity for EMA. (*B*) Diffuse and strong immunoreactivity for S-100 protein, seen in red.

and terminal deoxynucleotidyl transferase (TdT) should be obtained to exclude this possibility. Rhabdomyosarcoma is immunoreactive for desmin, muscle-specific actin. and nuclear myogenin.

DIAGNOSIS

Ancillary studies are essential to make the diagnosis. A panel of immunohisotchemical stains, such as CD99, FLI-1, keratin, chromogranin, synaptophysin, S-100, myogenin, desmin, smooth muscle actin (SMA), TdT, and EMA, can be helpful to distinguish SES from other malignant small round cell tumors. If conventional cytogenetics is not successful in demonstrating a characteristic translocation, FISH or reverse transcription–polymerase chain reaction (RT-PCR) should be pursued for documenting the same. Of the SESs in which RT-PCR studies have been performed, a majority harbored the *EWSR1-FLI1* and rarely the *EWSR1-ERG* gene fusion.[25]

PROGNOSIS

SES is associated with an indolent course and a favorable prognosis. Patients tend to present with a small tumor and localized disease and rarely with nodal disease or distant metastasis.[19] Relapse rate is approximately 15% compared with 30% for nonmetastatic osseous or deep-seated counterparts.[22] Three SES patients have reportedly died from disease, 2 of which occurred in the finger.[18] Standard treatment entails complete surgical resection followed by chemotherapy. SES has a 10-year survival rate of 91%.

Key features
OF SUPERFICIAL EWING SARCOMA

- Skin and subcutaneous tissue
- Histopathology similar to that of ES of bone and deep soft tissue, including atypical variants
- Diffuse and strong membranous expression for CD99

Pitfalls
IN DIAGNOSIS OF SUPERFICIAL EWING SARCOMA

! Occasionally has pigmented appearance
! Multinucleated giant tumor cells may be present
! Pseudoendotheliomatous spaces with hemosiderin deposition
! Can have fascicular pattern with spindled cell morphology
! Can show EMA and S-100 protein expression

Differential diagnosis
OF SUPERFICIAL EWING SARCOMA

Merkel cell carcinoma
- Rare in the pediatric age group
- Cytokeratin 20 immunopositivity
- Lack of *EWSR1* gene rearrangement

Cellular blue nevus and malignant melanoma
- Express HMB-45 and Melan-A
- Lack of *EWSR1* gene rearrangement

Clear cell sarcoma of soft tissue
- Expresses HMB-45 and Melan-A
- *EWSR1-ATF1* translocation

Myoepithelial tumors
- Express EMA and S-100 protein
- Absence of membranous CD99 immunoreactivity
- Loss of nuclear INI1 expression in 40% of cases
- *ESWR1-POU5F1* translocation

Angiomatoid fibrous histiocytoma
- Pseudovascular spaces and hemosiderin deposition
- Biphasic pattern with small cell and myofibroblastic components
- Characteristic peripheral lymphoid infiltrate
- Focal immunoreactivity for desmin, EMA, and membranous CD99
- *EWSR1-ATF1* or *EWSR1-CREB1* translocation

Neuroblastoma
- Children younger than 5 years
- Characteristic neuropil and ganglionic differentiation
- Synaptophysin, chromogranin, and PGP 9.5 expression
- Lack of CD99 immunoreactivity
- *EWSR1* gene rearrangement.

Lymphoblastic lymphoma
- Expression of lymphoid markers and TdT
- Diffuse membranous CD99 expression
- Lack of *EWSR1* gene rearrangement

Rhabdomyosarcoma
- Immunoreactivity for desmin, muscle-specific actin, and nuclear myogenin
- Lack of *EWSR1* gene rearrangement

POORLY DIFFERENTIATED CHORDOMA

OVERVIEW

Chordoma is a rare, slowly-growing, and locally aggressive neoplasm of the axial spine, primarily clivus and sacrum, thought to arise from notochordal remnants. In children and adolescents, chordoma has a predilection for the spheno-occipital and cervical regions. Pediatric chordomas comprise less than 5% of all chordomas.[26–28] Although chordomas in children are reported to be more aggressive than in adults, a distinct subtype of chordoma, the so-called poorly differentiated chordoma (PDC), occurs at a very young age, often presents as a soft tissue mass, and has unusual histologic features, a more aggressive behavior, and a greater incidence of metastasis. PDC accounts for 8% to 50% of pediatric chordomas.[26,27,29] PDC is also known in the literature as atypical, anaplastic, sarcomatoid, and dedifferentiated chordoma. Recently, it has been shown that PDCs have loss of nuclear INI1 inmunoreactivity and usually deletion of SMARCB1/INI1 gene.[29]

GROSS FEATURES

Chordomas are lobulated gelatinous, gray, and soft with areas of hemorrhage. Generally tumor ranges in size from 5 to 15 cm. In most cases it is associated with extension into the surrounding tissue. The gross appearance of PDC has not been described. Imaging characteristics on MRI suggesting high cellularity have been reported in PDC in contrast to conventional chordoma (Fig. 6).[30,31]

MICROSCOPIC FEATURES

In contrast to conventional chordoma, PDC consists of cellular nodules or sheets of small or large epithelioid or spindled cells with a variable amount of eosinophilic cytoplasm and absent or rare cytoplasmic vacuoles (Fig. 7). The cytoplasm may also be clear or have rhabdoid features. The nuclei are often larger and pleomorphic with prominent nucleoli. Some tumors are composed predominantly of spindled cells imparting a sarcomatoid appearance. The myxoid matrix is sparse or absent. PDC has mitotic activity and often areas of necrosis.

Both conventional chordoma and PDC are immunoreactive for keratin, EMA, S-100, vimentin, and brachyury (Figs. 8 and 9).[32] PDCs, however, more frequently lack nuclear expression of INI1 and some have deletion of the SMARCB1/INI1 gene (see Fig. 9).[29,33] This molecular aberration is suspected of playing a role in the morphology and aggressive behavior of PDC. A greater MIB1 proliferative index and a more frequent p53 expression have been reported in PDC.[33]

DIFFERENTIAL DIAGNOSIS

PDC, particularly when metastatic, is to be differentiated from mimics, such as epithelioid hemangioendothelioma (EHE), epithelioid sarcoma, pseudomyogenic EHE (PMEHE), poorly

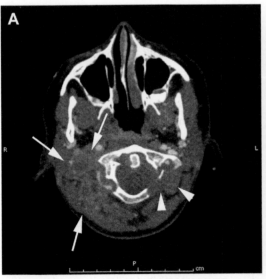
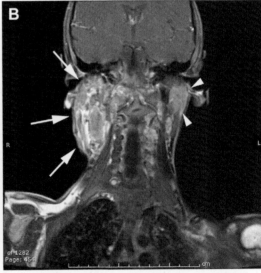

Fig. 6. PDC. Imaging. (*A*) Ill-defined, heterogeneous, soft tissue mass in right neck demonstrated by CT scan (*arrows*). Contralateral mass in left skull base with erosion of the C1 ring (*arrowheads*). (*B*) Mass on right shows irregular nodular enhancement (*arrows*) and mass on left is more attenuated and uniform (*arrowheads*).

Fig. 7. PDC. Light microscopy. (*A*) Cellular nodule of small and large epithelioid cells with variable amount of eosinophilic cytoplasm. (*B*) Large and pleomorphic nuclei, some with prominent nucleoli and occasional cytoplasmic vacuolization (hematoxylin-eosin).

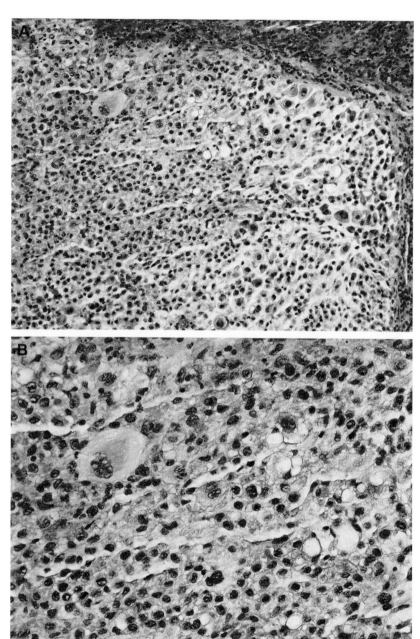

differentiated carcinoma, myoepithelial carcinoma, and malignant rhabdoid tumor (MRT).

Approximately 25% of EHEs express keratin, but reactivity is usually focal and less intense. Lesional cells express endothelial markers CD31 and CD34, which are absent in PDC, and lack nuclear brachyury.

Proximal-type epithelioid sarcoma is typically seen in adolescents and young adults. Similar to chordoma, it consists of solid or multinodular masses of epithelioid cells, usually with prominent necrosis. Tumor cells are immunopositive for cytokeratin, EMA, vimentin, nuclear FLI-1, and sometimes focally for S-100. Epithelioid sarcoma has loss of nuclear SMARCB1/INI1, but nuclear expression of brachyury is absent.

PMEHE, also known as epithelioid sarcoma-like hemangioendothelioma, has tumor cells with

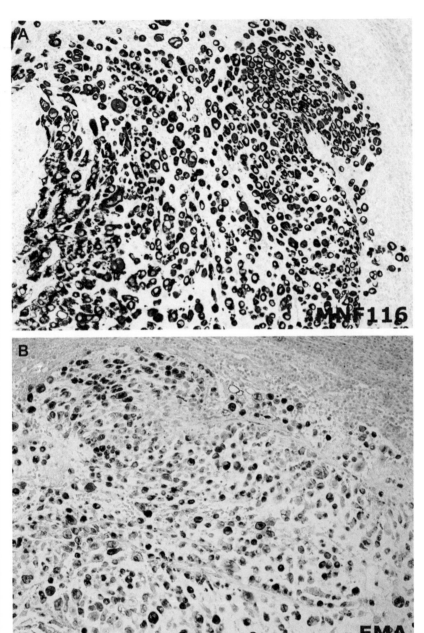

characteristic glassy eosinophilic cytoplasm. There is consistent expression of FLI-1, ERG, CD31, and cytokeratin AE1/AE3. Nuclear SMARCB1/INI1 is intact and brachyury is absent.

MRT presents at a younger age and tumor cells are smaller, less epithelioid, and almost always lack brachyury nuclear expression. Focal nuclear expression of brachyury has been reported in 2 atypical teratoid/rhabdoid tumors of the brain.[33]

Poorly differentiated carcinoma, including the nuclear protein in testis (NUT) midline carcinoma, is an important differential diagnosis. It does not, however, exhibit nuclear brachyury and SMARCB1/INI1 expression is expected to be present. NUT midline carcinomas show nuclear expression of NUT.

Myoepithelial carcinoma shows significant morphologic and immunohistochemical overlap with PDC with respect to immunoreactivity for

Fig. 9. PDC. Immunohistochemistry. (*A*) Diffuse and intense nuclear immunoreactivity for brachyury. (*B*) Loss of nuclear INI1 expression in tumor cells in contrast to surrounding inflammatory and endothelial cells.

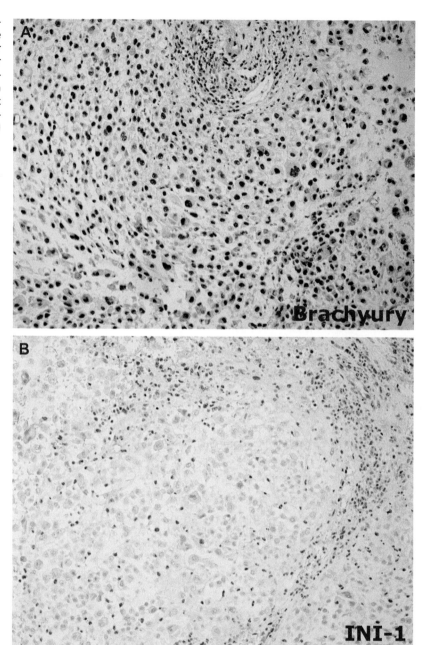

cytokeratin and S-100 protein. Additionally, there is loss of SMARCB1/INI1 in 40% of them. Immunonegativity for brachyury may be helpful.

Chondrosarcoma may on occasion enter the differential diagnosis with PDC because they share S-100 immunopositivity, but the former has abundant myxoid-to-chondroid matrix and is negative for keratin and brachyury.

DIAGNOSIS

Integration of clinical and imaging information is important in arriving at a diagnosis of PDC. Imaging characteristics on MRI suggesting high cellularity have been reported in PDC in contrast to conventional chordoma.[30,31] Immunohistochemical staining for brachyury and SMARCB1/INI1 is routinely performed to help distinguish chordoma from its mimics.

PROGNOSIS

PDC occurs at a very young age and is associated with a worse prognosis and a high rate of metastases compared with conventional chordoma.[34] The prognosis has been improved with the introduction of new surgical techniques and proton beam radiation therapy.[27,35,36]

Key features
OF POORLY DIFFERENTIATED CHORDOMA

- Cellular nodules or sheets of small or large epithelioid or spindled cells with variable amount of eosinophilic cytoplasm and absent or sparse cytoplasmic vacuoles
- The cytoplasm may have clear or rhabdoid appearance
- Nuclei often larger and pleomorphic with prominent nucleoli
- Sparse or absent myxoid matrix
- Frequent mitotic activity and necrosis
- Immunoreactivity for keratin, EMA, S-100, and brachyury, and loss of nuclear INI1
- Deletion of *SMARCB1/INI1* gene

Pitfalls
IN DIAGNOSIS OF POORLY DIFFERENTIATED CHORDOMA

! Lacks histologic features of conventional chordoma

! May have rhabdoid features

! Nuclei often larger and pleomorphic with prominent nucleoli

! Sometimes spindled cells imparting sarcomatoid appearance

! Loss of nuclear INI1 immunoreactivity and deletion of *SMARCB1/INI1* gene

⚠⚠ Differential diagnosis
OF POORLY DIFFERENTIATED CHORDOMA

Epithelioid hemangioendothelioma
- Expresses endothelial markers CD31, CD34, and ERG
- 25% express keratin (focal and weak)
- Lack nuclear brachyury expression
- *WWTR1-CAMTA1* or *YAP1-TFE3* translocation

Proximal-type epithelioid sarcoma
- Solid or multinodular masses of epithelioid cells with prominent necrosis
- Immunopositive for cytokeratin, EMA, nuclear FLI-1, and sometimes focally for S-100.
- Loss of nuclear INI1 expression
- Lacks nuclear brachyury expression

Pseudomyogenic epithelioid hemangioendothelioma
- Also known as epithelioid sarcoma-like hemangioendothelioma
- Characteristic glassy eosinophilic cytoplasm
- Expression of FLI-1, ERG, CD31, and cytokeratin AE1/AE3
- Nuclear INI1 expression intact
- Lacks nuclear brachyury expression.

Poorly differentiated carcinoma (including the NUT midline carcinoma)
- Nuclear INI1 expression intact
- NUT midline carcinoma shows nuclear expression of NUT
- Lacks nuclear brachyury expression

Myoepithelial carcinoma
- Cytokeratin and S-100 protein expression
- Loss of nuclear INI1 expression in 40% of pediatric cases
- Lacks nuclear brachyury expression

Malignant rhabdoid tumor
- Younger age
- Tumor cells smaller and less epithelioid
- Loss of nuclear INI1 expression
- Lacks nuclear brachyury expression

Chondrosarcoma
- Abundant myxoid/chondroid matrix
- S-100 protein expression
- Cytokeratin negativity
- Lacks nuclear brachyury expression

NASAL CHONDROMESENCHYMAL HAMARTOMA

OVERVIEW

Nasal chondomesenchymal hamartoma (NCMH) is a rare benign lesion of the nasal cavity, paranasal sinuses, and upper nasopharynx, described primarily in infants and children (Fig. 10).[37–43] Recent reports have indicated a strong association with the pleuropulmonary blastoma (PPB) tumor predisposition disorder characterized by germline and somatic mutations of DICER1.[44–46] NCMHs associated with PPB have

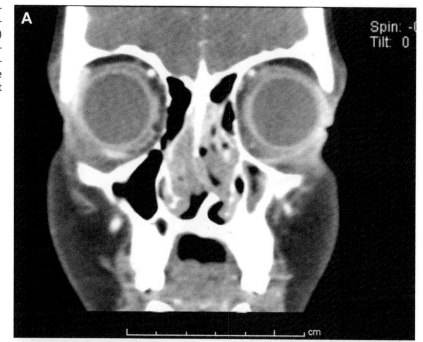

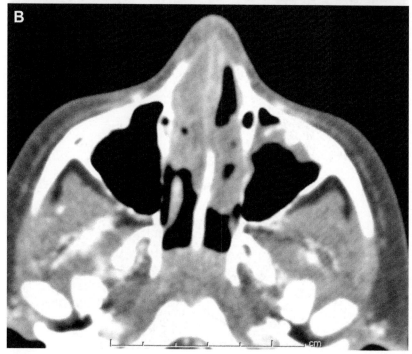

Fig. 10. Nasal chondromesenchymal hamartoma. Imaging. (*A*) Sagittal view (*B*) Horizontal view, CT scan demonstrating soft tissue masses in right and left nasal cavities.

occurred in older children (median age of 10 years) and were frequently bilateral. A novel translocation t(12;17) (q24.1;q21) in NCMH as the sole anomaly has been reported in a child with PPB.[47] In all patients with PPB, the NCMH was discovered after the diagnosis of PPB. It is uncertain if NCMH in infants and NCMH in the PPB-setting are the same entity.

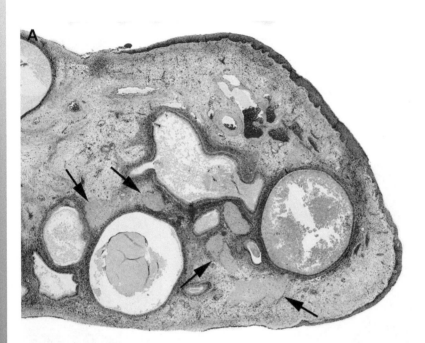

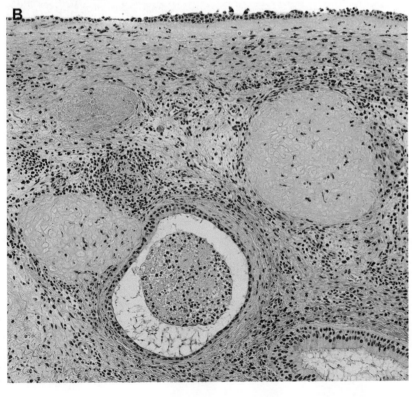

Fig. 11. Nasal chondro-mesenchymal hamartoma. Light microscopy. (*A*) Polypoid mass surfaced predominantly by squamous epithelium and containing cystic structures lined by respiratory-type epithelium and nodules of cartilage (*arrows*). (*B*) Epithelial cystic elements, partially devitalized cartilaginous nodules and chronic inflammation (hematoxylin-eosin).

GROSS FEATURES

NCMH most often are submitted as multiple fragments from an endoscopic procedure. The fragments are irregular and sometimes polypoid white-tan and rubbery. The texture is varied from firm with an obvious cartilaginous appearance to soft fleshy and tan in color. The cut surface is solid and firm-to-mucoid with cystic changes. Foci of hemorrhage and calcifications can be seen.

MICROSCOPIC FEATURES

NCMHs are cystic and solid polypoid masses of variably immature stromal and chondroid elements

(**Fig. 11**). The cysts vary in size and are lined by respiratory epithelium. Nodules of hyaline cartilage are almost invariably present; most are well demarcated from the surrounding stroma but occasionally ill defined (**Figs. 12** and **13**). The stroma is variably cellular and composed of bland spindled cells and inflammatory cells loosely embedded in a myxoid or fibrous matrix (**Fig. 14**). In hypercelluar areas a storiform pattern may be observed. A subepithelial cambium layer of immature stroma or cartilage is sometimes seen (see **Fig. 14**A). There may be minor atypia of stromal or cartilaginous cells. Mononuclear cells, osteoclast-like multinucleated giant cells, bone, calcification, and blood-filled cystic spaces may bring to mind entities

Fig. 12. NCMH. Light microscopy. (*A*) Irregular nodules of hyaline cartilage. (*B*) Variation in cellularity and appearance of mature chondrocytes, some of which are necrotic (hematoxylineosin).

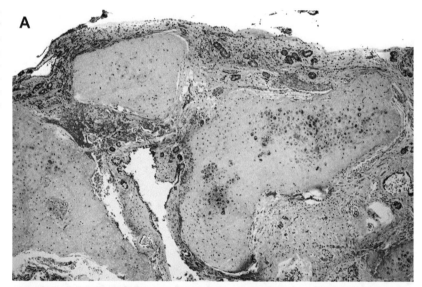

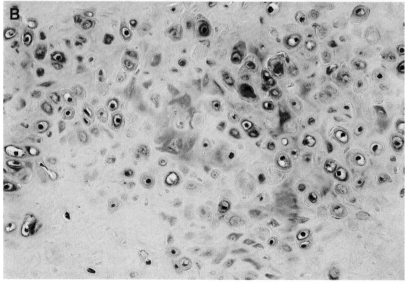

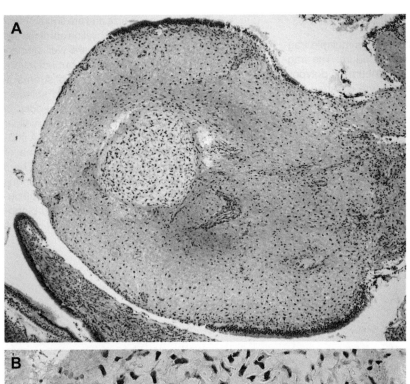

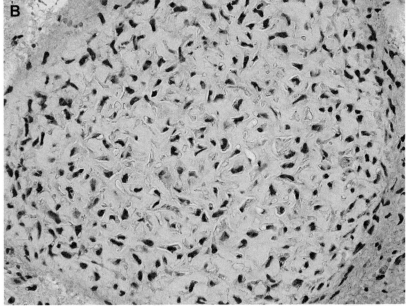

Fig. 13. Nasal chondro-mesenchymal hamartoma. Light microscopy. (*A*) Polyp with abundant primitive mesenchymal stroma and small nodule of cellular cartilage. (*B*) Immature appearing chondrocytes (hematoxylin-eosin).

such as nonossifying fibroma, fibrous dysplasia, and aneurysmal bone cyst. The histology of NCMH has been compared with that of mesenchymal hamartoma of the chest wall in infants. NCMH, however, lacks the characteristic endochondral ossification or epiphyseal platelike structures. S-100 protein is expressed in the chondroid elements and focally and weakly in the stromal spindled cells. The spindled cell component is also immunoreactive for smooth muscle actin.

Fig. 14. NCMH. Light microscopy. (*A*) Cambium layer with subepithelial band of primitive chondroid stroma. (*B*) In areas, the stroma is loose and composed of bland spindled cells (hematoxylin-eosin).

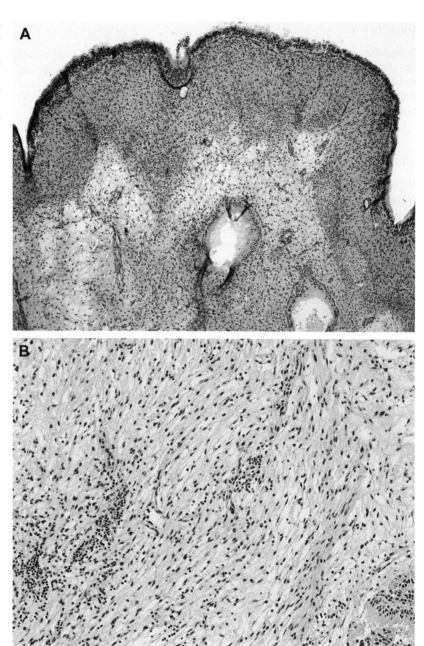

DIFFERENTIAL DIAGNOSIS

Immature stromal and chondroid elements help in distinguishing NCMH from an inflammatory polyp, schneiderian papilloma, respiratory epithelial adenomatoid hamartoma, or myxoma. Because of the chondroid elements, cartilaginous neoplasms also enter the differential diagnosis. The lack of mitoses, significant pleomorphism, or overt malignant features argues against chondrosarcoma and mesenchymal chondrosarcoma. Lack of rhabdomyoblasts and nuclear immunoreactivity for myogenin excludes rhabdomyosarcoma.

DIAGNOSIS

Integration of clinical, radiological, and unique morphologic findings is of major importance in arriving at the diagnosis, which conveys significant implications for tumor surveillance and genetic counseling.

PROGNOSIS

NCMH is a benign, often bilateral tumor with limited growth potential and is treated by complete local resection through functional endoscopic sinus surgery. Recurrence usually develops after incomplete resection. Adjuvant therapy is not required.

Pitfalls
IN DIAGNOSIS OF NASAL CHONDROMESENCHYMA HAMARTOMA

! Botryoid rhabdomyosarcoma-like subepithelial cambium layer

! Minor atypia of stromal or cartilaginous cells

! Mononuclear cells, osteoclast-like multinucleated giant cells, bone, calcification, and blood-filled cystic spaces

Differential diagnosis
OF NASAL CHONDROMESENCHYMAL HAMARTOMA

Inflammatory polyp, schneiderian papilloma, respiratory epithelial adenomatoid hamartoma, and myxoma

- Lack immature stromal and chondroid elements

Cartilaginous neoplasms (chondrosarcoma and mesenchymal chondrosarcoma)

- More cellular with frequent mitoses and nuclear atypia

- Infiltrative growth pattern

Rhabdomyosarcoma

- Characteristic rhabdomyoblasts

- Myogenin and desmin immunoreactivity

Key features
OF NASAL CHONDROMESENCHYMAL HAMARTOMA

- Cystic and solid polypoid masses of epithelial cysts and variably immature stromal and chondroid elements

- Cysts lined by respiratory epithelium

- Nodules of variably cellular cartilage

- Variably cellular, myxoid, or fibrous stroma and bland spindled cells

- Storiform pattern may be observed

- Subepithelial cambium layer of immature chondroid stroma sometimes seen

- Mononuclear cells, osteoclast-like multinucleated giant cells, bone, calcification, and blood-filled cystic spaces

- Lacks endochondral ossification

- S-100 protein expressed in the chondroid elements and focally and weakly in stromal spindled cells

- Spindled cell component immunoreactive for smooth muscle actin

- Association with the PPB tumor predisposition disorder characterized by germline and somatic mutations of *DICER1*

REFERENCES

1. Demetri GD, Antonia S, Benjamin RS, et al. Soft tissue sarcoma. J Natl Compr Canc Netw 2010;8:630–74.
2. McGrory JE, Pritchard DJ, Arndt CA, et al. Nonrhabdomyosarcoma soft tissue sarcomas in children. The Mayo Clinic Experience. Clin Orthop Relat Res 2000;4:247–58.
3. Meyer WH, Spunt SL. Soft tissue sarcomas of childhood. Cancer Treat Reb 2004;30:269–80.
4. Mariño-Enríquez A, Fletcher CD. Round cell sarcomas – Biologically important refinements in subclassification. Int J Biochem Cell Biol 2014;53:493–504.
5. Sangüeza OP, Sangüeza P, Valda LR, et al. Multiple primitive neuroectodermal tumors. J Am Acad Dermatol 1994;31(2 Pt 2):356–61.
6. Lee CS, Southey MC, Slater H, et al. Primary cutaneous Ewing's sarcoma/peripheral primitive neuroectodermal tumors in childhood. A molecular,

cytogenetic, and immunohistochemical study. Diagn Mol Pathol 1995;4(3):174–81.

7. Sexton CW, White WL. Primary cutaneous Ewing's family sarcoma. Report of a case with immunostaining for glycoprotein p30/32 mic2. Am J Dermatopathol 1996;18(6):601–5.

8. Hasegawa SL, Davison JM, Rutten A, et al. Primary cutaneous Ewing's sarcoma: immunophenotypic and molecular cytogenetic evaluation of five cases. Am J Surg Pathol 1998;22(3):310–8.

9. Chow E, Merchant TE, Pappo A, et al. Cutaneous and subcutaneous Ewing's sarcoma: an indolent disease. Int J Radiat Oncol Biol Phys 2000;46(2): 433–8.

10. Kourda M, Chatti S, Sfia M, et al. Primary cutaneous extraskeletal Ewing's sarcoma. Ann Dermatol Venereol 2005;132(12 Pt 1):986–9.

11. Ehrig T, Billings SD, Fanburg-Smith JC. Superficial primitive neuroectodermal tumor/Ewing sarcoma (PN/ES): same tumor as deep PN/ES or new entity? Ann Diagn Pathol 2007;11(3):153–9.

12. Terrier-Lacombe MJ, Guillou L, Chibon F, et al. Superficial primitive Ewing's sarcoma: a clinicopathologic and molecular cytogenetic analysis of 14 cases. Mod Pathol 2009;22(1):87–94.

13. Shingde MV, Buckland M, Busam KJ, et al. Primary cutaneous Ewing sarcoma/primitive neuroectodermal tumour: a clinicopathological analysis of seven cases highlighting diagnostic pitfalls and the role of FISH testing in diagnosis. J Clin Pathol 2009; 62(10):915–9.

14. Kalra S, Gupta R, Singh S, et al. Primary cutaneous ewing's sarcoma/primitive neuroectodermal tumor: report of the first case diagnosed on aspiration cytology. Acta Cytol 2010;54(2):193–6.

15. Bahk WJ, Chang ED, Bae JM, et al. Primary cutaneous Ewing's sarcoma/primitive neuroectodermal tumor manifesting numerous small and huge ulcerated masses: its complete remission by chemotherapy and magnetic resonance imaging findings. Skeletal Radiol 2010;39(6):595–600.

16. Bruno M, D'antona GI, Vita G, et al. Subcutaneous Ewing sarcoma/PNET as a second cancer in a previously irradiated young patient. an uncommon type of post-irradiation soft tissue sarcoma. Pathologica 2011;103(2):43–5.

17. Delaplace M, Mélard P, Perrinaud A, et al. Primitive cutaneous Ewing's sarcoma: a diagnostic and therapeutic dilemma. Ann Dermatol Venereol 2011; 138(5):395–8.

18. Machado I, Llombart B, Calabuig-Fariñas S, et al. Superficial Ewing's sarcoma family of tumors: a clinicopathological study with differential diagnoses. J Cutan Pathol 2011;38(8):636–43.

19. Collier AB 3rd, Simpson L, Monteleone P. Cutaneous Ewing sarcoma: report of 2 cases and literature review of presentation, treatment, and outcome of 76 other reported cases. J Pediatr Hematol Oncol 2011;33(8):631–4.

20. Delaplace M, Lhommet C, de Pinieux G, et al. Primary cutaneous Ewing sarcoma: a systematic review focused on treatment and outcome. Br J Dermatol 2012;166(4):721–6.

21. Machado I, Traves V, Cruz J, et al. Superficial small round-cell tumors with special reference to the Ewing's sarcoma family of tumors and the spectrum of differential diagnosis. Semin Diagn Pathol 2013; 30(1):85–94.

22. Oliveira Filho Jd, Tebet AC, Oliveira AR, et al. Primary cutaneous Ewing sarcoma–case report. An Bras Dermatol 2014;89(3):501–3.

23. Arnold MA, Ballester LY, Pack SD, et al. Primary subcutaneous spindle cell Ewing sarcoma with strong S100 expression and EWSR1-FLI1 fusion: a case report. Pediatr Dev Pathol 2014;17(4):302–7.

24. Fisher C. The diversity of soft tissue tumours with EWSR1 gene rearrangements: a review. Histopathology 2014;64(1):134–50.

25. Wei S, Siegal GP. Round cell tumors of bone: an update on recent molecular genetic advances. Adv Anat Pathol 2014;21:359–72.

26. Hoch BL, Nielsen GP, Liebsch NJ, et al. Base of skull chordomas in childrens and adolescents a clinicopathologic study of 73 cases. Am J Surg Pathol 2006;30(7):811–8.

27. Chavez JA, Din NU, Memon A, et al. Anaplstic chordoma with loss of INI1 and brachyury expression in a 2-year-old girl. Clin Neuropathol 2014;33(6): 418–20.

28. Coffin CM, Swanson PE, Wick MR, et al. Chordoma in childhood and adolescence. A clinicopathologic analysis of 12 cases. Arch Pathol Lab Med 1993; 117(9):927–33.

29. Mobley BC, McKenney JK, Bangs CD, et al. Loss of SMARCB1/INI1 expression in poorly differentiated chordomas. Acta Neuropathol 2010;120(6): 745–53.

30. Larson TC 3rd, Houser OW, Laws ER Jr. Imaging of cranial chordomas. Mayo Clin Proc 1987;62(10): 886–93.

31. Machida T, Aoki S, Sasaki Y, et al. Magnetic resonance imaging of clival chordomas. Acta Radiol Suppl 1986;369:167–9.

32. Vujovic S, Henderson S, Presneau N, et al. Brachyury, a crucial regulator of notochordal development, is a novel biomarker for chordomas. J Pathol 2006;209(2):157–65.

33. Yadav R, Sharma MC, Malgulwar PB, et al. Prognostic value of MIB-1, p53, epidermal growth factor receptor, and INI1 in childhood chordomas. Neuro Oncol 2014;16(3):372–81.

34. Borba LA, Al-Mefty O, Mrak RE, et al. Cranial chordomas in children and adolescents. J Neurosurg 1996;84(4):584–91.

35. Rombi B, Ares C, Hug EB, et al. Spot-scanning proton radiation therapy for pediatric chordoma and chondrosarcoma: clinical outcome of 26 patients treated at paul scherrer institute. Int J Radiant Oncol Biol Phys 2013;86(3):578–84.

36. Amichetti M, Cianchetti M, Amelio D, et al. Proton therapy in chordoma of the base of the skull: a systematic review. Neurosurg Rev 2009;32(4): 403–16.

37. Ozolek JA, Carrau R, Barnes EL, et al. Nasal chondromesenchymal hamartoma in older children and adults: series and immunohistochemical analysis. Arch Pathol Lab Med 2005;129(11):1444–50.

38. McDermott MB, Ponder TB, Dehner LP. Nasal chondromesenchymal hamartoma: an upper respiratory tract analogue of the chest wall mesenchymal hamartoma. Am J Surg Pathol 1998;22(4):425–33.

39. Terris MH, Billman GF, Pransky SM. Nasal hamartoma: case report and review of the literature. Int J Pediatr Otorhinolaryngol 1993;28(1):83–8.

40. Ludemann JP, Tewfik TL, Meagher-Villemure K, et al. Congenital mesenchymoma transgressing the cribriform plate. J Otolaryngol 1997;26(4):270–2.

41. Kim DW, Low W, Billman G, et al. Chondroid hamartoma presenting as a neonatal nasal mass. Int J Pediatr Otorhinolaryngol 1999;47(3):253–9.

42. Kato K, Ijiri R, Tanaka Y, et al. Nasal chondromesenchymal hamartoma of infancy: the first Japanese case report. Pathol Int 1999;49(8):731–6.

43. Hsueh C, Hsueh S, Gonzalez-Crussi F, et al. Nasal chondromesenchymal hamartoma in children: report of 2 cases with review of the literature. Arch Pathol Lab Med 2001;125(3):400–3.

44. Johnson C, Nagaraj U, Esguerra J, et al. Nasal chondromesenchymal hamartoma: radiographic and histopathologic analysis of a rare pediatric tumor. Pediatr Radiol 2007;37(1):101–4.

45. Priest JR, Williams GM, Mize WA, et al. Nasal chondromesenchymal hamartoma in children with pleuropulmonary blastoma—A report from the International Pleuropulmonary Blastoma Registry registry. Int J Pediatr Otorhinolaryngol 2010;74(11):1240–4.

46. Stewart DR, Messinger Y, Williams GM, et al. Nasal chondromesenchymal hamartomas arise secondary to germline and somatic mutations of DICER1 in the pleuropulmonary blastoma tumor predisposition disorder. Hum Genet 2014;133(11):1443–50.

47. Behery RE, Bedrnicek J, Lazenby A, et al. Translocation t(12;17)(q24.1;q21) as the sole anomaly in a nasal chondromesenchymal hamartoma arising in a patient with pleuropulmonary blastoma. Pediatr Dev Pathol 2012;15(3):249–53.

Chondro-Osseous Lesions of Soft Tissue

Soo-Jin Cho, MD, PhD, Andrew Horvai, MD, PhD*

KEYWORDS

- Myositis ossificans • Ossifying fibromyxoid tumor • Osteosarcoma • Chondroma
- Synovial chondromatosis

ABSTRACT

Soft tissue lesions can contain bone or cartilage matrix as an incidental, often metaplastic, phenomenon or as a diagnostic feature. The latter category includes a diverse group ranging from self-limited proliferations to benign neoplasms to aggressive malignancies. Correlating imaging findings with pathology is mandatory to confirm that a tumor producing bone or cartilage, in fact, originates from soft tissue rather than from the skeleton. The distinction can have dramatic diagnostic and therapeutic implications. This content focuses on the gross, histologic, radiographic, and clinical features of bone or cartilage-producing soft tissue lesions. Recent discoveries regarding tumor-specific genetics are discussed.

OVERVIEW

A diverse group of somatic soft tissue lesions, reactive and neoplastic, may contain skeletal matrix (osteoid, bone and/or cartilage) and can be classified into 2 main categories (Box 1). First, bone or cartilage may be a secondary, incidental feature but its presence is not definitional. Variants of some neoplasms (eg, melanoma,[1,2] carcinoma,[3] "dedifferentiated" liposarcoma,[4,5] low-grade fibromyxoid sarcoma,[6] and schwannoma[7]) can contain bone or cartilage produced by the neoplastic component or as a metaplastic feature. The second category consists of soft tissue lesions that are *defined* by the presence of skeletal matrix and is the subject of this review. This group spans a wide clinical spectrum from self-limited mesenchymal proliferations to high-grade malignancies. Interpretation of gross, microscopic, clinical, and radiographic findings, together,

is critical for accurate diagnosis. The unraveling of the genetics of some of these tumors has refined classification schemes and provided diagnostic adjuncts.[8–10]

Imaging correlation is indispensable if a soft issue tumor contains bone or cartilage. Foremost, imaging confirms that the lesion, in fact, *arises from soft tissue*. Serious diagnostic errors can be avoided by reviewing the imaging firsthand or, at least, discussing the findings with the radiologist or treating clinician. For example, a cartilage tumor that originates in soft tissue is almost certainly benign, whereas a cartilage tumor of bone that *invades* soft tissue is probably malignant. If imaging is unavailable, the pathologist should render a descriptive diagnosis with a reasonable differential, refining with imaging correlation later, rather than a specific, but potentially incorrect diagnosis.

Osteoid is an organic extracellular matrix composed predominantly of type 1 collagen with smaller amounts of glycosaminoglycans and other proteins producing a waxy eosinophilic quality on routine hematoxylin-eosin histology. *Bone* contains both the organic osteoid component and a mineral component known as hydroxyapatite: $Ca_{10}(PO_4)_6(OH)_2$. Soft tissue lesions, like their skeletal counterparts, can contain 2 histologic forms of bone: woven and lamellar. Polarized optics can be helpful to distinguish the 2 types of bone (Fig. 1). Lamellar bone is always produced by benign osteoblasts, although they may be a secondary component in other malignancies. Woven bone is produced by both benign and malignant osteoblasts and reflects less organized collagen and rapid synthesis. *Cartilage* is an extracellular matrix composed of predominantly water and smaller amounts of proteoglycan and collagen (type 2). Neoplasms often contain these components in

Disclosures: The authors have no conflicts of interest to disclose.
Pathology, UCSF Medical Center Mission Bay, 1825 4th Street, Room M2354, San Francisco, CA 94158, USA
* Corresponding author.
E-mail address: andrew.horvai@ucsf.edu

surgpath.theclinics.com

Box 1
Categories of soft tissue lesions with skeletal matrix

Skeletal matrix is not definitional

Bone-forming melanoma

"Dedifferentiated" sarcomas

   Liposarcoma

   Leiomyosarcoma

   Malignant peripheral nerve sheath tumor

Tenosynovial giant cell tumor

Lipoma (chondrolipoma)

Fat necrosis

Nuchal fibrocartilaginous pseudotumor

Osteoma cutis

Fibroma of tendon sheath

Low-grade fibromyxoid sarcoma

Carcinoma

Schwannoma

Skeletal matrix is definitional

Myositis ossificans

   Soft tissue aneurysmal bone cyst

   Florid reactive periositis

Bizarre parosteal osteochondromatous proliferation

Subungual exostosis

Ossifying fibromyxoid tumor

Soft tissue osteosarcoma

Soft tissue chondroma

Synovial chondromatosis

Chest wall hamartoma

Chondro-osseous loose body

Chondroid syringoma

Mesenchymal chondrosarcoma

Extraskeletal myxoid chondrosarcoma

abnormal ratios, resulting in a "liquefied" or myxoid matrix. The cartilage in soft tissue neoplasms is typically the hyaline type; fibrocartilage and elastic cartilage are exceptionally rare in this setting.

Reactive and neoplastic soft tissue lesions can also contain amorphous or crystalline stromal calcifications that may raise the differential of skeletal matrix. Examples include calcifying aponeurotic fibroma, synovial sarcoma, crystal deposition diseases, and phosphaturic mesenchymal tumor.[11–13] Space limitations preclude a full discussion of each of these entities.

MYOSITIS OSSIFICANS AND RELATED TUMORS

Myositis ossificans represents the prototypical example of a family of tumors that (1) are composed of a population of fibroblastic-myofibroblastic cells; (2) produce osteoid, bone, and, less frequently, cartilage, in a reactive pattern; (3) often, but not invariably, arise after trauma; and (4) have a self-limited clinical course.[14] The group (summarized in **Table 1**) contains analogous tumors that differ

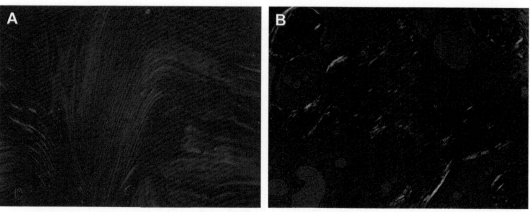

Fig. 1. Polarized optics is useful to discriminate (*A*) mature osteoid from rapidly produced, (*B*) woven osteoid. Note the distinctly parallel arrays of collagen in (*A*) compared with the short, haphazard lines in (*B*) (Hematoxylin-eosin, original magnification [*A*] ×100; [*B*] ×100).

from myositis by anatomic location (fibro-osseous pseudotumor of the digits, mesenteric ossification), or arise from periosteum (florid reactive periostitis).[15,16] Furthermore, recent genetic evidence suggests a link between a subset of myositis ossificans and soft tissue aneurysmal bone cyst (ABC).[10] Alternatively, ABC may be a secondary phenomenon within an existing myositis ossificans. Whereas all of the previously mentioned lesions were once considered reactive, recent molecular-genetic evidence shows that some tumors contain clonal genetic abnormalities (Table 1 and described later in this article), indicating that at least a subset represent self-limited neoplasms.

RADIOGRAPHIC FEATURES

The radiographic findings depend on the age of the lesion. Myositis initially manifests as a nonspecific soft tissue density that evolves into a nodule with a peripherally calcified rim (Fig. 2). Myositis is not connected to the skeleton, whereas florid reactive periostitis is attached to the underlying cortex. Soft tissue ABC contains fluid-fluid levels on cross-sectional imaging.

GROSS FEATURES

Myositis and soft tissue ABC typically measure less than 5 cm. The lesions of the digits (fibro-osseous pseudotumor, florid reactive periostitis) come to clinical attention when they are 1 to 2 cm. Mesenteric ossification is the largest of the group, sometimes up to 10 cm or larger. Myositis is unencapsulated although circumscribed and contains fleshy, hemorrhagic, and myxoid areas as well as gritty calcifications at the periphery (Fig. 3). Mature tumors consist entirely of hard

bone. Soft tissue ABC contains hemorrhagic cysts separated by fibrous and calcified septa.

MICROSCOPIC FEATURES

The histologic features of myositis ossificans depend on the age of the lesion (Fig. 4A–D). Early in its evolution, myositis resembles nodular fasciitis. Namely, it consists of myofibroblastic cells in a loose fascicular or "tissue culture" growth pattern. The stroma is myxoid with chronic inflammation, extravasated erythrocytes, and capillaries (see Fig. 4A). Subsequently, deposits of woven osteoid and bone form irregular trabeculae at the periphery (see Fig. 4B, C). The osteoblasts associated with the bone are large with prominent nucleoli but lack pleomorphism and only form a monolayer attached to seams of osteoid. They do not form sheets. Multinucleated osteoclasts may be present at any stage. Mitotic activity may be prominent, but atypical mitoses are not observed. As the lesion becomes fully mature, the bone is remodeled into lamellar bone with inactive-appearing osteocytes (see Fig. 4D). Rarely, cartilage undergoing endochondral ossification, reminiscent of fracture callus, may be present. Acute inflammation and necrosis are notably absent.

Myositis ossificans can contain areas resembling ABC, including hemorrhagic cysts lined by fibrous septa containing fibroblasts, osteoclasts, and chronic inflammatory cells, as well as densely mineralized bone ("blue bone") (Fig. 4E). If the entire lesion shows such features, it can be classified as a soft tissue ABC.

Immunohistochemistry has little utility in the diagnosis of these lesions. The spindle-cell component may be positive for smooth muscle actin and desmin.[14]

Table 1
Benign/self-limited chondro-osseous tumors of soft tissue

Tumor	Location	Age	Attached to Bone	Prognosis	Genetics
Myositis ossificans	Proximal extremity	Young adults	No	Local excision curative	(subset) t(17p13); *USP6* rearrangements
Soft tissue aneurysmal bone cyst	Proximal extremity	Young adults	No	Local excision curative	t(17p13); *USP6* rearrangements
Mesenteric ossification	Intra-abdominal	Mid-older adults	No	Local excision curative	Unknown
Fibro-osseous pseudotumor of digits	Hands, feet	Young adults	No	Local excision curative	Unknown
Florid reactive periostitis	Hands, feet	Young adults	Yes	Rare nondestructive recurrence	Unknown
Bizarre parosteal osteochondromatous proliferation	Hands, feet	Young adults	Yes	Nondestructive recurrence ~ 50%	t(1;17)(q32;q21), inv(7)
Subungual exostosis	Subungual, periungual	Young adults	Yes	Rare nondestructive recurrence	t(X;6)(q13-14;q22); *COL12A1*, *COL4A5* rearrangements

Differential Diagnosis

Nodular fasciitis

- Correlation with imaging is helpful; plain radiographs will demonstrate the calcified component of myositis that is absent in nodular fasciitis

- The distinction is not clinically significant because both are self-limited tumors

Soft tissue osteosarcoma (Table 2)

- Patients in sixth decade and older

- Tumors may arise in previously irradiated field

- Osteoid and calcification central or haphazard, which can be demonstrated radiographically

- Large (>10 cm)

- Sheets of cells with pleomorphism, nuclear hyperchromasia, and atypical mitoses

- Genetically complex, *USP6* rearrangement absent

Subungual exostosis

- Subungual or periungual

- Purely soft tissue initially, attached to cortex as lesion evolves

- Zonal, arrangement from superficial to deep: fibrous tissue → cartilage → bone

- t(X;6) (q13–14;q22) translocation resulting in rearrangements of the *COL12A1* and *COL4A5* genes[9]

Bizarre parosteal osteochondromatous proliferation (BPOP, Nora lesion)

- Exclusively involves digits

- Imaging shows attachment to underlying cortex

- Cartilage is definitional (vs only occasionally present in myositis) and highly cellular with enlarged chondrocytes

- t(1;17)(q32;q21) or inv(7)[8,17]

PROGNOSIS

Regardless of whether they are "true" neoplasms or purely reactive processes, myositis ossificans, florid reactive periostitis, and fibro-osseous pseudotumor are uniformly self-limited processes. If discovered incidentally, and a diagnosis can be made with combined imaging, and clinical and biopsy findings, these lesions can be followed without intervention. Otherwise, conservative excision is curative. Rarely, if incompletely excised, tumors may recur or persist, but nondestructively. Metastasis and malignant transformation are the essentially nonexistent. One series suggests that myositis ossificans with a *USP6* rearrangement and soft tissue ABC may have a more protracted, although still benign, clinical course.[10]

GENETIC FEATURES

As mentioned previously, a subset of myositis ossificans is characterized by gene fusions involving the *USP6* gene on chromosome 17p13. Intriguingly, this same gene is rearranged in nodular fasciitis.[18] The combination of histologic and genetic similarities between these tumors supports a biological relationship.

Key Features
MYOSITIS OSSIFICANS AND RELATED TUMORS

- Presents in young adults frequently at sites of trauma

- Histology shows zonal pattern with nodular fasciitis-like center and maturing bone peripherally

- Myofibroblasts and osteoblasts may have large nuclei with prominent nucleoli and mitotic activity, but pleomorphism, nuclear hyperchromasia, and necrosis are absent

- Florid reactive periostitis and soft tissue aneurysmal bone cyst are closely related lesions

- Most important differential diagnosis is soft tissue osteosarcoma (see Table 1)

- *USP6* rearrangements may be present in subset of cases

OSSIFYING FIBROMYXOID TUMOR

Ossifying fibromyxoid tumor (OFMT) is a rare soft tissue neoplasm of uncertain histotype characterized by bland ovoid to round cells in a fibromyxoid matrix rimmed by a thin, incomplete shell of lamellar bone.[19] Most examples are of

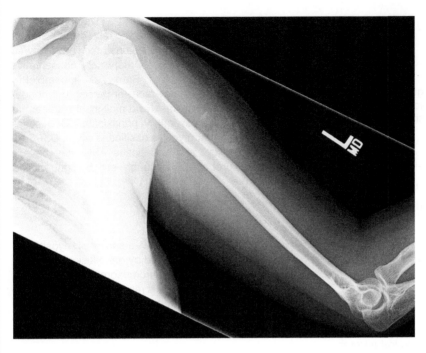

Fig. 2. Plain anterior-posterior radiograph of the left arm shows a peripherally calcified mass in the vicinity of the biceps. The circumscription and pattern of calcification is consistent with myositis ossificans.

intermediate malignant potential (hence the term "tumor" rather than "sarcoma"). The tumors are 1.5- to 2.0-fold more common in men than women, primarily in middle age, and present as a small, painless mass of many years' duration. Soft tissues of the proximal extremities are the most common sites, where the tumors may be attached to tendons. Less common locations include the head, neck, and trunk.

RADIOGRAPHIC FEATURES

Plain films demonstrate a circumscribed soft tissue mass separate from the underlying bone or

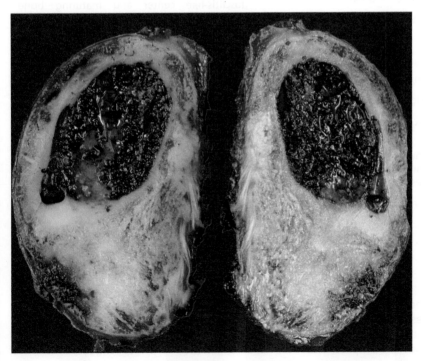

Fig. 3. Grossly, myositis ossificans consists of a fleshy to fibrous circumscribed mass, usually with a peripheral calcified zone. This example has an eccentric hemorrhagic cavity suggesting a component of ABC, which can be seen in myositis ossificans (see text).

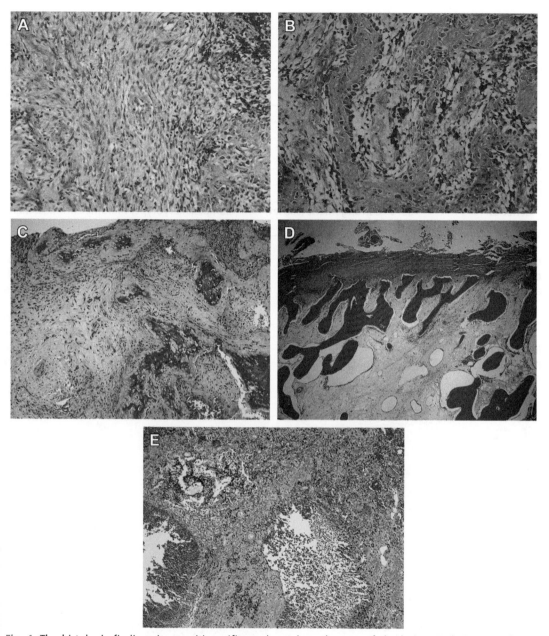

Fig. 4. The histologic findings in myositis ossificans depend on the age of the lesion. Early in its evolution, myositis contains areas resembling nodular fasciitis (*A*) and plump, "active" osteoblasts begin to form osteoid (*B*). Eventually this osteoid calcifies into woven (*C*) and lamellar (*D*) bone. Note the accentuation of the mature lamellar bone at the periphery of the lesion (*top of panel D*). Occasionally, features of aneurysmal bone cyst (*E*) may be present (Hematoxylin-eosin, original magnification [*A*] ×100; [*B*] ×100; [*C*] ×40; [*D*] ×20; [*E*] ×40).

joint. Depending on the extent of calcification, the lesion may contain irregular mineral signal. Cross-sectional imaging (computed tomography [CT]) shows a thin (<1 cm), partial rim of mineralization and a soft tissue density that enhances with intravenous contrast.[20] MRI shows low to intermediate signal and heterogeneous high signal on T1 and fat-suppressed T2 sequences, respectively.[21]

GROSS FEATURES

Most OFMT are circumscribed and smaller than approximately 4 cm. A 0.1-cm to 1.0-cm thick, "egg shell" rim of bone partially encapsulates a fleshy, firm to gelatinous homogeneous center. Exceptional cases may be up to 10 cm, with a thicker shell of bone. Approximately 20% of cases lack bone entirely. Malignant forms (see Prognosis)

Table 2
Clinicopathologic, radiologic comparison of myositis ossificans and extraskeletal osteosarcoma

	Myositis Ossificans	Extraskeletal Osteosarcoma
Demographics	Young adults	Older adults
Clinical history	Trauma	Radiation
Growth	Rapid (months)	Slow (years)
Size	<5 cm	>10 cm
Location of bone within lesion	Periphery	Center
Pleomorphism	Absent	Present
Mitotic activity	Present	Present, atypical forms
Genetics	*USP6* rearrangement (subset)	Complex karyotype, multiple chromosomal gains, losses and rearrangements

may have infiltrative margins with the fleshy component extending outside the bony capsule and entrapping surrounding connective tissue.

MICROSCOPIC FEATURES

In 80% of cases, a rim of lamellar bone, variably mineralized, encapsulates the tumor (Fig. 5A).

The bone can be confined as a shell only, or protrude centripetally. Osteoblasts are usually absent, or small and inactive. The central portion consists of lobules of fibromyxoid matrix separated by fibrous septae and evenly distributed round to ovoid cells (see Fig. 5B, C). The cells show a variety of growth patterns: anastomosing cords, trabeculae, or haphazard. They have pale, slightly

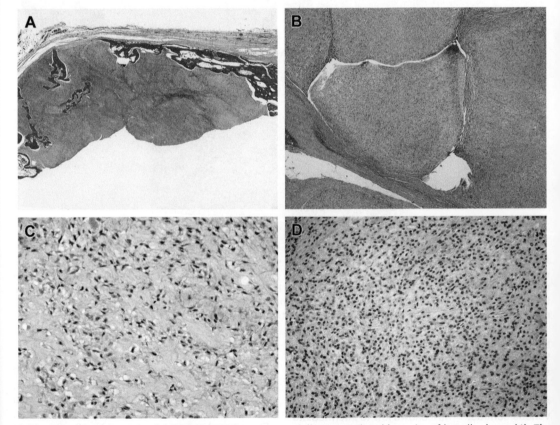

Fig. 5. Microscopic features of OFMT. Most tumors are partially encapsulated by a rim of lamellar bone (*A*). The center of the tumor consists of lobules of fibromyxoid stroma (*B*) with cords, trabeculae, or sheets (*C, D*) of monotonous round to ovoid cells without pleomorphism or significant mitotic activity (Hematoxylin-eosin, original magnification [*A*] ×20; [*B*] ×40; [*C*] ×200; [*D*] ×100).

eosinophilic cytoplasm, round nuclei with small nucleoli but lack pleomorphism (see **Fig. 5D**). Mitotic activity is low (typically <2 per 50 high-power fields [HPF]) and atypical mitoses are absent. Necrosis and satellite tumors have no prognostic significance.

Malignant OFMT is controversial. Although examples with diffuse hypercellularity, central ossification, and high nuclear grade have been classified as malignant OFMT (**Fig. 6**),[19] a subset may represent other sarcomas with metaplastic bone.[22]

Immunohistochemistry for S100 protein is positive in approximately 90% of benign OFMT.[23] Desmin is positive in about half of cases. Loss of INI1 (SMARCB1) has been reported in a mosaic pattern.[24] Rare examples (<10%) express smooth muscle actin, neuron-specific enolase, or glial fibrillary acidic protein (GFAP).

PROGNOSIS

Most OFMT have a protracted course, with local recurrence possible decades after initial excision. Predictors of local recurrence are few, but mitotic activity greater than 2 per 50 HPF increases risk.[19,23] OFMT with frankly malignant features (diffuse hypercellularity, high mitotic rate, high nuclear grade) is at higher risk of local recurrence and metastasis,[19] although, as mentioned previously, some of these may represent other high-grade sarcomas with bone production.

GENETIC FEATURES

Recurrent rearrangement of chromosome 6p21 mapping to the *PHF1* locus has been demonstrated in conventional OFMT.[28–31] Malignant OFMT shows *PHF1* rearrangement and may show loss of chromosome 22q, possibly leading to *SMARCB1 (INI1)* loss.[24,30]

Differential Diagnosis

Low-grade fibromyxoid sarcoma (LGFMS) and hyalinizing spindle-cell tumor with giant rosettes

- Occasionally demonstrates a bony capsule[6,25–27]

- Cells typically spindled to stellate

- Immunohistochemistry: S100 negative, MUC4 positive

- *CREB3L1* or *CREB3L2* fusion supports LGFMS

- LGFMS is generally more aggressive than OFMT and can metastasize

Epithelioid schwannoma

- Similar cytomorphology and growth pattern as OFMT, and shared S100 positivity

- Schwannoma can occasionally contain interspersed or peripheral ossification[7]

- Fibrillar stroma, palisading, Antoni A and B areas favor schwannoma

- *PHF1* rearrangement supports OFMT

Soft tissue osteosarcoma

- Older adults, may be history of radiation

- Bone present centrally or as lacelike deposits

- Highly pleomorphic, often bizarre cells with atypical mitoses

- S100 usually negative

Key Features
OSSIFYING FIBROMYXOID TUMOR

- Low-grade mesenchymal neoplasm of uncertain histotype

- Characteristic lobular growth pattern, fibromyxoid stroma, ovoid to round cells growing in cords, singly or haphazardly

- Most cases have a thin, incomplete shell of woven or lamellar bone

- Most cases S100 positive

- Mitotic activity >2 per 10 HPF associated with higher risk of recurrence

- Malignant OFMT remains controversial

- Benign forms have rearrangement of *PHF1* locus on 6p21

EXTRASKELETAL OSTEOSARCOMA

INTRODUCTION

Extraskeletal osteosarcoma is a highly aggressive tumor defined by the presence of malignant cells producing osteoid or bone but arising from soft tissue rather than the skeleton. Unlike conventional intraosseous osteosarcoma, the extraskeletal variety presents later (mid to late adulthood) and is sometimes associated with previous radiation.[32] Clinical presentation is with a large, painless,

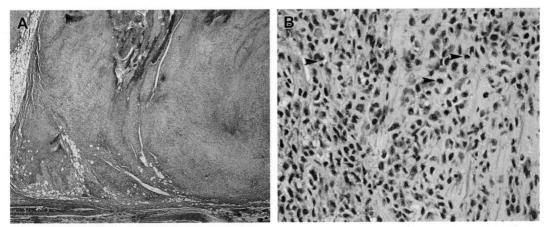

Fig. 6. Malignant OFMT shows bone formation toward the center of the lesion (*A, top of image*) and more diffuse hypercellularity, pleomorphism and increased mitotic activity (*B, arrowheads* point to mitoses) than the benign form (Hematoxylin-eosin, original magnification [*A*] ×40; [*B*] ×400).

deep soft tissue mass that grows over many months to a few years.

RADIOGRAPHIC FEATURES

Plain films reveal an ill-defined, large (>5 cm) soft tissue density. Mineralization, present in 50%, is usually central or diffuse (**Fig. 7**). CT images demonstrate displacement of fat planes with muscle attenuation.[33] The tumors are low signal intensity on T1-weighted and high signal intensity on T2-weighted MRI, respectively.[34] Tecnicium-99m scan may show uptake and may highlight metastases.

GROSS FEATURES

The tumors are large (5–15 cm), tan, fleshy and often contain hemorrhage and necrosis. Mineralization, if present, is concentrated centrally (**Fig. 8**) or haphazardly. Tumors may be circumscribed but are not encapsulated.

MICROSCOPIC FEATURES

Extraskeletal osteosarcomas are highly cellular and composed of polygonal, epithelioid, and/or spindled cells with marked pleomorphism (**Fig. 9**). Nuclei are hyperchromatic and vesicular with prominent nucleoli. Bizarre tumor giant cells are common. Mitotic activity is brisk (>10 mitotic figures per 10 HPF) including conspicuous atypical mitoses.

By definition, the tumor cells produce osteoid or bone (see **Fig. 9**A–D), although this finding can be focal. The matrix ramifies as delicate seams between individual tumor cells or groups of cells. Generally, bone is more abundant and more mineralized centrally, whereas the periphery of the tumor consists of a "front" of proliferating cells invading surrounding tissue (see **Fig. 9**A). Hyaline cartilage also may be present, usually containing atypical chondrocytes (see **Fig. 9**E). Osteoclasts, often present (see **Fig. 9**F), lack pleomorphism. Coagulative necrosis and hemorrhage are common.

Immunohistochemistry is usually not routinely necessary except to exclude other high-grade malignancies with incidental bone. An antibody against nuclear protein SATB2 marks osteoblasts, including malignant osteoblasts in soft tissue osteosarcoma.[35] In our experience, SATB2 is most useful if dense eosinophilic matrix is associated with malignant cells but cannot be definitively characterized as osteoid. In such cases, demonstration of SATB2 in the surrounding malignant cells confirms osteoblastic lineage, thus supporting the diagnosis of osteosarcoma (see **Fig. 9**G, H).

A minority of tumors may express S100, smooth muscle actin, desmin, or keratins, but usually only weakly and focally.

Differential Diagnosis

Conventional (skeletal) osteosarcoma with soft tissue extension

- Adolescents, most commonly involves distal femur and proximal tibia

- Distinction is based on correlation with imaging

- Better prognosis

Myositis ossificans and related lesions (see Table 1)

- Young adults, history of trauma

- Zonation with fasciitis-like center and mature bone at periphery

- No pleomorphism, nuclear hyperchromasia, atypical mitoses, or necrosis

- *USP6* rearrangement in some cases

Heterologous osteoblastic differentiation in other malignancies

- Metaplastic carcinoma: presence of invasive or in situ carcinoma elsewhere in tumor

- "Dedifferentiated" liposarcoma:

  ○ Presence of well-differentiated liposarcoma

  ○ Retroperitoneum is the most common site

  ○ 12q13–15 amplification

  ○ "Low-grade" extraskeletal osteosarcoma may represent dedifferentiated liposarcoma with a low-grade osteosarcoma component[4]

- Subungual melanoma

  ○ Can produce metaplastic bone[1,2]

  ○ Usually no cartilage

  ○ Nests and sheets of markedly anaplastic melanocytes with abundant mitoses

  ○ The presence of an associated in situ melanoma is diagnostic

  ○ Immunohistochemistry for melanoma markers (S100 protein, HMB45, Melan-A) is positive in the pleomorphic cells

PROGNOSTIC FEATURES

Soft tissue osteosarcoma shows a high rate of metastasis to lung and a 5-year survival rate of approximately 25%. This is in contrast to conventional intraosseous osteosarcoma, which, with localized disease and multimodal therapy, shows approximately 70% 5-year survival.[36] The difference is probably both patient and tumor related. Recall that soft tissue osteosarcoma presents in older adults, who are less able to tolerate aggressive chemotherapy, and at anatomic sites that render excision more challenging.[37] There also may be biological differences between skeletal and extraskeletal osteosarcomas that account for treatment response.

GENETIC FEATURES

No recurrent genetic abnormalities have been identified. Generally, tumors have multiple gains and losses and highly complex aberrations.

Key Features
SOFT TISSUE OSTEOSARCOMA

- High-grade malignancy of older adults, sometimes associated with previous radiation

- Defined by the presence of malignant cells producing osteoid or bone

- Excluding a primary skeletal osteosarcoma with soft tissue extension is essential and must be done with radiographic correlation

- SATB2 immunohistochemistry can confirm presence of osteoblasts

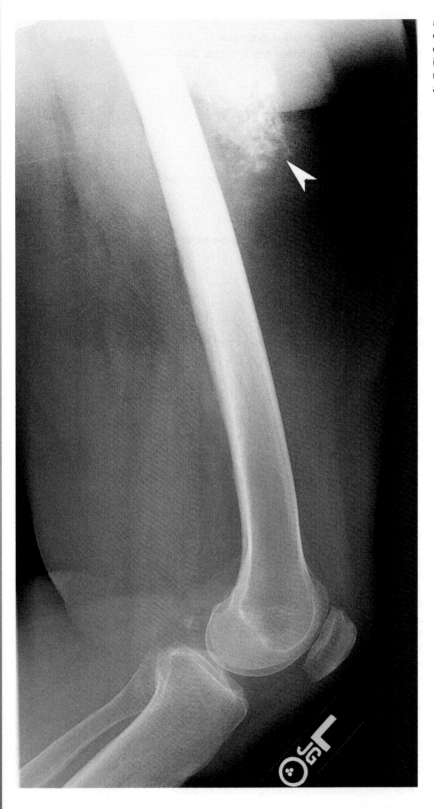

Fig. 7. Extraskeletal osteosarcoma of the thigh characterized by a large ill-defined soft tissue mass with central mineralization (*arrowhead*).

! Radiographic correlation is obligatory to establish that the tumor originates from soft tissue rather than from bone with soft tissue extension; this is especially true in soft tissue osteosarcoma

! Do not overdiagnose myositis ossificans as osteosarcoma because of high mitotic activity, rapid growth, and (reactive) nuclear atypia

! It may not be possible to distinguish between the benign bone-forming lesions on a small biopsy; a descriptive diagnosis is adequate if soft tissue osteosarcoma can be excluded

! A shell of bone in a soft tissue tumor can be seen in other neoplasms besides OFMT

! Do not misdiagnose a metaplastic carcinoma, bone-forming melanoma, or dedifferentiated liposarcoma as primary soft tissue osteosarcoma

SOFT TISSUE CHONDROMA

Soft tissue chondroma (STC) is a benign neoplasm composed of chondrocytes in a hyaline cartilage matrix that arises in extraosseous and extrasynovial tissues. Synonyms include chondroma of soft parts and extraskeletal chondroma. STC most commonly involves the digits, hands, and feet, with more than 80% occurring in the fingers.[38,39] Less common sites include the trunk and head and neck. They occur equally in men and women, with a peak age range in the 30s to 60s.[40] Almost all STCs are solitary lesions that present as slowly enlarging, painless masses. Multiple lesions are more likely to represent synovial chondromatosis.

RADIOGRAPHIC FEATURES

STC is a well-demarcated soft tissue lesion that does not involve the underlying bone, although it can cause compression or erosion of the bone. Focal ringlike or curvilinear calcifications can be seen on plain radiographs (Fig. 10).[41]

Fig. 8. Grossly, extraskeletal osteosarcoma consists of a central area of calcification (*arrowheads*) surrounded by a fleshy, hemorrhagic mass.

GROSS FEATURES

Tumors are circumscribed, small (usually <2 cm), and not attached to underlying bone. Cut surfaces are typically multinodular, pale blue, and may be calcified or myxoid (Fig. 11A).

MICROSCOPIC FEATURES

STC is composed of lobules of mature cartilage. The matrix is predominantly hyaline cartilage, but may have areas that are variably myxoid, fibrous, or ossified (see Fig. 11B–D). The chondrocytes are usually clustered (see Fig. 11B) and cytologically bland. So-called "atypical" features, such as hypercellularity, nuclear enlargement, and binucleation lack prognostic significance. Mitoses are rare or absent. Amorphous calcifications are common (see Fig. 11C). A foreign body giant-cell reaction may be present peripherally. Immunohistochemistry is not necessary for diagnosis, but the chondrocytes express S100 protein and ERG.[42]

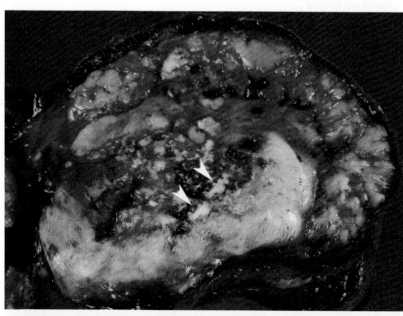

Differential Diagnosis

Synovial chondromatosis
- Involvement of large joints (eg, knee, hip, elbow, shoulder)
- Multiple small nodules attached to synovial membrane; can become detached as loose bodies in joint space
- Some experts suggest that STC and synovial chondromatosis are closely related, if not identical, entities

Extraskeletal myxoid chondrosarcoma
- Although extraskeletal myxoid chondrosarcoma histologically resembles cartilage, definite mature cartilage differentiation is not seen ultrastructurally or biochemically[43,44]
- Most common in deep soft tissue of proximal extremities compared with STC, which affects hands and feet
- Most cases characterized by t(9;22), which results in a *EWSR1-NR4A3* gene fusion

Myositis ossificans
- Presents at sites of trauma, deep soft tissue of proximal extremities
- Histologic zonation with nodular fasciitislike center and maturing bone peripherally
- Hyaline cartilage is an unusual finding

Periosteal or juxtacortical chondroma
- A benign cartilage-forming tumor arising on the peripheral surface of bone
- Radiographically characterized as a marginated lucency attached to the cortical surface of bone, with erosion of the underlying cortex that can cause a saucerlike depression with sclerosis of the interface
- Histologically indistinguishable from STC

Nuchal fibrocartilaginous tumor
- Rare benign proliferation of fibrocartilaginous nodules seen primarily in midline of posterior neck, originating within nuchal ligament, possibly related to previous trauma
- Histologically shows tendonlike fibrosis and fibrocartilage with bland fibroblasts and chondrocytes; focal myxoid change and calcification may be seen

Chondroid lipoma
- Very rare, benign adipocytic neoplasm with prominent myxoid-chondroid matrix and occasional lipoblasts
- More common in women, usually subcutaneous involvement in proximal limbs and limb girdles
- Matrix varies from chondroid to chondromyxoid, but true hyaline cartilage is rare
- Characterized by a t(11;16) (q13;p13) translocation, resulting in fusion of *MGC3032* and *MKL2* genes[45,46]

Calcifying aponeurotic fibroma
- Islands of calcification surrounded by palisaded epithelioid fibroblasts (resembling chondrocytes) are histologic hallmark
- Cartilage and osseous metaplasia may be present in long-standing lesions
- Most commonly in subcutaneous tissues of hands and feet
- Poorly circumscribed cellular fibroblastic component with fascicular growth pattern and infiltrative border

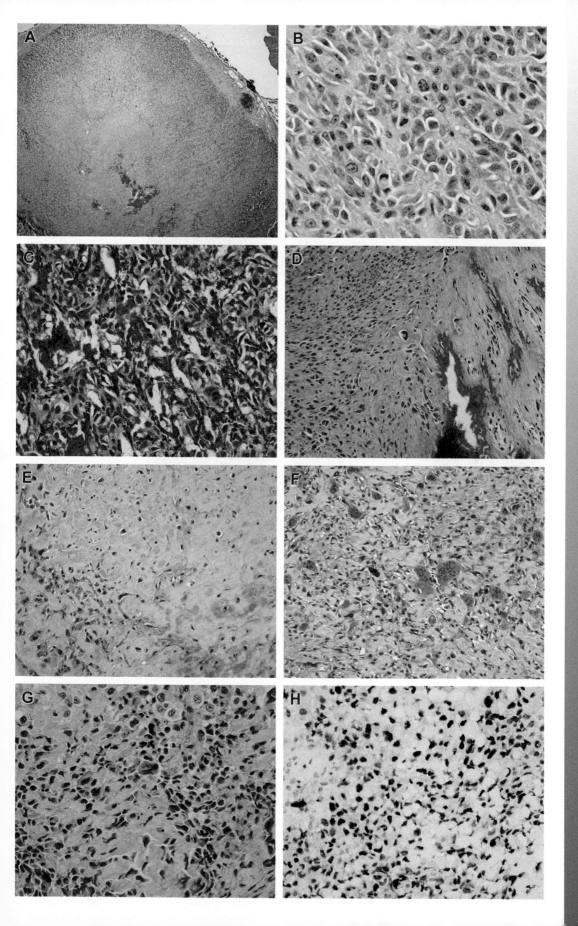

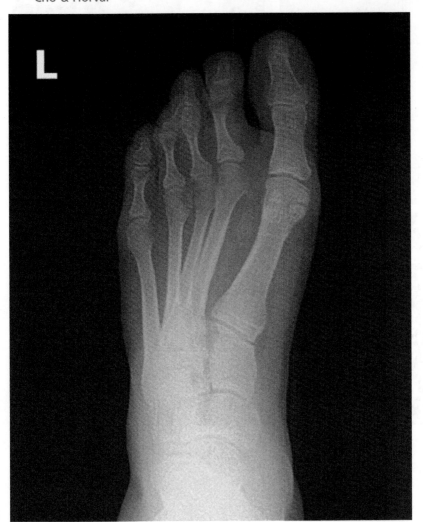

Fig. 10. Plain radiograph of a STC involving the left foot shows a purely soft tissue lesion between the first and second metatarsals without obvious joint involvement or cortical erosion of adjacent bone. This lesion shows curvilinear calcifications.

PROGNOSTIC FEATURES

Simple excision is curative. Local recurrence seen in 15% to 20% of cases, but malignant transformation is essentially nonexistent.

GENETIC FEATURES

Some cases of STC demonstrate clonal chromosomal abnormalities, including monosomy 6, trisomy 5, and rearrangements of chromosomes 11 and 12.[47,48]

Key Features
SOFT TISSUE CHONDROMA

- Benign cartilaginous tumor of soft tissue, most commonly involving the hands and feet

- Composed of mature hyaline cartilage; "atypical" histologic features are not prognostically significant

- May be histologically indistinguishable from synovial chondromatosis and periosteal chondroma; distinction requires clinical and radiographic correlation

Fig. 9. Microscopic features of extraskeletal osteosarcoma. Osteoid and bone (below center) is commonly present centrally with a peripheral front of cells that invade outward into soft tissue (*A*). Tumor cells are pleomorphic with conspicuous mitotic activity (*B*), producing osteoid and/or bone (*C, D*). Cartilage (*E*) and osteoclast-type giant cells (*F*) are occasionally present. When calcification is absent, it may be difficult to discriminate osteoid from other types of collagenous stroma (*G*). Immunostaining for SATB2 may be helpful in such cases (*H*) to confirm an osteoblastic lineage ([*A–G*] Hematoxylin-eosin, [*H*] SATB2; original magnification [*A*] ×20; [*B*] ×400; [*C*] ×200; [*D*] ×100; [*E*] ×100; [*F*] ×100; [*G*] ×200; [*H*] ×200).

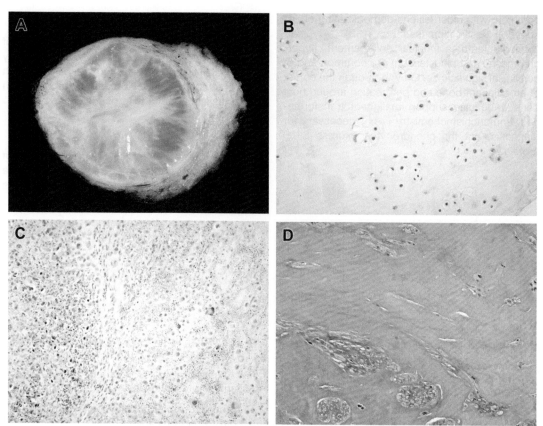

Fig. 11. STC. Grossly, STC consists of a well-circumscribed mass with pearly, pale blue cut surfaces, which can also show gelatinous, myxoid areas, as in this lesion (*A*). Sections show lobules of hyaline cartilage with cytologically bland chondrocytes that show characteristic clustering (*B*). The matrix may be "grungy" with amorphous calcifications (*C*) or show myxoid, degenerative features (*D*) (Hematoxylin-eosin, original magnification [*B*] ×100; [*C*] ×40; [*D*] ×100).

SYNOVIAL CHONDROMATOSIS

Synovial chondromatosis (SC) is a benign, extraosseous cartilaginous neoplasm composed of nodules of varying size in subsynovial tissue and attached to the synovial membrane of a joint, tendon sheath, or bursa. SC most commonly involves large joints of the limbs, most commonly the knee (approximately two-thirds of cases), as well as hip, elbow, shoulder, and axial joints, such as the temporomandibular joint.[38] SC can be entirely extra-articular (tenosynovial chondromatosis).[38] SC is more common in men, with a peak age range of 20s to 40s. Common presenting symptoms include pain, stiffness, swelling, decreased range of motion, or joint locking.

RADIOGRAPHIC FEATURES

If calcified, plain films demonstrate nodules within the joint space (**Fig. 12**). Unmineralized examples are detectable by MRI as lobulated masses bright on T2-weighted sequences and limited to the joint space or extending into the surrounding soft tissue.[49] A joint effusion may be present.

GROSS FEATURES

SC consists of multiple discrete nodules of cartilage that involve the synovium. Cut surfaces are pale blue, often with central calcification. Nodules may become detached and form loose bodies within the joint space or become embedded within fat or muscle.

MICROSCOPIC FEATURES

SC is composed of nodules of hyaline cartilage (**Fig. 13**A), with a synovial lining at the periphery that may be focal. The chondrocytes show characteristic clustering (see **Fig. 13**). Calcifications are common, with older lesions demonstrating endochondral ossification (see Fig. 13B). "Atypical" cytologic features (nuclear enlargement, hyperchromasia, and binucleation) are common and of no clinical significance. Growth through the cortex of an adjacent bone and permeation around host bone trabeculae support malignant transformation. Immunohistochemistry is not necessary for diagnosis, but the chondrocytes express S100 protein.

Differential Diagnosis

Soft tissue chondroma

- Solitary mass that occurs in the hands and feet; no synovial lining microscopically

- Histologic features similar to SC with clustering and occasional "atypical" chondrocytes

- Some experts suggest that STC and synovial chondromatosis are closely related, if not identical, entities

Chondro-osseous loose bodies ("joint mice")

- Non-neoplastic, reactive process consisting of free-floating osteocartilaginous fragment(s) within a joint space or embedded in synovium

- Most cases associated with trauma/mechanical injury (osteochondral fracture), osteoarthritis, epiphyseal osteonecrosis, or previous involvement of the joint by infection or inflammatory arthritis

- Peripheral hyaline and fibrocartilage concentrically layered around central necrotic bone

- Tidemark (indicative of articular origin) is diagnostic, if present

- Chondrocytes usually evenly distributed rather than clustered

Chondrosarcoma of bone extending into joint space

- Radiographic findings critical to determine site of origin

- Grade 1 chondrosarcoma of bone may have less nuclear atypia and lower cellularity than SC

- Chondrocytes evenly distributed compared with clustered in SC

- Primary soft tissue chondrosarcoma is virtually nonexistent in conventional hyaline form

---

PROGNOSTIC FEATURES

Local recurrence is seen in 15% to 20% of cases.[38] Malignant transformation is extremely rare, but has been reported associated with long-standing, multiply recurrent tumors, with metastasis in about a third of such cases.[50,51]

GENETIC FEATURES

Chromosome 6 anomalies, rearrangements of chromosome 1, and extra copies of chromosome 5 have been reported.[52] IDH1 and IDH2 mutations are absent.[53]

Key Features
SYNOVIAL CHONDROMATOSIS

- Cartilaginous tumor of synovial/subsynovial tissue, most commonly in large joints

- Composed (usually) of multiple nodules of hyaline cartilage surrounded by synovium

- "Atypical" histologic features do not necessarily imply malignancy

- Although exceptionally rare, malignant transformation exists

- Clinical and radiographic correlation necessary to distinguish from soft tissue chondroma, chondro-osseous loose bodies, and primary chondrosarcoma of bone that is secondarily involving the joint

---

MESENCHYMAL CHONDROSARCOMA

Mesenchymal chondrosarcoma (MCS) is a biphasic, high-grade malignant neoplasm that consists of primitive round cells and hyaline cartilage. MCS represents fewer than 3% of all chondrosarcomas. Although most arise in bone, 30% are primary soft tissue tumors.[54–56] The genders are affected equally, with peak incidence in the teens and 20s. The meninges are one of the most common sites of extraskeletal involvement[56,57]; rarely, viscera are involved. Presenting signs and symptoms are nonspecific, with pain and a tender mass noted.

RADIOGRAPHIC FEATURES

MCS is often seen as a circumscribed mass within the soft tissue with variable amounts of calcification and foci of low signal intensity within contrast-enhancing lobules on CT or MRI.[58]

Fig. 12. A plain radiograph of the right shoulder shows multiple radio-opaque nodules surrounding the glenohumeral joint. When calcified, as in this case, SC can be seen on plain films.

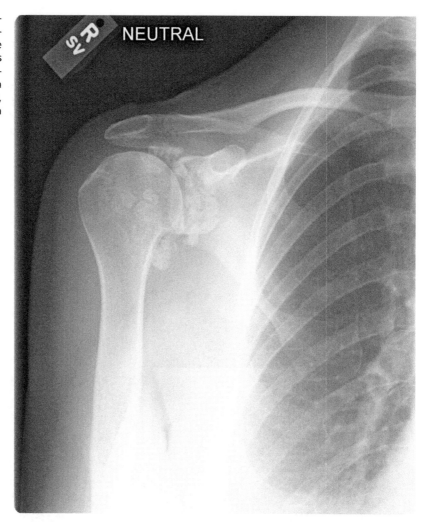

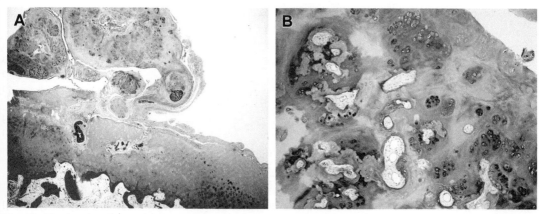

Fig. 13. SC arises in subsynovial tissue and is attached to the synovial membrane (*A*). It is composed of multiple nodules of hyaline cartilage that, similar to STC, show characteristic clustering of chondrocytes, with calcifications and sometimes endochondral ossification (*B*) (Hematoxylin-eosin, original magnification [*A*] ×20; [*B*] ×40).

GROSS FEATURES

The tumor consists of a mixture of pale blue carti-lage and fleshy soft tissue, often with cystic areas, necrosis, and hemorrhage (Fig. 14A). Calcifica-tions may be seen.

MICROSCOPIC FEATURES

The tumor is biphasic: composed of benign hya-line cartilage and primitive, small round blue cells (see Fig. 14B, C). The cartilage can be discrete and focal or the entire tumor may be variegated with alternating zones of cartilage and round cells. The cartilage component is usually low grade and may show calcification or endochondral

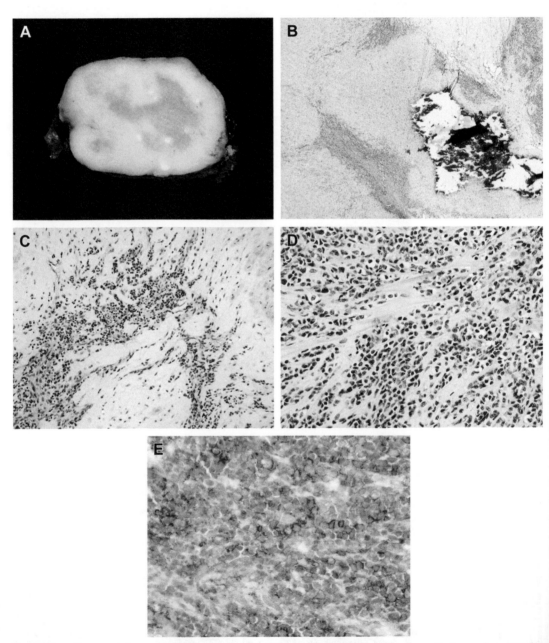

Fig. 14. Grossly, cut sections of MCS demonstrate cartilaginous as well as fleshy areas that may be cystic (*A*). Microscopically, a biphasic tumor is seen, with hyaline cartilage and primitive round cells (*B, C*). Focal calcification may be present (*B*). The round-cell component can be round to spindled (*D*) and show variable positivity for CD99 (*E*) ([*B–D*] Hematoxylin-eosin, [*E*] CD99; original magnification [*B*] ×40; [*C*] ×100; [*D*] ×200; [*E*] ×400).

ossification (see **Fig. 14**B). The round-cell component has a high nuclear:cytoplasmic ratio, and can be variably round to spindled (see **Fig. 14**D). A branching, so-called "hemangiopericytomatous," vascular pattern may be present in the round-cell component.

The cartilage component is positive for S100 protein.[56] The round cell component of MCS can demonstrate variable membrane positivity for CD99 (see **Fig. 14**E),[59–61] nuclear SOX9,[56] and cytoplasmic desmin,[57,61] but is negative for Fli-1.[62]

Differential Diagnosis

Ewing sarcoma family tumors (ESFTs)
- The small round-cell component of MCS, like ESFT, expresses CD99, but is negative for Fli1 and characteristic translocations involving the *EWSR1* gene (eg, t[11;22] and *EWSR1-FLI1* gene fusion) are not seen in MCS
- Cartilage is not a feature of ESFT
- ESFTs do not demonstrate *HEY1-NCOA2* fusions found in MCS

Dedifferentiated chondrosarcoma involving soft tissue
- Radiographic correlation is essential to establish skeletal origin
- Although biphasic, dedifferentiated chondrosarcoma composed of large, discrete foci of grade 1 chondrosarcoma and a second, high-grade component (osteosarcoma, fibrosarcoma, or undifferentiated sarcoma); small round-cell component is unusual
- Affects older adults

Extraskeletal chondroblastic osteosarcoma
- Affects older adults, often with previous radiation
- Malignant osteogenic component is definitional
- Chondrocytes and osteoblasts have high-grade, pleomorphic cytologic features
- A small round-cell component is unusual

PROGNOSTIC FEATURES

The clinical course is variable. Some patients may progress rapidly, whereas others can present with recurrence and metastasis decades after complete resection.[55]

GENETIC FEATURES

A recurrent *HEY1-NCOA2* fusion transcript was recently identified in MCS and appears to be absent in other chondrosarcomas.[63] *IDH1* and *IDH2* point mutations are absent in MCS.[53,64]

Key Features
MESENCHYMAL CHONDROSARCOMA

- 30% of MCS present as a primary soft tissue tumor, the remainder arise in bone
- Biphasic tumor composed of hyaline cartilage and primitive round cells, with multiple abrupt transitions between the 2 components
- The primitive round-cell component can raise a broad differential diagnosis, including many small round blue cell tumors (SRBCTs), but neoplastic cartilage is not a feature seen in other SRBCTs

---

EXTRASKELETAL MYXOID CHONDROSARCOMA

Although definite mature cartilage differentiation is not observed in extraskeletal myxoid chondrosarcoma (EMC),[43,44] it is included here given that the myxoid matrix histologically and histochemically resembles cartilage and EMC is often included as a cartilaginous tumor based on historical assertions.

EMC is a rare malignant neoplasm composed of spindled or epithelioid cells within a myxoid matrix. It presents in mid to late adulthood with a painless mass within the deep soft tissue, most commonly in the proximal extremities and rarely in the trunk or head and neck.[65,66] It more commonly affects men and is very rare in children.

RADIOGRAPHIC FEATURES

Imaging findings are often nonspecific. Calcifications may be seen on plain films and CT. On CT and MRI, peripheral and septal contrast-enhancement can be seen.[67]

GROSS FEATURES

EMCs are large (average 7 cm), circumscribed, and encapsulated masses that on cut section show multilobulated architecture with fibrous septa surrounding gelatinous areas (**Fig. 15**A).

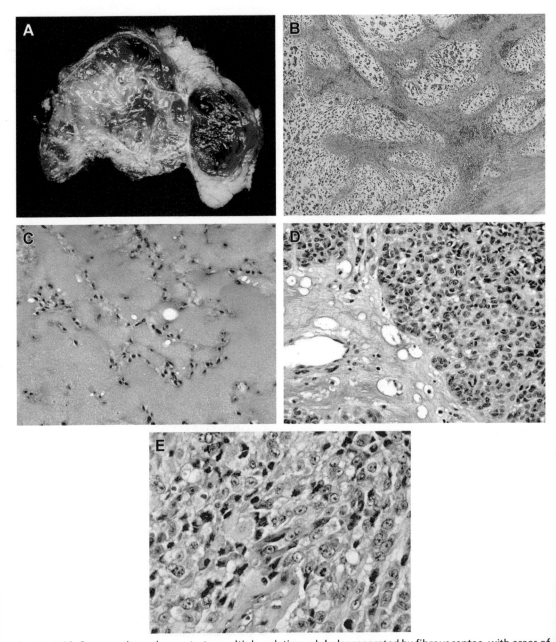

Fig. 15. EMC. Gross specimen demonstrates multiple gelatinous lobules separated by fibrous septae, with areas of hemorrhage (*A*). Microscopically, the tumor consists of spindled and epithelioid cells in a trabecular or reticular arrangement in myxoid stroma (*B,C*). The cellular variant can show larger clusters or sheets of cells (*D*). High-grade tumors show increased cellularity and cellular pleomorphism (*E*) (Hematoxylin-eosin, original magnification [*B*] ×40; [*C*] ×200; [*D*] ×200; [*E*] ×400).

Hemorrhage may be seen (see **Fig. 15**A), but necrosis is unusual. Cellular variants may have a more fleshy appearance.

MICROSCOPIC FEATURES

EMC is composed of spindled and epithelioid cells arranged in cords and chains, resulting in a trabecular or reticular pattern, embedded within multiple nodules of myxoid stroma that are separated by fibrous septa (see **Fig. 15**B). The tumor cells typically have uniform, round to oval, hyperchromatic nuclei without nucleoli, and eosinophilic cytoplasm (see **Fig. 15**C). The cellular variant shows sheets of epithelioid cells and only scant myxoid stroma (see **Fig. 15**D). Mitotic activity is typically low (<2 mitotic figures per 10 HPF).

High-grade features include high cellularity, cellular pleomorphism (including rhabdoid cytomorphology), high mitotic activity, and larger tumor size (see **Fig. 15E**).[66,68]

The tumor cells are positive for S100 protein in up to 50% of cases and some studies suggest neuroendocrine differentiation by immunohistochemistry and ultrastructure.[44,69–71] Keratins and smooth muscle markers are negative. Tumors with rhabdoid cytomorphology can show loss of staining for INI1 (SMARCB1).[72]

Differential Diagnosis

Soft tissue chondroma and synovial chondromatosis

- Soft tissue chondroma affects distal extremities

- Matrix may be myxoid, but typical hyaline cartilage invariably present at least focally

- Chondrocytes in well-defined, clear, lacunae with clustering

- Trabecular and reticular growth patterns distinctly unusual

- *NR4A3* gene rearrangements absent

Soft tissue mixed tumor/myoepithelioma

- Anastomosing cords of epithelioid, plasmacytoid, clear, or spindled cells

- Cytokeratin, EMA, and S-100 protein positive; many positive for calponin, GFAP, and smooth muscle actin

- *NR4A3* gene rearrangements absent (although a subset have *EWSR1* gene rearrangement)[73]; consequently fluorescence in situ hybridization results need to be interpreted with caution

Chordoma

- Typically involves clivus, sacrococcygeum

- Very rarely can be entirely extraosseous and intradural or metastasize to somatic soft tissue

- "Chondroid" variant can have features suggestive of EMC

- Positive for keratins, EMA, and brachyury

- *NR4A3* gene rearrangements absent

- Poorly differentiated variant shows loss of INI1 (SMARCB1)

PROGNOSTIC FEATURES

Histologically, higher-grade tumors follow a more aggressive clinical course. Tumors can recur or metastasize decades after initial resection. Metastasis, usually to lung, is seen in up to 50% of patients, although long survival is possible despite metastases.[66]

GENETIC FEATURES

Most (90%) cases show a reciprocal t(9;22)(q22;q12) translocation, resulting in a *EWSR1-NR4A3* gene fusion, or less commonly, a t(9;17)(q22;q11) translocation, resulting in a *RPB56-NR4A3* gene fusion.[74] Non-*EWSR1-NR4A3* variant fusions may correlate with high-grade morphology.[75]

Key Features
EXTRASKELETAL MYXOID CHONDROSARCOMA

- Despite the name, no mature hyaline cartilage is seen within the tumor, but the prominent myxoid matrix can resemble cartilage

- Low-grade lesions contain myxoid tumor nodules separated by fibrous bands, with spindled and epithelioid cells arranged in cords and chains embedded within the myxoid stroma

- Higher-grade examples show increasing cellularity, mitotic activity, and cellular pleomorphism, including rhabdoid morphology

- Can show recurrence and metastasis decades after initial resection

Pitfalls
OF CARTILAGE-PRODUCING TUMORS OF SOFT TISSUE

! Radiographic correlation is obligatory to establish origin of the tumor from soft tissue rather than from bone with secondary soft tissue extension.

! Primary hyaline-type chondrosarcoma is virtually nonexistent in soft tissue and should prompt a search for a preexisting lesion, such as synovial chondromatosis, a primary intraosseous tumor with soft tissue extension, or metastasis.

! Do not misinterpret "atypical" cytologic features of chondrocytes in soft tissue chondroma and synovial chondromatosis as evidence of malignancy.

REFERENCES

1. Emanuel PO, Idrees MT, Leytin A, et al. Aggressive osteogenic desmoplastic melanoma: a case report. J Cutan Pathol 2007;34:423–6.
2. Lucas DR, Tazelaar HD, Unni KK, et al. Osteogenic melanoma. A rare variant of malignant melanoma. Am J Surg Pathol 1993;17:400–9.
3. Carter MR, Hornick JL, Lester S, et al. Spindle cell (sarcomatoid) carcinoma of the breast: a clinicopathologic and immunohistochemical analysis of 29 cases. Am J Surg Pathol 2006;30:300–9.
4. Yoshida A, Ushiku T, Motoi T, et al. Well-differentiated liposarcoma with low-grade osteosarcomatous component: an underrecognized variant. Am J Surg Pathol 2010;34:1361–6.
5. Horvai AE, DeVries S, Roy R, et al. Similarity in genetic alterations between paired well-differentiated and dedifferentiated components of dedifferentiated liposarcoma. Mod Pathol 2009;22:1477–88.
6. Thway K, Chisholm J, Hayes A, et al. Pediatric low-grade fibromyxoid sarcoma mimicking ossifying fibromyxoid tumor: adding to the diagnostic spectrum of soft tissue tumors with a bony shell. Hum Pathol 2015;46(3):461–6.
7. Graham DI, Bond MR. Intradural spinal ossifying schwannoma. Case report. J Neurosurg 1972;36:487–9.
8. Nilsson M, Domanski HA, Mertens F, et al. Molecular cytogenetic characterization of recurrent translocation breakpoints in bizarre parosteal osteochondromatous proliferation (Nora's lesion). Hum Pathol 2004;35:1063–9.
9. Storlazzi CT, Wozniak A, Panagopoulos I, et al. Rearrangement of the COL12A1 and COL4A5 genes in subungual exostosis: molecular cytogenetic delineation of the tumor-specific translocation t(X;6)(q13-14;q22). Int J Cancer 2006;118:1972–6.
10. Sukov WR, Franco MF, Erickson-Johnson M, et al. Frequency of USP6 rearrangements in myositis ossificans, brown tumor, and cherubism: molecular cytogenetic evidence that a subset of "myositis ossificans-like lesions" are the early phases in the formation of soft-tissue aneurysmal bone cyst. Skeletal Radiol 2008;37:321–7.
11. Fetsch JF, Miettinen M. Calcifying aponeurotic fibroma: a clinicopathologic study of 22 cases arising in uncommon sites. Hum Pathol 1998;29:1504–10.
12. Milchgrub S, Ghandur-Mnaymneh L, Dorfman HD, et al. Synovial sarcoma with extensive osteoid and bone formation. Am J Surg Pathol 1993;17:357–63.
13. Ishida T, Dorfman HD, Bullough PG. Tophaceous pseudogout (tumoral calcium pyrophosphate dihydrate crystal deposition disease). Hum Pathol 1995;26:587–93.
14. Rosenberg AE, Oliveira AM. Myositis ossificans and fibro-osseous pseudotumor of digits. In: Fletcher CD, Bridge JA, Hogendoorn PC, et al, editors. WHO classification of tumours of soft tissue and bone. Lyon (France): IARC Press; 2013. p. 50–1.
15. Ostrowski ML, Spjut HJ. Lesions of the bones of the hands and feet. Am J Surg Pathol 1997;21:676–90.
16. Patel RM, Weiss SW, Folpe AL. Heterotopic mesenteric ossification: a distinctive pseudosarcoma commonly associated with intestinal obstruction. Am J Surg Pathol 2006;30:119–22.
17. Broehm CJ, M'Lady G, Bocklage T, et al. Bizarre parosteal osteochondromatous proliferation: a new cytogenetic subgroup characterized by inversion of chromosome 7. Cancer Genet 2013;206:402–5.
18. Erickson-Johnson MR, Chou MM, Evers BR, et al. Nodular fasciitis: a novel model of transient neoplasia induced by MYH9-USP6 gene fusion. Lab Invest 2011;91:1427–33.
19. Folpe AL, Weiss SW. Ossifying fibromyxoid tumor of soft parts: a clinicopathologic study of 70 cases with emphasis on atypical and malignant variants. Am J Surg Pathol 2003;27:421–31.
20. Schaffler G, Raith J, Ranner G, et al. Radiographic appearance of an ossifying fibromyxoid tumor of soft parts. Skeletal Radiol 1997;26:615–8.
21. Ideta S, Nishio J, Aoki M, et al. Imaging findings of ossifying fibromyxoid tumor with histopathological correlation: a case report. Oncol Lett 2013;5:1301–4.
22. Miettinen M, Fetsch JF, Antonescu CR, editors. AFIP atlas of tumor pathology: tumors of the soft tissues. Silver Spring (MD): ARP Press; 2014. p. 374–7.
23. Miettinen M, Finnell V, Fetsch JF. Ossifying fibromyxoid tumor of soft parts–a clinicopathologic and immunohistochemical study of 104 cases with long-term follow-up and a critical review of the literature. Am J Surg Pathol 2008;32:996–1005.
24. Graham RP, Dry S, Li X, et al. Ossifying fibromyxoid tumor of soft parts: a clinicopathologic, proteomic, and genomic study. Am J Surg Pathol 2011;35:1615–25.
25. Doyle LA, Moller E, Dal Cin P, et al. MUC4 is a highly sensitive and specific marker for low-grade fibromyxoid sarcoma. Am J Surg Pathol 2011;35:733–41.
26. Lee AF, Yip S, Smith AC, et al. Low-grade fibromyxoid sarcoma of the perineum with heterotopic ossification: case report and review of the literature. Hum Pathol 2011;42:1804–9.
27. Hisaoka M, Matsuyama A, Aoki T, et al. Low-grade fibromyxoid sarcoma with prominent giant rosettes and heterotopic ossification. Pathol Res Pract 2012;208:557–60.
28. Kawashima H, Ogose A, Umezu H, et al. Ossifying fibromyxoid tumor of soft parts with clonal chromosomal aberrations. Cancer Genet Cytogenet 2007;176:156–60.

29. Gebre-Medhin S, Nord KH, Moller E, et al. Recurrent rearrangement of the PHF1 gene in ossifying fibromyxoid tumors. Am J Pathol 2012;181:1069–77.
30. Graham RP, Weiss SW, Sukov WR, et al. PHF1 rearrangements in ossifying fibromyxoid tumors of soft parts: a fluorescence in situ hybridization study of 41 cases with emphasis on the malignant variant. Am J Surg Pathol 2013;37:1751–5.
31. Antonescu CR, Sung YS, Chen CL, et al. Novel ZC3H7B-BCOR, MEAF6-PHF1, and EPC1-PHF1 fusions in ossifying fibromyxoid tumors–molecular characterization shows genetic overlap with endometrial stromal sarcoma. Genes Chromosomes Cancer 2014;53:183–93.
32. Chung EB, Enzinger FM. Extraskeletal osteosarcoma. Cancer 1987;60:1132–42.
33. Bane BL, Evans HL, Ro JY, et al. Extraskeletal osteosarcoma. A clinicopathologic review of 26 cases. Cancer 1990;65:2762–70.
34. Varma DG, Ayala AG, Guo SQ, et al. MRI of extraskeletal osteosarcoma. J Comput Assist Tomogr 1993;17:414–7.
35. Conner JR, Hornick JL. SATB2 is a novel marker of osteoblastic differentiation in bone and soft tissue tumours. Histopathology 2013;63:36–49.
36. Geller DS, Gorlick R. Osteosarcoma: a review of diagnosis, management, and treatment strategies. Clin Adv Hematol Oncol 2010;8:705–18.
37. Lee JS, Fetsch JF, Wasdhal DA, et al. A review of 40 patients with extraskeletal osteosarcoma. Cancer 1995;76:2253–9.
38. Fetsch JF, Vinh TN, Remotti F, et al. Tenosynovial (extraarticular) chondromatosis: an analysis of 37 cases of an underrecognized clinicopathologic entity with a strong predilection for the hands and feet and a high local recurrence rate. Am J Surg Pathol 2003;27:1260–8.
39. Khedhaier A, Maalla R, Ennouri K, et al. Soft tissues chondromas of the hand: a report of five cases. Acta Orthop Belg 2007;73:458–61.
40. Pollock L, Malone M, Shaw DG. Childhood soft tissue chondroma: a case report. Pediatr Pathol Lab Med 1995;15:437–41.
41. Hondar Wu HT, Chen W, Lee O, et al. Imaging and pathological correlation of soft-tissue chondroma: a serial five-case study and literature review. Clin Imaging 2006;30:32–6.
42. Shon W, Folpe AL, Fritchie KJ. ERG expression in chondrogenic bone and soft tissue tumours. J Clin Pathol 2015;68:125–9.
43. Aigner T, Oliveira AM, Nascimento AG. Extraskeletal myxoid chondrosarcomas do not show a chondrocytic phenotype. Mod Pathol 2004;17:214–21.
44. Goh YW, Spagnolo DV, Platten M, et al. Extraskeletal myxoid chondrosarcoma: a light microscopic, immunohistochemical, ultrastructural and immuno-ultrastructural study indicating neuroendocrine differentiation. Histopathology 2001;39:514–24.
45. Ballaux F, Debiec-Rychter M, De Wever I, et al. Chondroid lipoma is characterized by t(11;16)(q13;p12-13). Virchows Arch 2004;444:208–10.
46. Huang D, Sumegi J, Dal Cin P, et al. C11orf95-MKL2 is the resulting fusion oncogene of t(11;16)(q13;p13) in chondroid lipoma. Genes Chromosomes Cancer 2010;49:810–8.
47. Dahlen A, Mertens F, Rydholm A, et al. Fusion, disruption, and expression of HMGA2 in bone and soft tissue chondromas. Mod Pathol 2003;16:1132–40.
48. Buddingh EP, Naumann S, Nelson M, et al. Cytogenetic findings in benign cartilaginous neoplasms. Cancer Genet Cytogenet 2003;141:164–8.
49. Walker EA, Murphey MD, Fetsch JF. Imaging characteristics of tenosynovial and bursal chondromatosis. Skeletal Radiol 2011;40:317–25.
50. Davis RI, Hamilton A, Biggart JD. Primary synovial chondromatosis: a clinicopathologic review and assessment of malignant potential. Hum Pathol 1998;29:683–8.
51. Campanacci DA, Matera D, Franchi A, et al. Synovial chondrosarcoma of the hip: report of two cases and literature review. Chir Organi Mov 2008;92:139–44.
52. Buddingh EP, Krallman P, Neff JR, et al. Chromosome 6 abnormalities are recurrent in synovial chondromatosis. Cancer Genet Cytogenet 2003;140:18–22.
53. Amary MF, Bacsi K, Maggiani F, et al. IDH1 and IDH2 mutations are frequent events in central chondrosarcoma and central and periosteal chondromas but not in other mesenchymal tumours. J Pathol 2011;224:334–43.
54. Guccion JG, Font RL, Enzinger FM, et al. Extraskeletal mesenchymal chondrosarcoma. Arch Pathol 1973;95:336–40.
55. Nakashima Y, Unni KK, Shives TC, et al. Mesenchymal chondrosarcoma of bone and soft tissue. A review of 111 cases. Cancer 1986;57:2444–53.
56. Fanburg-Smith JC, Auerbach A, Marwaha JS, et al. Reappraisal of mesenchymal chondrosarcoma: novel morphologic observations of the hyaline cartilage and endochondral ossification and beta-catenin, Sox9, and osteocalcin immunostaining of 22 cases. Hum Pathol 2010;41:653–62.
57. Fanburg-Smith JC, Auerbach A, Marwaha JS, et al. Immunoprofile of mesenchymal chondrosarcoma: aberrant desmin and EMA expression, retention of INI1, and negative estrogen receptor in 22 female-predominant central nervous system and musculoskeletal cases. Ann Diagn Pathol 2010;14:8–14.
58. Hashimoto N, Ueda T, Joyama S, et al. Extraskeletal mesenchymal chondrosarcoma: an imaging review

of ten new patients. Skeletal Radiol 2005;34:785–92.

59. Abbas M, Ajrawi T, Tungekar MF. Mesenchymal chondrosarcoma of the thyroid–a rare tumour at an unusual site. APMIS 2004;112:384–9.

60. Brown RE, Boyle JL. Mesenchymal chondrosarcoma: molecular characterization by a proteomic approach, with morphogenic and therapeutic implications. Ann Clin Lab Sci 2003;33:131–41.

61. Hoang MP, Suarez PA, Donner LR, et al. Mesenchymal chondrosarcoma: a small cell neoplasm with polyphenotypic differentiation. Int J Surg Pathol 2000;8:291–301.

62. Lee AF, Hayes MM, Lebrun D, et al. FLI-1 distinguishes Ewing sarcoma from small cell osteosarcoma and mesenchymal chondrosarcoma. Appl Immunohistochem Mol Morphol 2011;19:233–8.

63. Wang L, Motoi T, Khanin R, et al. Identification of a novel, recurrent HEY1-NCOA2 fusion in mesenchymal chondrosarcoma based on a genome-wide screen of exon-level expression data. Genes Chromosomes Cancer 2012;51:127–39.

64. Damato S, Alorjani M, Bonar F, et al. IDH1 mutations are not found in cartilaginous tumours other than central and periosteal chondrosarcomas and enchondromas. Histopathology 2012;60:363–5.

65. Enzinger FM, Shiraki M. Extraskeletal myxoid chondrosarcoma. An analysis of 34 cases. Hum Pathol 1972;3:421–35.

66. Meis-Kindblom JM, Bergh P, Gunterberg B, et al. Extraskeletal myxoid chondrosarcoma: a reappraisal of its morphologic spectrum and prognostic factors based on 117 cases. Am J Surg Pathol 1999;23:636–50.

67. Tateishi U, Hasegawa T, Nojima T, et al. MRI features of extraskeletal myxoid chondrosarcoma. Skeletal Radiol 2006;35:27–33.

68. Lucas DR, Fletcher CD, Adsay NV, et al. High-grade extraskeletal myxoid chondrosarcoma: a high-grade epithelioid malignancy. Histopathology 1999;35:201–8.

69. Harris M, Coyne J, Tariq M, et al. Extraskeletal myxoid chondrosarcoma with neuroendocrine differentiation: a pathologic, cytogenetic, and molecular study of a case with a novel translocation t(9;17)(q22;q11.2). Am J Surg Pathol 2000;24:1020–6.

70. Oliveira AM, Sebo TJ, McGrory JE, et al. Extraskeletal myxoid chondrosarcoma: a clinicopathologic, immunohistochemical, and ploidy analysis of 23 cases. Mod Pathol 2000;13:900–8.

71. Okamoto S, Hisaoka M, Ishida T, et al. Extraskeletal myxoid chondrosarcoma: a clinicopathologic, immunohistochemical, and molecular analysis of 18 cases. Hum Pathol 2001;32:1116–24.

72. Kohashi K, Oda Y, Yamamoto H, et al. SMARCB1/INI1 protein expression in round cell soft tissue sarcomas associated with chromosomal translocations involving EWS: a special reference to SMARCB1/INI1 negative variant extraskeletal myxoid chondrosarcoma. Am J Surg Pathol 2008;32:1168–74.

73. Antonescu CR, Zhang L, Chang NE, et al. EWSR1-POU5F1 fusion in soft tissue myoepithelial tumors. A molecular analysis of sixty-six cases, including soft tissue, bone, and visceral lesions, showing common involvement of the EWSR1 gene. Genes Chromosomes Cancer 2010;49:1114–24.

74. Panagopoulos I, Mertens F, Isaksson M, et al. Molecular genetic characterization of the EWS/CHN and RBP56/CHN fusion genes in extraskeletal myxoid chondrosarcoma. Genes Chromosomes Cancer 2002;35:340–52.

75. Agaram NP, Zhang L, Sung YS, et al. Extraskeletal myxoid chondrosarcoma with non-EWSR1-NR4A3 variant fusions correlate with rhabdoid phenotype and high-grade morphology. Hum Pathol 2014;45:1084–91.

Myoepithelial Tumors
An Update

Vickie Y. Jo, MD

KEYWORDS

• Mixed tumor • Myoepithelioma • Myoepithelial carcinoma • Cutaneous • Soft tissue • Bone

ABSTRACT

Primary myoepithelial neoplasms of soft tissue are uncommon, and have been increasingly characterized by clinicopathologic and genetic means. Tumors are classified as mixed tumor/chondroid syringoma, myoepithelioma, and myoepithelial carcinoma, and they share morphologic, immunophenotypic, and genetic features with their salivary gland counterparts. However, soft tissue myoepithelial tumors are classified as malignant based on the presence of cytologic atypia, in contrast to the criterion of invasive growth in salivary gland sites. This review discusses the clinicopathologic and morphologic characteristics, distinct variants, and currently known genetic alterations of myoepithelial neoplasms of soft tissue, skin, and bone.

OVERVIEW

The clinicopathologic, morphologic, and genetic features of myoepithelial neoplasms arising in soft tissue have been increasingly characterized over the past 10 to 15 years. In contrast to myoepithelial neoplasms in the salivary gland, primary myoepithelial tumors in soft tissue and skin (with the exception of some cutaneous lesions) lack any known normal cellular counterpart, which has likely contributed to their underrecognition in the past. Myoepithelial tumors affect male and female individuals equally over a wide age range, with peak incidence between the third and fifth decades; approximately 20% of cases occur in pediatric patients, in whom they are frequently malignant.[1-3] Tumors most commonly arise in the subcutis of the extremities and proximal limb girdles; however, they may occur over a broad anatomic distribution (including deep-seated, visceral, and bone locations).[4-6] Cutaneous lesions are confined to the dermis and arise frequently in the extremities, trunk, and head and neck regions.[7-9]

Tumors are classified as mixed tumor/chondroid syringoma, myoepithelioma, and myoepithelial carcinoma. Similar to their salivary gland counterparts, myoepithelial tumors of soft tissue, skin, and bone demonstrate heterogeneous morphologic and immunohistochemical features, but are notably distinct in their histologic criteria for malignancy. Cytologic atypia is the solely known predictor of aggressive behavior in soft tissue tumors; in contrast, malignancy in salivary gland tumors is based on the presence of invasive growth. Myoepithelial neoplasms show coexpression of epithelial markers (cytokeratin and/or epithelial membrane antigen [EMA]) and S-100 protein.[1-3,7,8,10] *EWSR1* gene rearrangement has been identified in nearly half of all myoepitheliomas and myoepithelial carcinomas in soft tissue, skin, and bone, as well as rare alternate *FUS* gene rearrangement[4-6,11-14]; likewise, *EWSR1* gene rearrangement is present in a subset of primary salivary myoepithelial neoplasms (many of which are characterized by clear-cell morphology).[15] At least two-thirds of mixed tumors harbor pleomorphic adenoma gene 1 (*PLAG1*) gene rearrangement,[16-18] similarly *PLAG1* gene alterations are present in up to 88% of pleomorphic adenoma[19] and 63% to 75% of carcinoma ex pleomorphic adenoma.[19,20] Mixed tumors and soft tissue myoepithelioma/myoepithelial carcinoma are thus likely related to their respective primary salivary counterparts based on shared morphologic, immunophenotypic, and genetic features.

MYOEPITHELIOMA AND MYOEPITHELIAL CARCINOMA

OVERVIEW

Myoepithelioma and myoepithelial carcinoma of soft tissue and skin exhibit a wide range of

Department of Pathology, Brigham and Women's Hospital, Harvard Medical School, 75 Francis Street, Boston, MA 02115, USA
E-mail address: vjo@partners.org

Surgical Pathology 8 (2015) 445–466
http://dx.doi.org/10.1016/j.path.2015.05.005

surgpath.theclinics.com

cytologic and architectural features, both within a given lesion and between different tumors. Tumors arise most frequently in the subcutis of the extremities, but may be deep-seated and can arise in nearly any anatomic site, including trunk, head and neck, and visceral locations.[1–3,8,10] Patients are affected over a wide age range spanning childhood to the elderly, and there is no sex predilection.[1–3,8,10] Notably, malignant tumors represent more than half of myoepithelial tumors in pediatric patients.[2,3] Most patients present with a painless, slow-growing, nontender cutaneous or subcutaneous mass. Larger masses (which are more likely malignant) may be associated with pain and local mass effects.

GROSS FEATURES

Grossly, tumors are generally well-circumscribed and lobulated, but frequently show infiltrative growth. Myoepithelioma ranges in size from 0.5 to 2.5 cm (mean, 0.7 cm) for dermal lesions[8] and 0.7 to 12 cm (mean, 3.8 cm) in soft tissue.[2] Myoepithelial carcinomas are often larger, with average size from 4.7 to 5.9 cm with a range of 1.3 to 20 cm.[2,3] Tumors are tan/white to yellow and variably firm, fleshy, myxoid, gritty, or calcified; hemorrhage and necrosis may be present in malignant tumors.

MICROSCOPIC FEATURES

Both benign and malignant tumors are multinodular or lobular, and despite being well-circumscribed often show infiltrative growth. A wide range of cytologic and architectural features characterize myoepithelial tumors. Spindled, ovoid, or epithelioid tumor cells are arranged in a combination of reticular, trabecular, or nested growth patterns in association with a variably chondromyxoid or hyalinized stroma (Fig. 1). Foci of solid growth or singly infiltrating cells are common. Some tumors may show a dominant single growth pattern, such as solid growth of spindle cells (Fig. 2A). In pediatric patients, an epithelioid morphology predominates in most cases.[3] Other occasional morphologic appearances include plasmacytoid "hyaline cells" with densely eosinophilic cytoplasm (see Fig. 2B), tumor cells with copious clear vacuolated cytoplasm (formerly identified in so-called "parachordoma") (see Fig. 2C), and rhabdoid morphology.[21] Up to 15% of cases show heterologous differentiation, including chondro-osseous (most common, in 10%–15% of tumors) (see Fig. 2D), adipocytic, and squamous.[1–3,8,12]

The spindled, ovoid, or epithelioid tumor cells have variable eosinophilic or clear cytoplasm,

and have ovoid-to-round nuclei. Myoepitheliomas lack cytologic atypia, and if present is mild at most (Fig. 3). Nucleoli are small or inconspicuous, and hyperchromasia and vesicular nuclear changes are absent. Mitotic activity may be present, but atypical mitotic figures should not be present. Rare examples have perineural invasion, and tumor necrosis is rare.

Cytologic atypia is the sole criterion for malignancy, as it is the best predictor for malignant behavior.[2,3] Myoepithelial carcinomas have moderate-to-severe nuclear atypia, and nuclei are often vesicular with a coarse chromatin pattern and prominent nucleoli. Currently no standard criteria exist, but myoepithelial carcinoma are graded (somewhat subjectively) as low, intermediate, and high, based on the degree of nuclear atypia and additional presence of mitotic activity and necrosis (Fig. 4). The histologic grade does not appear to have prognostic significance, and high mitotic rates and necrosis alone are not predictive of aggressive behavior.[2,3] Unlike carcinoma ex pleomorphia adenoma, soft tissue myoepithelial carcinoma rarely has areas of morphologically benign mixed tumor or myoepithelioma.[2,3] In pediatric patients, many myoepithelial carcinomas show a prominent population of epithelioid cells with variably eosinophilic cytoplasm, and approximately 30% of cases show a sheetlike growth of round cells with scant cytoplasm[3] (Fig. 5).

Myoepithelial neoplasms show co-expression of epithelial markers and S-100 protein (Fig. 6A, B). Cytokeratin (pan-keratin, AE1/AE3, Cam5.2) is positive in most cases (93%–100%), whereas EMA positivity is more variable (19%–79%).[1–3,7,8,10] S-100 protein is frequently positive (72%–100%), although the frequency of glial fibrillary acidic protein (GFAP) staining is lower (27%–54%).[1–3,7,8,10] Expression of myogenic markers is variable (and thus not often used in routine evaluation): calponin is most likely to be positive (86%–100%), in comparison with smooth muscle actin (SMA) (36%–64%), HHF-35 (20%–60%), and desmin (0%–20%).[1–3,7,8,10] The frequency of p63 positivity ranges from 23% to 70% in myoepithelioma and 7% to 40% in myoepithelial carcinomas[2,8,22,23] (see Fig. 6C). SOX10 positivity is present in most (82%) myoepitheliomas and in 30% of malignant tumors.[24] A subset of myoepithelial carcinomas exhibit loss of nuclear expression of SMARCB1/INI1 (9%–22%)[3,25] (see Fig. 6D), likely owing to functional loss of material on chromosome 22q11.2.

Rearrangement of the EWSR1 gene, encoded on chromosome 22q, is present in up to 45% of all myoepitheliomas and myoepithelial carcinoma of skin and soft tissue; a subset have alternate FUS rearrangement.[4–6,11–14,21,23,26] Documented

Fig. 1. Myoepithelial neoplasms are characterized by multinodular growth (*A*) and are architecturally and cytologically heterogeneous, with frequent trabecular (*B*), reticular (*C*), and nested (*D*) growth patterns in association with a hyalinized or chondromyxoid stroma.

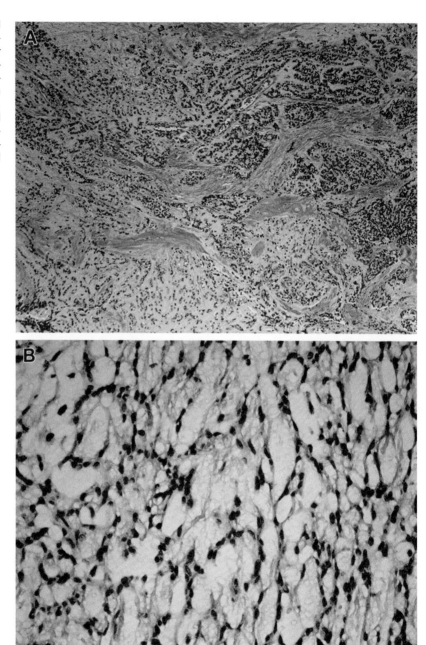

fusion partners thus far include *POU5F1* (6p21), *PBX1* (1q23), *ZNF444* (19q23), *ATF1* (12q13), *PBX3* (9q33), and *KLF17* (1p34).[4,9,11,26] Homozygous deletions of the *SMARCB1* gene have recently been reported in myoepithelial carcinomas lacking *EWSR1* gene rearrangement.[27]

Although the biologic significance of the fusion gene products is unknown, there may be some correlation between specific gene fusions and morphology based on preliminary observations.

In several large series, Antonescu and colleagues[4] observed that tumors with *EWSR1-POU5F1* fusion had the distinctive appearance of nests of epithelioid cells with clear cytoplasm (**Fig. 7**); tumors with *EWSR1-PBX1* fusion had a deceptively bland-appearing spindle-cell proliferation with a predominant sclerotic stroma[4]; tumors with *EWSR1-PBX3* demonstrated spindle-to-epithelioid cells arranged in nests and fascicles within a myxoid and collagenous stroma[26]; and tumors with

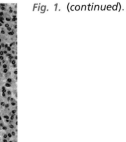

Fig. 1. (continued).

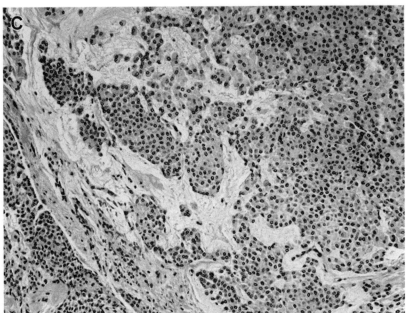

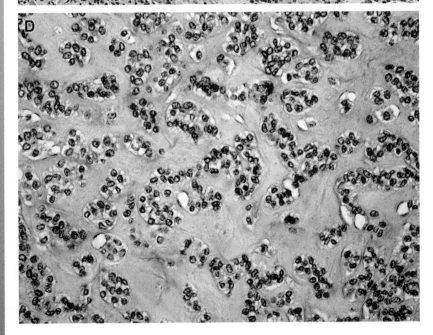

FUS-KLF17 fusion showed a trabecular growth pattern of ovoid-to-epithelioid cells in a myxohyaline stroma.[11]

DIAGNOSIS AND DIFFERENTIAL DIAGNOSIS

Owing to their characteristic wide morphologic spectrum, the differential diagnosis of myoepithelial neoplasms may be broad. However, the architectural and cytologic heterogeneity within a given tumor is a distinctive feature of myoepithelial tumors. The diagnosis of myoepithelioma or myoepithelial carcinoma typically requires an inclusive immunohistochemical panel, and confirmation of EWSR1 gene rearrangement may be helpful in certain contexts.

Extraskeletal myxoid chondrosarcoma (EMC) may resemble a myoepithelial tumor on both

Fig. 2. Occasionally, my-oepithelial tumors can also show foci of solid spindle cells (*A*), plasma-cytoid cells with abundant dense eosinophilic cyto-plasm ("hyaline bodies") (*B*), abundant clear vacuo-lated cytoplasm (*C*), and heterologous metaplasia, most commonly osseous (*D*) and/or cartilaginous.

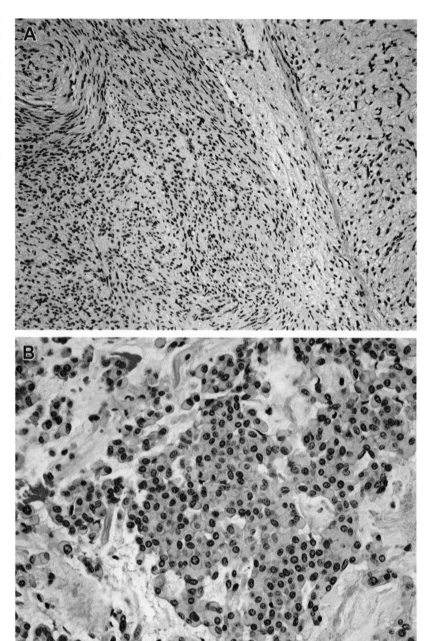

morphologic and immunohistochemical grounds. EMC is characterized by multinodular growth of uniform ovoid tumor cell population arranged in a distinctly reticular growth pattern within a myx-oid stroma. Tumor cells have uniform round nuclei with small to indistinct nucleoli and eosinophilic cytoplasm that extends into bipolar and stellate processes that appear to "reach out" to one another. The tumor nodules are overall hypocellu-lar but show more hypercellular growth at the periphery of the nodules. Rare high-grade vari-ants of EMC show diffuse hypercellularity, epithe-lioid cytomorphology, and higher nuclear grade, which may resemble myoepithelial carcinoma. Myoepithelial neoplasms tend to show more het-erogeneous cytologic features and architectural patterns, although some cases may show a pre-dominance of reticular architecture. Immunohisto-chemistry is often helpful: EMC shows rare focal S-100 or EMA positivity, but is consistently

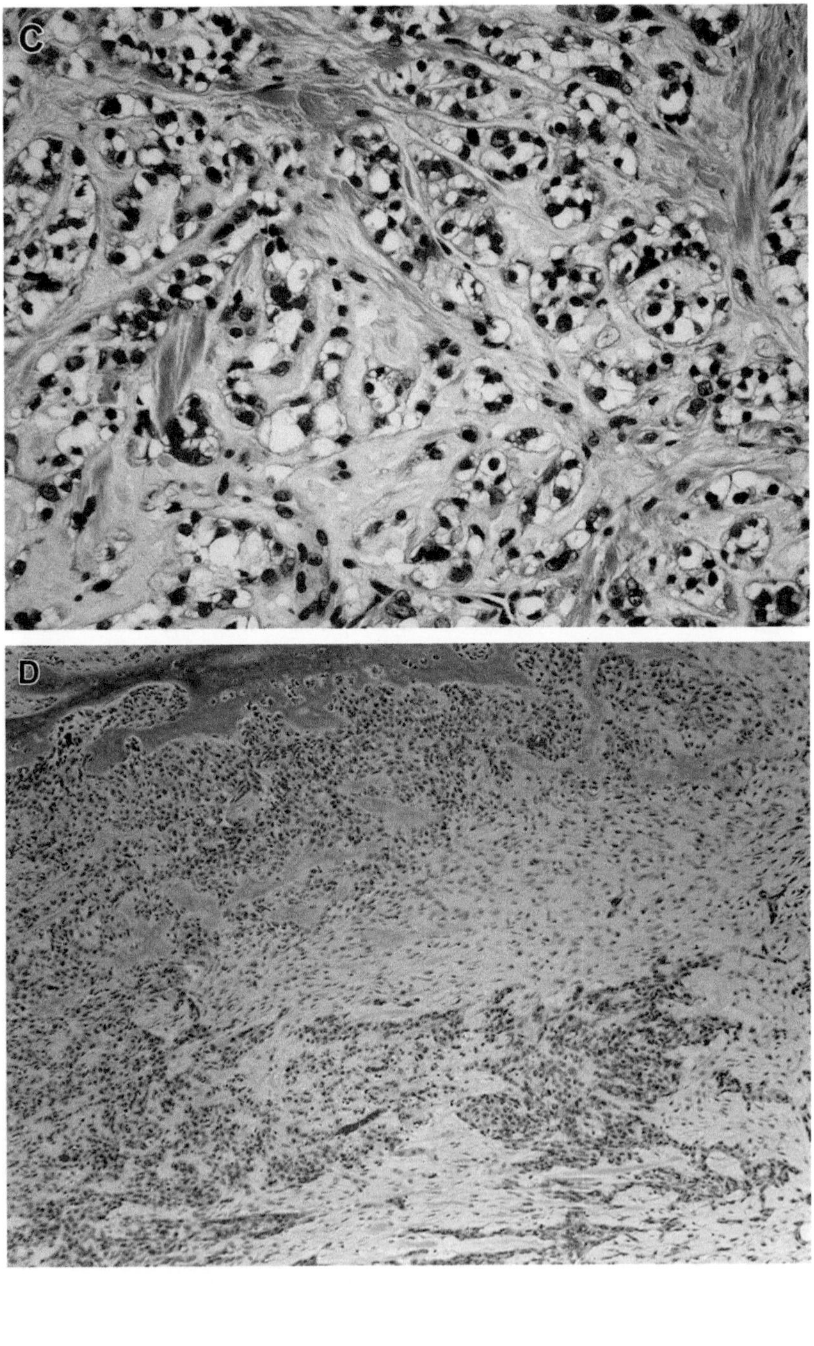

Fig. 2. (*continued*).

negative for cytokeratin, GFAP, and p63. EMC harbors the translocation t(9;22) (q22;q11) resulting in *NR4A3-EWSR1* fusion. Although SMARCB1/INI1 loss and *EWSR1* translocation are features of both EMC and myoepithelial tumors, detection of *NR4A3* rearrangement is diagnostic of EMC.[28]

Ossifying fibromyxoid tumor (OFMT) has many overlapping morphologic and immunohistochemical features with myoepithelial tumors. OFMT is characterized by multilobular growth of ovoid tumor cells arranged in cords and trabeculae in a variable fibromyxoid stroma. Tumor cells are uniformly ovoid to round with delicate nucleoli and palely eosinophilic cytoplasm. Most tumors have a peripheral shell of metaplastic bone (which is frequently "incomplete"). However, some OFMTs lack the peripheral bony shell, and heterologous osseous differentiation is present in some myoepithelial tumors. Malignant variants of OFMT remain

Fig. 3. Myoepithelioma has little or at most mild cytologic atypia; nuclei have fine chromatin, smooth contours, and inconspicuous-to-small nucleoli.

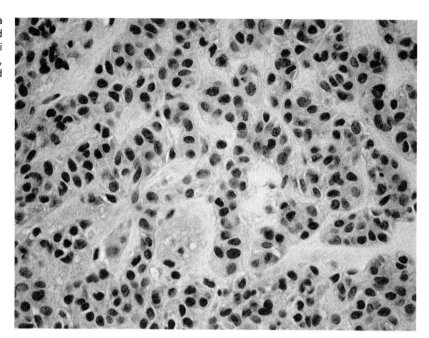

to be well defined, but convincing examples show high nuclear grade, solid growth, hypercellularity, mitotic counts of greater than 2 per 50 high-power fields (HPF), and irregular distribution of bone within the tumor lobules and cells. OFMT shows positivity for S-100 and variable positivity for cytokeratin and GFAP; however, desmin is frequently positive in OFMT and rarely in myoepithelial tumors. Myoepithelial tumors show more architectural and cytologic heterogeneity compared with OFMT, including cells with variably clear and eosinophilic cytoplasm and varying nested and solid growth patterns. Challenging cases may require molecular studies to confirm either *EWSR1* gene rearrangement in myoepithelioma and *PHF1* rearrangement in OFMT.[29,30]

Myoepithelial carcinoma may need to be distinguished from metastatic carcinoma in older patients, and clinical correlation is necessary (including whether a patient has a history of a salivary gland tumor). Extensive myxoid stroma and multinodular growth is a feature more typical of myoepithelial carcinoma. S-100 and GFAP positivity will favor myoepithelial carcinoma, although S-100 positivity may be seen in breast carcinoma. Immunohistochemistry, to include differentiation-specific markers based on the clinical context, should be helpful, such as estrogen receptor (ER) for breast, thyroid transcription factor 1 (TTF-1) for lung, and CDX-2 for gastrointestinal primaries, depending on the clinical context.

Proximal-type epithelioid sarcoma is also a diagnostic consideration, given its characteristic appearance of sheets of epithelioid cells with copious eosinophilic cytoplasm and large vesicular nuclei with distinct nucleoli. However, proximal-type epithelioid sarcoma is characterized by more cytologic uniformity than seen in myoepithelial carcinoma, and myxoid stromal changes are not typical. Epithelioid sarcoma is positive for cytokeratin and EMA and shows nuclear SMARCB1/INI1 loss, but CD34 is positive in approximately 50% of cases and S-100 is negative. Confirmation of *EWSR1* gene rearrangement will distinguish myoepithelial carcinoma from epithelioid sarcoma.

Myoepithelial carcinoma in pediatric patients raises a broader differential diagnosis, and includes malignant rhabdoid tumor and round cell sarcomas. Extrarenal rhabdoid tumor is rare in patients older than 3 years, and is characterized by sheets of large polygonal cells with round nuclei, prominent nucleoli, and abundant eosinophilic cytoplasm (often having hyaline inclusions). Extrarenal rhabdoid tumor shows variable positivity for epithelial markers and S-100, and consistent loss of INI1 secondary to alterations in the *SMARCB1/INI1* gene.[31] Fluorescence in situ hybridization (FISH) for *EWSR1* gene rearrangement and cytologic and architectural heterogeneity are features that help identify myoepithelial carcinoma.

Poorly differentiated synovial sarcoma is characterized by round cell morphology and shows frequent expression of epithelial markers and occasional S-100 positivity; however, in most cases, foci of conventional synovial sarcoma with spindle-cell morphology are present. Tumors can be distinguished from myoepithelial neoplasms by a lack of lobular architecture and absence of trabecular, nested, and reticular growth patterns. TLE1 is a sensitive and specific marker for synovial sarcoma, including most poorly differentiated tumors[32]; confirmation of the translocation t(X;18) (p11;q11), resulting in SS18-SSX1 fusion, is also diagnostic. Numerous other round cell sarcomas may enter the differential diagnosis, especially in biopsy specimens. Immunohistochemical and molecular studies can distinguish most entities, such as desmin and myogenin positivity and FOXO1 gene rearrangement in alveolar rhabdomyosarcoma. Ewing sarcoma may be a diagnostic pitfall, as it also harbors EWSR1 gene rearrangement and shows cytokeratin positivity in up to 30% of cases.

However, Ewing sarcoma is more cytologically uniform than myoepithelial carcinoma and is negative for S-100.

PROGNOSIS

Overall, myoepithelioma typically follows a benign clinical course with complete resection.[1,2,7–10] Up to 18% of myoepitheliomas are known to recur, and the risk appears higher with incomplete surgical resection.[2,8] Distant metastasis of morphologically benign myoepithelial neoplasms is rare.[2,8,10]

Myoepithelial carcinoma shows more aggressive behavior (irrespective of histologic grade or margin status), with a recurrence rate of 39% to 42% and the development of distant metastasis in 32% to 52% of affected patients.[2,3] Commonly reported sites of metastasis are lung, bone, lymph node, liver, brain, and soft tissue. The reported frequencies of disease-related deaths in several large series ranged from 13% to 43%.[2,3]

Pathologic Key Features
MYOEPITHELIOMA AND MYOEPITHELIAL CARCINOMA

- Most frequently arise as subcutaneous masses in the extremities, but may occur at any anatomic site

- Patients affected at all ages; no sex predilection

- Characterized by a wide range of cytologic and architectural features, both within a given lesion and between different tumors

- Tumors are multinodular or lobular, appear well circumscribed but are often infiltrative

- Variable reticular, trabecular, or nested growth patterns in association with a chondromyxoid or hyalinized stroma

- Spindled, ovoid, or epithelioid tumor cells with ovoid-to-round nuclei and eosinophilic-to-clear cytoplasm

- Other appearances include solid growth of spindle cells, plasmacytoid "hyaline cells," copious clear vacuolated cytoplasm, and heterologous differentiation (most frequently chondroid and/or osseous)

- Myoepitheliomas are cytologically benign and atypia is absent (or mild at most)

- Myoepithelial carcinomas have moderate-to-severe nuclear atypia, with vesicular nuclei having course chromatin pattern and prominent nucleoli; mitotic activity and necrosis are often present

- Co-expression of cytokeratin (pan-keratin, AE1/AE3, Cam5.2), EMA, and S-100; variable positivity for GFAP, p63, Sox-10

- A subset of myoepithelial carcinomas exhibit nuclear loss of expression of SMARCB1/INI1

- EWSR1 gene rearrangement is present in up to half of all myoepitheliomas and myoepithelial carcinoma (and alternate FUS rearrangement in seen in a small subset)

- A subset of myoepithelial carcinomas have homozygous deletions of the SMARCB1 gene

- Distinctive morphologic appearances appear associated with specific gene fusions (eg, tumors with EWSR1-POU5F1 show nested growth of epithelioid cells with clear cytoplasm)

MIXED TUMORS OF SOFT TISSUE AND SKIN

OVERVIEW

Mixed tumor (also known as chondroid syringoma in the skin) refers to benign myoepithelial tumors that show tubuloductal differentiation, and are morphologically identical to mixed tumor/pleomorphic adenoma of the salivary gland. Men and women are equally affected, most frequently in adulthood. Mixed tumors arise most commonly in the subcutis on the extremities, although cutaneous lesions are also frequent in the head and neck region.[7,8] Patients typically present with a firm, nontender slow-growing superficial papule or mass.

GROSS FEATURES

Tumors are grossly well circumscribed, and most measure less than 5.0 cm in greatest dimension, although they may be as large as 12 cm in soft tissue sites.[2] The cut surface is yellow/white to tan with variable firm, myxoid, or glistening appearance. Lesions are nodular or lobulated, and lack gross hemorrhage or necrosis.

MICROSCOPIC FEATURES

Mixed tumors are unencapsulated, and despite appearing well circumscribed they are often infiltrative. Tumors are multinodular or lobular with variably myxoid, hyalinized, or chondroid stroma. Spindled, ovoid, and epithelioid tumor cells are arranged in reticular, trabecular, and nested growth patterns, with occasional areas of solid growth. Tubuloductal differentiation is present, but may be focal (**Fig. 8**). Tumor cells have uniformly sized ovoid-to-round nuclei with a fine chromatin pattern and small or inconspicuous nucleoli, and variably eosinophilic-to-clear cytoplasm. Tumors with abundantly clear and vacuolated cytoplasm or plasmacytoid cells with densely eosinophilic cytoplasm ("hyaline cells") may occur.[1] Chondroid syringomas are morphologically subclassified as apocrine (most common) and eccrine.[7,33] Heterologous differentiation is present in 15% of cases, and is most frequently cartilaginous and/or osseous and less commonly adipocytic or squamous.[1,7]

Myoepithelial differentiation can be demonstrated by an immunohistochemical panel of cytokeratin, EMA, S-100, and GFAP. EMA is more likely to be positive in ductal cells.[1,7–9,16] p63 is positive in 27% to 45% of all benign myoepithelial neoplasms[8,22]; interestingly, p63 is more uniformly positive in nearly all salivary pleomorphic adenomas.[34,35] Frequent expression of PLAG1

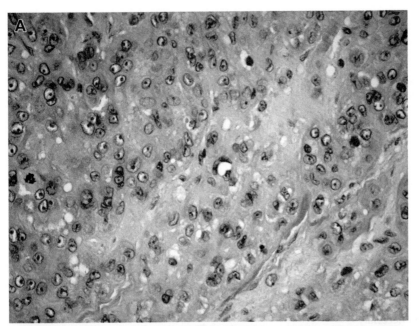

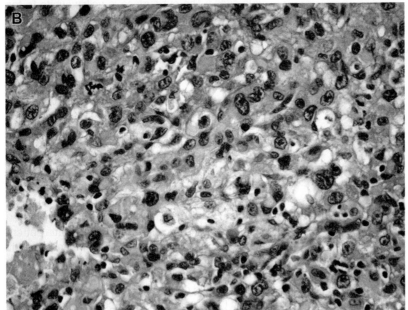

Fig. 4. Myoepithelial carcinoma is defined by cytologic atypia. Low-grade tumors show moderate cytologic atypia with vesicular nuclei and prominent nuclei (A), whereas high-grade myoepithelial carcinoma shows severe cytologic atypia, mitotic activity, and necrosis (B).

(58%–100%) is observed in mixed tumors in soft tissue and skin (Fig. 9), and has been shown to be absent in myoepithelioma.[17,18]

A subset of mixed tumor in skin and soft tissue show rearrangement of the *PLAG1* gene encoded on chromosome 8q12.[16,17] Using FISH, Bahrami and colleagues[17] first reported *PLAG1* gene rearrangement in 8 (72%) of 11 cases of cutaneous and soft tissue mixed tumors. A subsequent study by Antonescu and colleagues[16] demonstrated *PLAG1* gene rearrangement in 13 (37%) of 35 soft tissue and skin myoepithelial tumors with ductal differentiation; *PLAG1-LIFR* fusion was subsequently detected by rapid amplification of cDNA ends and reverse-transcriptase polymerase chain reaction.

Fig. 5. A subset of myoepithelial carcinoma in pediatric patients shows a round cell component.

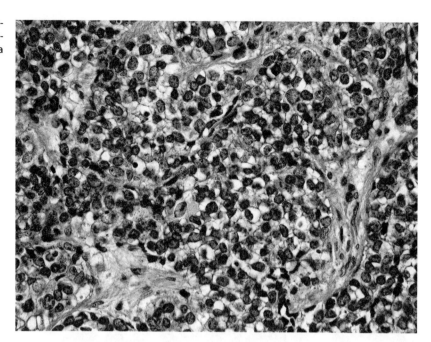

DIAGNOSIS AND DIFFERENTIAL DIAGNOSIS

Despite the morphologic heterogeneity of myoepithelial neoplasms, the diagnosis of mixed tumor is typically straightforward with the identification of tubuloductal differentiation. The main diagnostic pitfalls are distinction from a primary salivary neoplasm and the rare occurrence of "benign metastasizing pleomorphic adenoma."

Salivary pleomorphic adenoma and mixed tumors of skin and soft tissue show identical morphologic and immunohistochemical features, and harbor *PLAG1* gene rearrangements. Pleomorphic adenoma is the most common tumor of major and minor salivary glands. For lesions arising in the head and neck, connection with salivary gland must be excluded before classifying a mixed tumor as a cutaneous or soft tissue primary. Recurrence after incomplete resection of a pleomorphic adenoma is common, and any previous history of a salivary gland tumor in the region of a new lesion should be investigated. Rarely, a patient with pleomorphic adenoma may develop distant metastases after resection of a benign tumor, referred to as "benign metastasizing pleomorphic adenoma/mixed tumor," which is often associated with high morbidity and mortality secondary to multiple metastases over a protracted time course. Tumors that metastasize seem to be associated with previous recurrences of the primary tumor; however, no histologic predictors for recurrence or metastasis have yet been identified.[36] Metastases may occur at nearly any anatomic site; thus, clinical correlation is essential.

PROGNOSIS

Soft tissue and cutaneous mixed tumors are benign and follow an indolent clinical course. Recurrence is observed in up to 18% of all benign myoepithelial neoplasms, and distant metastasis is exceptionally rare.[2,8,10] Malignant transformation of skin and soft tissue mixed tumors has not been well characterized; areas of morphologically benign myoepithelioma or mixed tumor are rare within myoepithelial carcinoma of soft tissue.[2,3]

Pathologic Key Features
MIXED TUMOR/CHONDROID SYRINGOMA

- Men and women are equally affected, most frequently in adulthood

- Most common in the subcutis on the extremities; cutaneous lesions are also frequent in the head and neck region

- Unencapsulated and appear well circumscribed, but are often infiltrative

- Show the typical architectural and cytologic heterogeneity of myoepithelial tumors

- Tubuloductal differentiation is present

- Immunohistochemical expression of cytokeratin, EMA, S-100, and GFAP

- A subset harbor *PLAG1* gene rearrangement and are immunoreactive for PLAG1

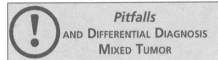

Pitfalls
AND DIFFERENTIAL DIAGNOSIS
MIXED TUMOR

! Tubuloductal differentiation may be focal

! Clinical correlation is required to exclude metastatic, recurrent, or locally aggressive pleomorphic adenoma of the salivary gland

CUTANEOUS SYNCYTIAL MYOEPITHELIOMA

OVERVIEW

Cutaneous syncytial myoepithelioma is a distinct benign variant that arises most frequently on the limbs. Tumors arise in patients of all ages, and male individuals are more frequently affected than female individuals. The typical clinical presentation is a painless polyploid or papular skin lesion.

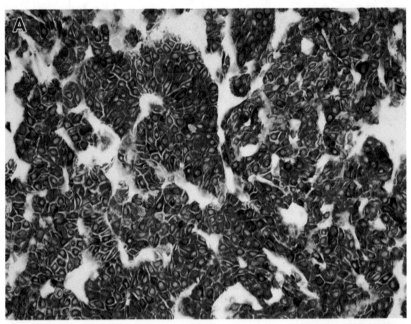

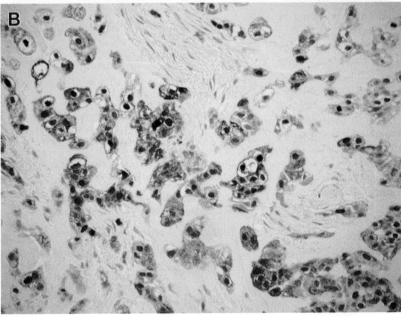

Fig. 6. Myoepithelial neoplasms express epithelial markers cytokeratin (pankeratin, *A*) or EMA and S-100 (*B*).

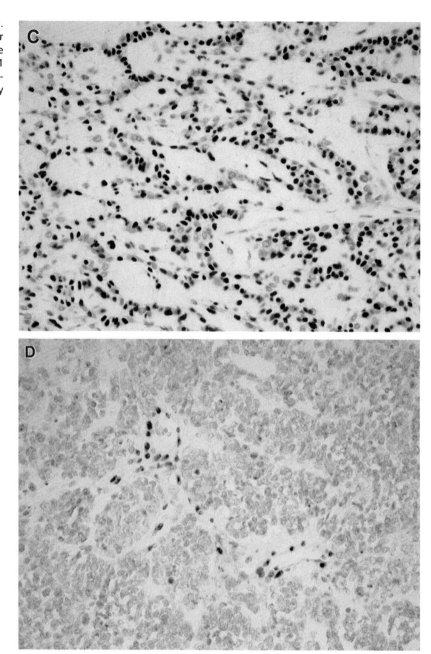

Fig. 6. (continued). Frequent positivity for GFAP and p63 (*C*) are observed. SMARCB1/INI1 is lost in a subset of tumors, most frequently carcinoma (*D*).

GROSS FEATURES

Tumors are described as well-circumscribed tan-white, firm dermal lesions, ranging in size from 0.3 to 2.7 cm (median, 0.8 cm).[12]

MICROSCOPIC FEATURES

Cutaneous syncytial myoepithelioma is characterized by a solid syncytial sheetlike growth of ovoid, spindled, or histiocytoid cells. Lesions are centered in the dermis and are unencapsulated, and are overall well circumscribed, but may show focally infiltrative growth. Tumor cells are uniformly sized, with pale vesicular nuclei with fine chromatin and small or inconspicuous nucleoli (Fig. 10). The cytoplasm is palely eosinophilic and cell borders are poorly defined. Nuclear atypia is minimal to absent, and mitotic activity is usually low (rarely exceeding 4 per 10 HPFs). Adipocytic

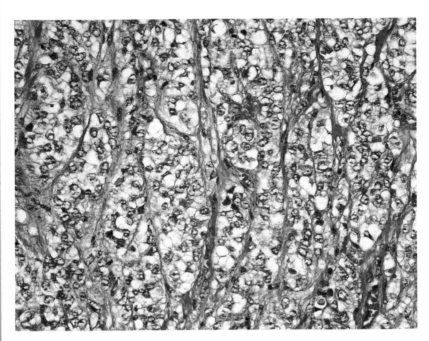

Fig. 7. There appears to be some correlation between certain morphologic features and fusion genes; tumors with *EWSR1-POU5F1* are characterized by a nested growth of epithelioid cells with clear cytoplasm.

and chondro-osseous differentiation has been observed.[8,12] A lymphocytic infiltrate may be present, both within and at the periphery of the tumor and around blood vessels. Significant cytologic atypia, necrosis, and lymphovascular invasion are absent.

The immunophenotype of cutaneous syncytial myoepithelioma is distinctive, with consistent positivity for EMA and S-100 protein.[8,12] In contrast to most myoepithelial tumors, cytokeratin is focally positive in only rare cases (12%). Variable positivity is seen for GFAP (42%), SMA (70%), and p63 (54%).

EWSR1 gene rearrangement is present in cutaneous syncytial myoepithelioma; however, no fusion partners have been identified to date. The known fusion partners in myoepithelial neoplasms, including *PBX1*, *ZNF444*, *POU5F1*, *DUX4*, *ATF1*, *CREB1*, *NR4A3*, *DDIT3*, and *NFATc2*, have been excluded.[12]

DIAGNOSIS AND DIFFERENTIAL DIAGNOSIS

The differential diagnosis of cutaneous syncytial myoepithelioma includes epithelioid fibrous histiocytoma, melanocytic lesions (most commonly Spitz nevi), and epithelioid sarcoma.

Epithelioid fibrous histiocytoma is a dermal tumor that commonly arises on the lower extremities in adult patients. Tumors appear as a well-circumscribed nodular proliferation of bland epithelioid cells with palely eosinophilic cytoplasm embedded in a collagenous and usually vascular stroma. Frequent binucleated tumor cells are seen, which is not a feature of cutaneous syncytial myoepithelioma. EMA positivity is seen in approximately 60% of epithelioid fibrous histiocytoma and cytokeratin is negative, but S-100, GFAP, and p63 staining is consistently negative.[37] *ALK* gene fusions and ALK overexpression have very recently been identified in epithelioid fibrous histiocytoma, and ALK immunohistochemistry may be used to help in the differential diagnosis, as cutaneous syncytial myoepithelioma lacks expression of ALK.[38,39]

Melanocytic lesions showing little cytologic atypia and pleomorphism may also be considered in the differential diagnosis, especially when a junctional component is not present or visualized. Spitz nevi are well circumscribed and are occasionally completely intradermal. Most Spitz nevi can be identified by careful examination for the presence of a junctional component, nested growth pattern, Kamino body formation, and downward "maturation" into deeper dermis. Although S-100 positivity is shared by both Spitz nevi (and other melanocytic neoplasms) and cutaneous syncytial myoepithelioma, the melanocytic

Fig. 8. Mixed tumor/chondroid syringoma show architectural and cytologic heterogeneity, and are defined by tubuloductal differentiation (*A*, *B*).

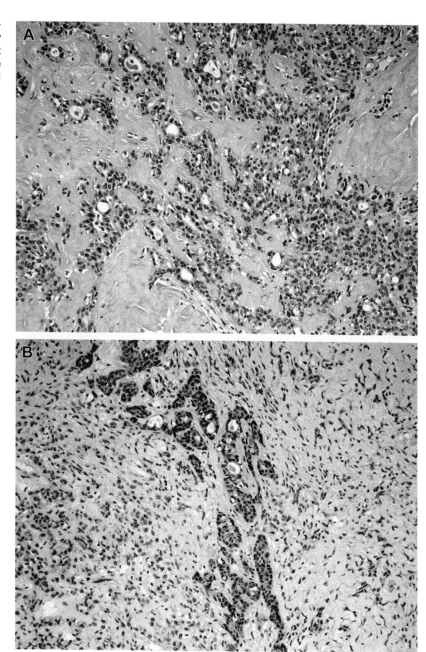

markers HMB-45, Melan-A, and MiTF, along with EMA, will be discriminatory.

Distal-type epithelioid sarcoma shows an infiltrative growth pattern and is often composed of poorly circumscribed, discontinuous nodules. In contrast, cutaneous syncytial myoepithelioma is usually a small, superficial, single nodule.

Epithelioid sarcoma is composed of an admixture of epithelioid and spindle cells with abundant eosinophilic cytoplasm and vesicular nuclei; tumor cells appear uniform but are characterized by mild-to-moderate nuclear atypia, although cases having solid growth and relatively less atypia may mimic cutaneous syncytial myoepithelioma.

Epithelioid sarcoma is also positive for EMA, but is positive for pan-keratin and CD34 and negative for S-100 and GFAP. Nuclear loss of expression of SMARCB1/INI1 is characteristic of epithelioid sarcoma, but has not been examined in cutaneous syncytial myoepithelioma; however, *EWSR1* rearrangement is diagnostic of cutaneous syncytial myoepithelioma.

PROGNOSIS

These are benign tumors and simple excision is curative in the vast majority of cases, with local recurrence observed in only rare cases after incomplete resection and no known risk of metastasis.[12]

> **Pathologic Key Features**
> CUTANEOUS SYNCYTIAL
> MYOEPITHELIOMA
>
> • Most commonly arise on the lower extremities in male adults
>
> • Unencapsulated well-circumscribed, but frequently infiltrative, dermal tumors
>
> • Solid syncytial sheetlike growth of ovoid, spindled, or histiocytoid cells
>
> • Uniform tumor cells with pale vesicular nuclei with fine chromatin, small or inconspicuous nucleoli, and palely eosinophilic syncytial cytoplasm
>
> • Minimal to absent nuclear atypia
>
> • Adipocytic and chondro-osseous differentiation may be seen
>
> • Positive for EMA and S-100 protein, but are typically negative for cytokeratin
>
> • Harbors *EWSR1* gene rearrangement

> **Pitfall**
> CUTANEOUS SYNCYTIAL
> MYOEPITHELIOMA
>
> ! Cytokeratin is negative or focal, in contrast to most myoepithelial neoplasms

> ▲▲ **Differential Diagnosis**
> CUTANEOUS SYNCYTIAL
> MYOEPITHELIOMA
>
> • Epithelioid benign fibrous histiocytoma
>
> • Spitz nevi and other melanocytic neoplasms
>
> • Distal-type epithelioid sarcoma

MYOEPITHELIAL TUMORS OF BONE

OVERVIEW

Primary myoepithelial neoplasms of bone are rare, with fewer than 30 cases reported in the literature to date.[4,6,26,40–48] Male and female individuals are equally affected over a wide age range from (14 to 55 years). Documented primary sites include craniofacial, sacroiliac, tibia, vertebral body L1, femur, humerus, and fibula. Most benign tumors demonstrate radiographic features suggestive of a slow-growing benign neoplasm, appearing well circumscribed and radiolucent with a thin sclerotic rim and occasional periosteal reaction or focal cortical erosion. Malignant tumors show a nonspecific permeative or destructive growth pattern on radiographs.

GROSS FEATURES

Tumors range in size between 3 and 18 cm, appear mucoid or chondroid, and have a variable white, red-gray, or pink cut surface with occasional focal hemorrhage.[5,46]

MICROSCOPIC FEATURES

Myoepithelial neoplasms in bone show similar morphologic features with soft tissue and skin tumors; most reported tumors are benign. Myoepitheliomas in bone are well-circumscribed multinodular and lobulated tumors with tumor cells arranged in solid and reticular growth patterns within a collagenous, myxoid, and hyalinized stroma (**Fig. 11**). As expected, tumors are positive for EMA and S-100 protein, and show variable reactivity for p63, GFAP, and keratin (AE1/AE3, Cam5.2).[5,41,42,44,46] *EWSR1* rearrangement has been demonstrated in up to 67% myoepithelioma of bone,[4,5,26] and one case with *FUS-POU5F1* has been reported.[6] Two of the 3 cases having *EWSR1-PBX3* fusion and the

Fig. 9. PLAG1 is frequently positive in mixed tumor/chondroid syringoma.

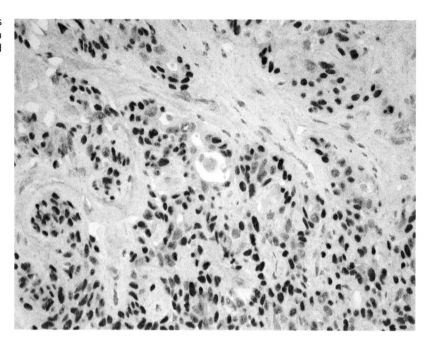

distinctive appearance of spindled to epithelioid cells arranged in fascicles embedded in a sclerotic and myxoid stroma were primary bone lesions.[26]

DIAGNOSIS AND DIFFERENTIAL DIAGNOSIS

Few primary bone tumors show morphologic features that overlap with myoepithelial tumors; chondromyxoid fibroma, chordoma, and chondrosarcoma are most likely to be considered in the differential diagnosis. Given the propensity for craniofacial sites, clinical and radiographic correlation is necessary to exclude a locally aggressive, recurrent, or metastatic pleomorphic adenoma.

Chondromyxoid fibroma is a rare benign cartilaginous tumor that most commonly arises in the metaphysis of long bones in patients during the second and third decades. These tumors show a multilobular growth of uniform spindle-to-stellate cells in a reticular growth pattern within a myxoid matrix; areas of more hypercellular growth are seen at the periphery of the lobules. The tumor cells have minimal eosinophilic cytoplasm that occasionally shows bipolar or multipolar extensions. Enlarged hyperchromatic nuclei are only occasionally seen, and mitotic activity is usually absent. The morphologic appearance may mimic myoepithelioma, but can be distinguished by immunohistochemistry: although S-100 is positive in chondromyxoid fibroma, cytokeratin and EMA are negative. In addition, identification of *EWSR1* gene rearrangement will identify most cases of myoepithelioma.

Chordoma is a notochordal tumor that most frequently arises in the axial skeleton (but may occur in extra-axial osseous and extra-osseous sites). Tumors are characterized by a multilobular growth of tumor cells arranged in cords and nests within a myxoid stroma, which may mimic a myoepithelial neoplasm. Tumor cells are also heterogeneous, with a population of cells with small round nuclei with abundant eosinophilic cytoplasm and other cells with abundant vacuolated cytoplasm (so-called "physaliferous" cells). Some examples of poorly differentiated chordoma, which have more solid growth, vesicular nucleoli, and abundant mitotic activity, may mimic myoepithelial carcinoma. Similar to myoepithelial tumors, chordoma is positive for cytokeratin, EMA, and S-100; however, brachyury is a sensitive and specific marker for chordoma (including poorly differentiated tumors).[49]

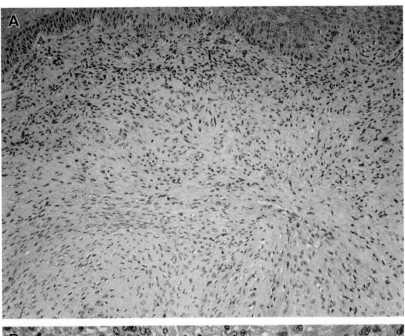

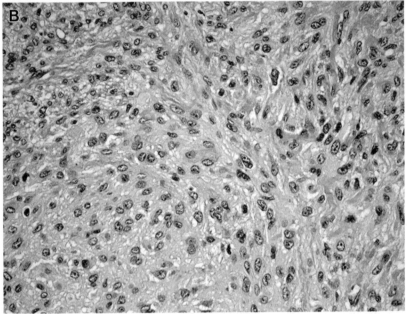

Fig. 10. Cutaneous syncytial myoepithelioma is characterized by an intradermal syncytial growth of benign-appearing ovoid, spindled, and histiocytoid tumor cells with pale eosinophilic cytoplasm (A, B).

Myxoid stromal change and hypercellularity are features of grade 2 or 3 chondrosarcomas, which are characterized by a lobular growth pattern of spindle and stellate chondrocytes with progressive cytologic atypia. Although S-100 is positive in chondrosarcoma, epithelial markers are usually negative. EWSR1 gene rearrangement is diagnostic of myoepithelial neoplasms; furthermore, molecular testing for IDH1/IDH2 mutations, which are present in nearly half of all central and periosteal chondrosarcomas,[50] may be helpful.

Fig. 11. Primary myoepithelial tumors have been recently described in bone. Myoepithelioma does not show infiltrative growth, and is well-demarcated from cortical and cancellous bone (*A, B*).

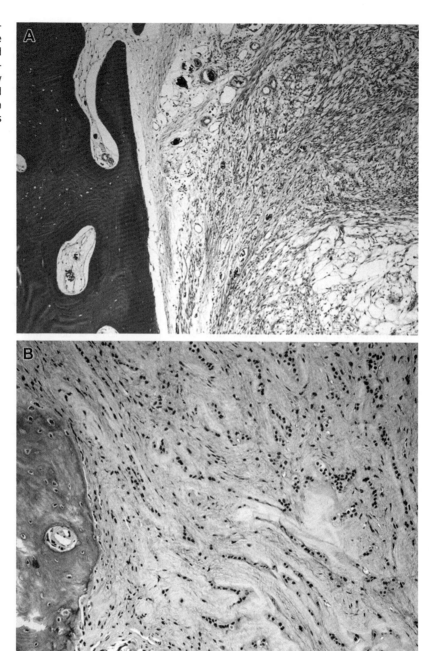

PROGNOSIS

Based on limited available data, myoepithelioma of bone shows benign behavior with no recurrence or metastasis after resection.[5,41–44,46] A more aggressive course for myoepithelial carcinoma is suggested by the few existing reports of one patient who presented with a satellite nodule[45] and another who developed lung metastasis at 13 months follow-up.[47]

Pathologic Key Features
MYOEPITHELIAL TUMORS IN BONE

- Most reported cases thus far have been benign, and documented sites include craniofacial, sacroiliac, tibia, vertebral body L1, femur, humerus, and fibula

- Male and female individuals equally affected over a wide age range

- Benign tumors demonstrate radiographic features suggestive of a slow-growing benign neoplasm; malignant tumors show nonspecific permeative or destructive growth

- Similar morphologic features with soft tissue and skin tumors

- Myoepithelioma is well circumscribed and multinodular, and does not show infiltrative growth

- Tumors are positive for EMA and S-100 protein, and show variable reactivity for p63, GFAP, and keratin (AE1/AE3, Cam5.2)

- *EWSR1* rearrangement (and alternate *FUS* rearrangement) are present in primary bone tumors

Pitfall
MYOEPITHELIAL TUMORS IN BONE

! A broad and inclusive panel is often necessary to identify myoepithelial differentiation

Differential Diagnosis
MYOEPITHELIAL TUMORS IN BONE

- Chondromyxoid fibroma

- Chordoma

- Chondrosarcoma, grade 2 or 3

- Metastatic or aggressive pleomorphic adenoma/carcinoma ex pleomorphic adenoma

REFERENCES

1. Kilpatrick SE, Hitchcock MG, Kraus MD, et al. Mixed tumors and myoepitheliomas of soft tissue: a clinicopathologic study of 19 cases with a unifying concept. Am J Surg Pathol 1997;21:13–22.

2. Hornick JL, Fletcher CD. Myoepithelial tumors of soft tissue: a clinicopathologic and immunohistochemical study of 101 cases with evaluation of prognostic parameters. Am J Surg Pathol 2003;27:1183–96.

3. Gleason BC, Fletcher CD. Myoepithelial carcinoma of soft tissue in children: an aggressive neoplasm analyzed in a series of 29 cases. Am J Surg Pathol 2007;31:1813–24.

4. Antonescu CR, Zhang L, Chang NE, et al. EWSR1-POU5F1 fusion in soft tissue myoepithelial tumors. A molecular analysis of sixty-six cases, including soft tissue, bone, and visceral lesions, showing common involvement of the EWSR1 gene. Genes Chromosomes Cancer 2010;49:1114–24.

5. Kurzawa P, Kattapuram S, Hornicek FJ, et al. Primary myoepithelioma of bone: a report of 8 cases. Am J Surg Pathol 2013;37:960–8.

6. Puls F, Arbajian E, Magnusson L, et al. Myoepithelioma of bone with a novel FUS-POU5F1 fusion gene. Histopathology 2014;65:917–22.

7. Mentzel T, Requena L, Kaddu S, et al. Cutaneous myoepithelial neoplasms: clinicopathologic and immunohistochemical study of 20 cases suggesting a continuous spectrum ranging from benign mixed tumor of the skin to cutaneous myoepithelioma and myoepithelial carcinoma. J Cutan Pathol 2003;30:294–302.

8. Hornick JL, Fletcher CD. Cutaneous myoepithelioma: a clinicopathologic and immunohistochemical study of 14 cases. Hum Pathol 2004;35:14–24.

9. Flucke U, Palmedo G, Blankenhorn N, et al. EWSR1 gene rearrangement occurs in a subset of cutaneous myoepithelial tumors: a study of 18 cases. Mod Pathol 2011;24:1444–50.

10. Michal M, Miettinen M. Myoepitheliomas of the skin and soft tissues. Report of 12 cases. Virchows Arch 1999;434:393–400.

11. Huang SC, Chen HW, Zhang L, et al. Novel FUS-KLF17 and EWSR1-KLF17 fusions in myoepithelial tumors. Genes Chromosomes Cancer 2015;54(5):267–75.

12. Jo VY, Antonescu CR, Zhang L, et al. Cutaneous syncytial myoepithelioma: clinicopathologic characterization in a series of 38 cases. Am J Surg Pathol 2013;37:710–8.

13. Brandal P, Panagopoulos I, Bjerkehagen B, et al. Detection of a t(1;22)(q23;q12) translocation leading to an EWSR1-PBX1 fusion gene in a myoepithelioma. Genes Chromosomes Cancer 2008;47:558–64.

14. Brandal P, Panagopoulos I, Bjerkehagen B, et al. t(19;22)(q13;q12) Translocation leading to the novel fusion gene EWSR1-ZNF444 in soft tissue myoepithelial carcinoma. Genes Chromosomes Cancer 2009;48:1051–6.

15. Skalova A, Weinreb I, Hyrcza M, et al. Clear cell myoepithelial carcinoma of salivary glands showing EWSR1 rearrangement: molecular analysis of 94 salivary gland carcinomas with prominent clear cell component. Am J Surg Pathol 2015;39:338–48.

16. Antonescu CR, Zhang L, Shao SY, et al. Frequent PLAG1 gene rearrangements in skin and soft tissue myoepithelioma with ductal differentiation. Genes Chromosomes Cancer 2013;52:675–82.

17. Bahrami A, Dalton JD, Krane JF, et al. A subset of cutaneous and soft tissue mixed tumors are genetically linked to their salivary gland counterpart. Genes Chromosomes Cancer 2012;51:140–8.

18. Matsuyama A, Hisaoka M, Hashimoto H. PLAG1 expression in cutaneous mixed tumors: an immunohistochemical and molecular genetic study. Virchows Arch 2011;459:539–45.

19. Martins C, Fonseca I, Roque L, et al. PLAG1 gene alterations in salivary gland pleomorphic adenoma and carcinoma ex-pleomorphic adenoma: a combined study using chromosome banding, in situ hybridization and immunocytochemistry. Mod Pathol 2005;18:1048–55.

20. Bahrami A, Dalton JD, Shivakumar B, et al. PLAG1 alteration in carcinoma ex pleomorphic adenoma: immunohistochemical and fluorescence in situ hybridization studies of 22 cases. Head Neck Pathol 2012;6:328–35.

21. Thway K, Bown N, Miah A, et al. Rhabdoid variant of myoepithelial carcinoma, with EWSR1 rearrangement: expanding the spectrum of EWSR1-rearranged myoepithelial tumors. Head Neck Pathol 2015;9(2):273–9.

22. Jo VY, Fletcher CD. P63 immunohistochemical staining is limited in soft tissue tumors. Am J Clin Pathol 2011;136:762–6.

23. Rekhi B, Sable M, Jambhekar NA. Histopathological, immunohistochemical and molecular spectrum of myoepithelial tumours of soft tissues. Virchows Arch 2012;461:687–97.

24. Miettinen M, McCue PA, Sarlomo-Rikala M, et al. Sox10-A marker for not only schwannian and melanocytic neoplasms but also myoepithelial cell tumors of soft tissue: a systematic analysis of 5134 tumors. Am J Surg Pathol 2015;39(6):826–35.

25. Hornick JL, Dal Cin P, Fletcher CD. Loss of INI1 expression is characteristic of both conventional and proximal-type epithelioid sarcoma. Am J Surg Pathol 2009;33:542–50.

26. Agaram NP, Chen HW, Zhang L, et al. EWSR1–PBX3: a novel gene fusion in myoepithelial tumors. Genes Chromosomes Cancer 2014;54(2):63–71.

27. Le Loarer F, Zhang L, Fletcher CD, et al. Consistent SMARCB1 homozygous deletions in epithelioid sarcoma and in a subset of myoepithelial carcinomas can be reliably detected by FISH in archival material. Genes Chromosomes Cancer 2014;53:475–86.

28. Flucke U, Tops BB, Verdijk MA, et al. NR4A3 rearrangement reliably distinguishes between the clinicopathologically overlapping entities myoepithelial carcinoma of soft tissue and cellular extraskeletal myxoid chondrosarcoma. Virchows Arch 2012;460:621–8.

29. Gebre-Medhin S, Nord KH, Moller E, et al. Recurrent rearrangement of the PHF1 gene in ossifying fibromyxoid tumors. Am J Pathol 2012;181:1069–77.

30. Graham RP, Weiss SW, Sukov WR, et al. PHF1 rearrangements in ossifying fibromyoxid tumors of soft parts: a fluorescence in situ hybridization study of 41 cases with emphasis on the malignant variant. Am J Surg Pathol 2013;37:1751–5.

31. Biegel JA, Tan L, Zhang F, et al. Alterations of the hSNF5/INI1 gene in central nervous system atypical teratoid/rhabdoid tumors and renal and extrarenal rhabdoid tumors. Clin Cancer Res 2002;8:3461–7.

32. Foo WC, Cruise MW, Wick MR, et al. Immunohistochemical staining for TLE1 distinguishes synovial sarcoma from histologic mimics. Am J Clin Pathol 2011;135:839–44.

33. Hassab-el-Naby HM, Tam S, White WL, et al. Mixed tumors of the skin. A histological and immunohistochemical study. Am J Dermatopathol 1989;11:413–28.

34. Bilal H, Handra-Luca A, Bertrand JC, et al. P63 is expressed in basal and myoepithelial cells of human normal and tumor salivary gland tissues. J Histochem Cytochem 2003;51:133–9.

35. Genelhu MC, Gobbi H, Soares FA, et al. Immunohistochemical expression of p63 in pleomorphic adenomas and carcinomas ex-pleomorphic adenomas of salivary glands. Oral Oncol 2006;42:154–60.

36. Wenig BM, Hitchcock CL, Ellis GL, et al. Metastasizing mixed tumor of salivary glands. A clinicopathologic and flow cytometric analysis. Am J Surg Pathol 1992;16:845–58.

37. Doyle LA, Fletcher CD. EMA positivity in epithelioid fibrous histiocytoma: a potential diagnostic pitfall. J Cutan Pathol 2011;38:697–703.

38. Jedrych J, Nikiforova M, Kennedy TF, et al. Epithelioid cell histiocytoma of the skin with clonal ALK gene rearrangement resulting in VCL-ALK and SQSTM1-ALK gene fusions. Br J Dermatol 2014;172(5):1427–9.

39. Doyle LA, Marino-Enriquez A, Fletcher CD, et al. ALK rearrangement and overexpression in epithelioid fibrous histiocytoma. Mod Pathol 2015;28:904–12.

40. Franchi A, Palomba A, Roselli G, et al. Primary juxtacortical myoepithelioma/mixed tumor of the bone: a report of 3 cases with clinicopathologic, immunohistochemical, ultrastructural, and molecular characterization. Hum Pathol 2013;44:566–77.

41. Cuesta Gil M, Bucci T, Navarro Cuellar C, et al. Intraosseous myoepithelioma of the maxilla: clinicopathologic features and therapeutic considerations. J Oral Maxillofac Surg 2008;66:800–3.

42. de Pinieux G, Beabout JW, Unni KK, et al. Primary mixed tumor of bone. Skeletal Radiol 2001;30:534–6.

43. Ferretti C, Coleman H, Altini M, et al. Intraosseous myoepithelial neoplasms of the maxilla: diagnostic and therapeutic considerations in 5 South African patients. J Oral Maxillofac Surg 2003;61:379–86.

44. Ghermandi R, Pala E, Gambarotti M, et al. Myoepithelioma of the spine: first case in the literature. Eur Rev Med Pharmacol Sci 2014;18:66–71.

45. Park JS, Ryu KN, Han CS, et al. Malignant myoepithelioma of the humerus with a satellite lesion: a case report and literature review. Br J Radiol 2010;83:e161–4.

46. Rekhi B, Amare P, Gulia A, et al. Primary intraosseous myoepithelioma arising in the iliac bone and displaying trisomies of 11, 15, 17 with del (16q) and del (22q11)–A rare case report with review of literature. Pathol Res Pract 2011;207:780–5.

47. Alberghini M, Pasquinelli G, Zanella L, et al. Primary malignant myoepithelioma of the distal femur. APMIS 2007;115:376–80.

48. Fritchie KJ, Bauman MD, Durward QJ. Myoepithelioma of the skull: a case report. Neurosurgery 2012;71:E901–4.

49. Tirabosco R, Mangham DC, Rosenberg AE, et al. Brachyury expression in extra-axial skeletal and soft tissue chordomas: a marker that distinguishes chordoma from mixed tumor/myoepithelioma/parachordoma in soft tissue. Am J Surg Pathol 2008;32:572–80.

50. Amary MF, Bacsi K, Maggiani F, et al. IDH1 and IDH2 mutations are frequent events in central chondrosarcoma and central and periosteal chondromas but not in other mesenchymal tumours. J Pathol 2011;224:334–43.

The New Kids on the Block
Recently Characterized Soft Tissue Tumors

Nicole N. Riddle, MD[a], Jerad M. Gardner, MD[b,c],*

KEYWORDS

• Soft tissue pathology • Sarcoma • Molecular • Liposarcoma • ALK

ABSTRACT

Soft tissue pathology is a rapidly changing subspecialty. New entities are described relatively often, and new molecular findings for soft tissue tumors are reported in the literature almost every month. This article summarizes the major features and diagnostic approach to several recently characterized entities: superficial CD34-positive fibroblastic tumor, fibrosarcoma-like lipomatous neoplasm, angiofibroma of soft tissue, low-grade sinonasal sarcoma with neural and myogenic features, malignant gastrointestinal neuroectodermal tumor, hemosiderotic fibrolipomatous tumor, and epithelioid inflammatory myofibroblastic sarcoma. Additionally, the article also provides a summary table of recent molecular findings in soft tissue tumors.

OVERVIEW

Soft tissue pathology is a rapidly changing subspecialty. Novel molecular findings are published monthly, rivaling even hematopathology in the speed with which the genetic underpinnings of neoplasia are probed. Tumors that were previously known under one rubric are reclassified with relative frequency. Lesions that for decades were thought to be reactive now are discovered to possess gene rearrangements (e.g. – nodular fasciitis), and the features of previously unknown or incompletely described tumors are coalesced and synthesized into new entities. The relative rarity of soft tissue tumors only adds to the challenge of keeping abreast of all of these advances. In this article, we attempt to highlight some of the more pertinent soft tissue tumors that have been recently characterized and to make them more accessible to the general surgical pathologist. We also provide a brief summary of significant molecular findings, not only in these newly described tumors, but also in older entities for which molecular abnormalities have only recently been elucidated.

SUPERFICIAL CD34-POSITIVE FIBROBLASTIC TUMOR

Carter and colleagues[1] characterized superficial CD34-positive fibroblastic tumor in 2013. They described 18 cases of a tumor with unique characteristics: striking nuclear pleomorphism, paradoxically rare mitotic activity, indolent behavior, and diffuse CD34 expression. All cases occurred in adults and all presented as a slow-growing supra-fascial mass of 10 cm or less (mean: 4.1 cm), most commonly in the lower extremity. Awareness of this entity is important, as there is a tendency for overdiagnosis as a pleomorphic sarcoma in light of the nuclear atypia, even though most cases do not recur or metastasize. Of 13 patients with follow-up (median: 24 months), there were no local recurrences, no distant metastases, and no death from disease; 1 patient had a regional lymph node metastasis 7 years after presentation. In light of this, Carter and colleagues[1] suggested this entity be considered as a lesion of borderline malignancy.

[a] Department of Pathology, University of Texas Health Science Center San Antonio, 7703 Floyd Curl Drive, MC7750, San Antonio, TX 78229, USA; [b] Department of Pathology, University of Arkansas for Medical Sciences, 4301 West Markham Street #517, Room S4/11, Little Rock, AR 72205, USA; [c] Department of Dermatology, University of Arkansas for Medical Sciences, 4301 West Markham Street #517, Room S4/11, Little Rock, AR 72205, USA

* Corresponding author. University of Arkansas for Medical Sciences, 4301 West Markham Street #517, Room S4/11, Little Rock, AR 72205.

E-mail address: JMGardnerMD@gmail.com

Surgical Pathology 8 (2015) 467–491
http://dx.doi.org/10.1016/j.path.2015.05.003
1875-9181/15/$ – see front matter © 2015 Elsevier Inc. All rights reserved.

PATHOLOGIC FEATURES

Superficial CD34-positive fibroblastic tumor is a subcutaneous mass with little or no involvement of the deep musculature. It is often relatively circumscribed, although it may show peripheral infiltrative growth. Most tumor cells display marked nuclear pleomorphism with hyperchromasia and multiple large inclusion-like nucleoli as well as cytoplasmic nuclear pseudoinclusions. The cells are spindled to epithelioid with abundant eosinophilic often granular cytoplasm and are arranged into hypercellular sheets or fascicles (Fig. 1A, B). Xanthomatous foamy tumor cells are commonly seen, and mixed inflammation is often present. Small vessels are arranged in a plexiform pattern in the background of the tumor, but large ectatic hyalinized vessels, like those of pleomorphic hyalinizing angiectactic tumor (PHAT), are not seen. Despite the extreme degree of nuclear atypia, mitotic figures

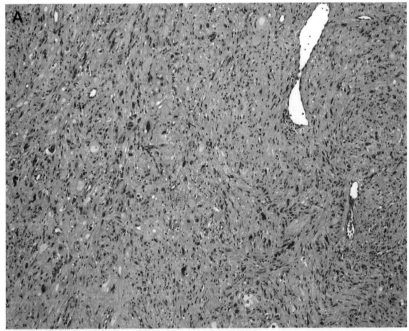

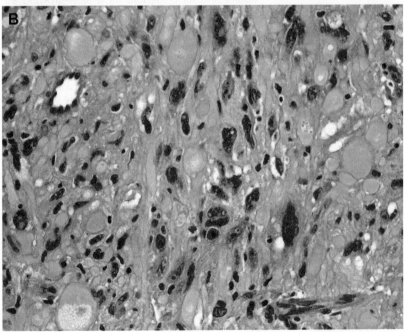

Fig. 1. (A) Superficial CD34-positive fibroblastic tumor is composed of sheets of pleomorphic spindle cells. (B) Superficial CD34-positive fibroblastic tumor: there is marked nuclear pleomorphism but mitoses are rare. Tumor cells display abundant eosinophilic cytoplasm.

Fig. 1. (continued). (C) Diffuse strong CD34 expression in tumor cells is a defining feature of superficial CD34-positive fibroblastic tumor. (D) Focal cytokeratin expression is present in most superficial CD34-positive fibroblastic tumors. (Courtesy of [A, B] Dr Scott Lauer, Omaha, NE; and [C, D] Dr Andrew Folpe, Rochester, MN.)

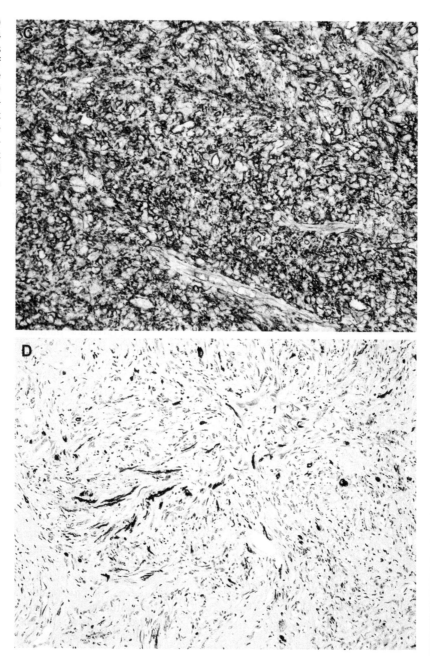

are very rare (<1/50 high-power fields [HPFs]) in most cases, and atypical forms are absent. Focal necrosis has been reported in only 1 case.[1]

By immunohistochemistry, this entity is diffusely and strongly positive for CD34 in all cases (see Fig. 1C). Most (69%) cases also display focal cytokeratin expression (see Fig. 1D). FLI-1, ERG, S100 protein, desmin, smooth muscle actin, and TP53 are all negative, Ki-67 proliferative index is less than 1%, and nuclear INI-1 (SMARCB1) expression is retained. Cases tested by fluorescence in situ hybridization (FISH) for TGFBR3 and/or MGEA5 rearrangements have all been negative.[1]

DIFFERENTIAL DIAGNOSIS

This entity may be easily confused with undifferentiated pleomorphic sarcoma (formerly "malignant fibrous histiocytoma"), myxofibrosarcoma, or atypical fibroxanthoma (AFX) because of the striking nuclear pleomorphism. Yet both the diffuse CD34 expression and the very low mitotic rate of superficial CD34-positive fibroblastic tumor would be distinctly unusual for those entities. Furthermore, AFX usually occurs in sun-exposed sites, such as the head and neck, rather than the lower extremity. Myxoinflammatory fibroblastic sarcoma (MIFS) has bizarre pleomorphism, large inclusion-like nucleoli, and relatively low mitotic activity, all features similar to superficial CD34-positive fibroblastic tumor. But in contrast, most MIFS occur in acral sites, lack diffuse CD34 expression, possess more abundant myxoid background, and display rearrangements of *TGFBR3* and/or *MGEA5* genes.[2] PHAT is also in the differential diagnosis, as it has marked nuclear pleomorphism but low mitotic activity, but the characteristic ectatic hyalinized blood vessels and abundant hemosiderin deposition that typify PHAT are lacking in superficial CD34-positive fibroblastic tumor. Other entities potentially in the differential, such as intermediate or malignant vascular tumors, epithelioid sarcoma, or malignant granular cell tumor can usually be easily excluded by immunohistochemistry.[1]

Key Pathologic Features

1. Supra-fascial mass, less than 10 cm

2. Striking pleomorphism but low mitotic rate (<1 per 50 HPFs)

3. Diffuse strong CD34 expression (always), focal cytokeratin expression (often)

Main Differential Diagnosis

1. Undifferentiated pleomorphic sarcoma

2. Myxofibrosarcoma

3. Atypical fibroxanthoma

4. Myxoinflammatory fibroblastic sarcoma

5. Pleomorphic hyalinizing angiectactic tumor

Pitfalls

! Marked pleomorphism mimics high-grade pleomorphic sarcomas

! CD34 and cytokeratin expression could lead to confusion with vascular and/or epithelial tumors

---

FIBROSARCOMA-LIKE LIPOMATOUS NEOPLASM

In 2013, Deyrup and colleagues[3] revisited the concept of "spindle cell liposarcoma," a term that in their opinion actually represents a heterogeneous group of tumors, including variants of well-differentiated liposarcoma, myxoid liposarcoma, and even spindle cell lipoma based on their analysis of previous publications on this topic. After excluding those entities by molecular analysis, they describe 12 cases of what they propose to represent a distinct group of low-grade adipocytic neoplasm with prominent spindle cell component that they termed "fibrosarcoma-like lipomatous neoplasm" in light of a tendency for parallel fascicular arrangement of the spindle cells. Most of these tumors arose in adults (mean age: 50 years), although 2 cases were in adolescents. They presented as superficial or deep soft tissue masses with a wide size range (mean: 7.5 cm) arising in the groin and paratesticular region, as well as the buttock, thigh, flank, and shoulder. No recurrence or metastasis was identified in any of these patients (mean follow-up time: 68 months), suggesting that perhaps "liposarcoma" is not an appropriate term for this tumor, based on current data.

PATHOLOGIC FEATURES

Fibrosarcoma-like lipomatous neoplasm is a vaguely multinodular tumor with variable cellularity (**Fig.** 2A). It is composed of relatively uniform fibroblast-like spindle cells arranged parallel to one another in a myxoid background with an arborizing capillary vasculature (see **Fig.** 2B, C). The characteristic finding is the presence of a wide range of adipocytic differentiation apparently recapitulating the various embryologic steps of fat development (see **Fig.** 2D). This includes preadipocyte-like cells that resemble bland fibroblasts with no obvious lipid droplet, as well as more differentiated spindle cells that display minute cytoplasmic lipid droplets. In some of these, the lipid droplets are larger and indent the nucleus, forming univacuolated ("ice cream cone") and bivacuolated ("hourglass") spindled lipoblasts (see **Fig.** 2E). Signet ring lipoblasts, similar to those of myxoid liposarcoma, also may be present. Variable amounts of these different lipoblasts are present in each case.[3] These lipoblasts have bland and uniform nuclei without significant atypia; pleomorphic lipoblasts are not seen.

DIFFERENTIAL DIAGNOSIS

The major differential diagnoses are well-differentiated liposarcoma/atypical lipomatous

Fig. 2. (*A*) Fibrosarcoma-like lipomatous neoplasm is a multinodular tumor with variable cellularity. (*B*) Fibrosarcoma-like lipomatous neoplasm is composed of relatively uniform fibroblast-like spindle cells in a myxoid background with an arborizing capillary vasculature. (*C*) The fibroblast-like spindle cells are often arranged parallel to one another in fibrosarcoma-like lipomatous neoplasm.

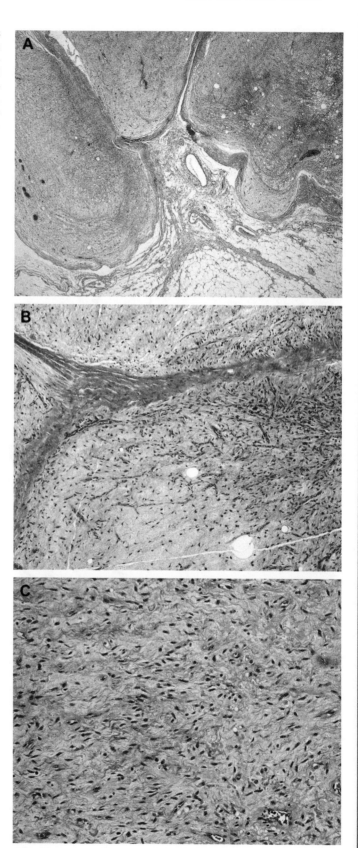

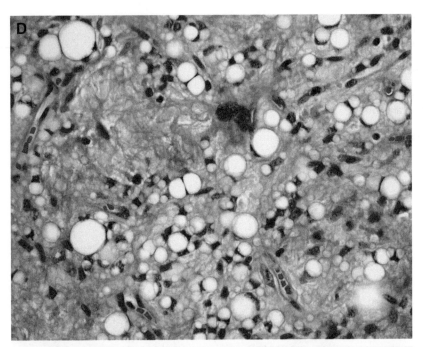

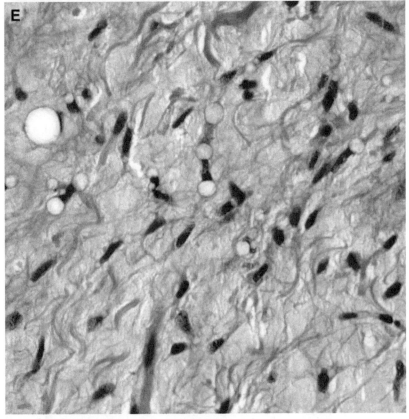

Fig. 2. (continued). (D) The characteristic finding in fibrosarcoma-like lipomatous neoplasm is the presence of a wide range of adipocytic differentiation recapitulating the various embryologic steps of fat development. *(E)* Univacuolated ("ice cream cone") and bivacuolated ("hourglass") spindled lipoblasts are often seen in fibrosarcoma-like lipomatous neoplasm.

tumor (WDL/ALT), myxoid liposarcoma, and spindle cell lipoma. Fibrosarcoma-like lipomatous neoplasm certainly may have overlapping morphologic features with all of these entities. Fortunately, molecular analysis can usually easily exclude these possibilities. WDL/ALT possesses amplification of 12q13-15, including the *MDM2* and *CDK4* genes. Myxoid liposarcoma has characteristic translocations resulting in rearrangement of *DDIT3*. Spindle cell lipoma displays uniform loss of chromosome 13 and frequent losses of chromosomes 16 and 6. FISH or other molecular techniques can detect these molecular signatures. In contrast, fibrosarcoma-like lipomatous neoplasm is negative for all of these molecular abnormalities and also displays a flat profile on array comparative genomic hybridization analysis with no identifiable chromosomal gains or losses.[3]

Key Pathologic Features

1. Uniform fibroblast-like spindle cells arranged in parallel

2. Myxoid background with arborizing thin vessels

3. Wide range of lipoblasts, including signet ring and spindled univacuolated/bivacuolated cells

Main Differential Diagnosis

1. Well-differentiated liposarcoma/atypical lipomatous tumor (WDL/ALT)

2. Myxoid liposarcoma

3. Spindle cell lipoma

Pitfalls

! Can be easily confused histologically with more aggressive entities (myxoid or well-differentiated liposarcomas)

! Literature regarding "spindle cell liposarcoma" can be confusing, as a variety of different tumors have been described under the same rubric

ANGIOFIBROMA OF SOFT TISSUE

Several entities are referred to as "angiofibroma" in pathology: nasopharyngeal angiofibroma, which typically occurs in the nasal cavity of adolescent males; cellular angiofibroma, which occurs in the genital region and is likely a close relative of spindle cell lipoma; and angiofibroma of the skin, which can either occur as solitary facial lesions in older adults (fibrous papule) or as multiple facial lesions in young patients with tuberous sclerosis (so-called by the misnomer "adenoma sebaceum"). In 2012, Mariño-Enríquez and Fletcher[4] described 37 cases of a previously undescribed soft tissue tumor composed of bland spindle cells and abundant branched vessels that they termed "angiofibroma of soft tissue." The tumors they described are clearly quite distinct histologically and molecularly from these other types of angiofibroma, and are also unlike any other previously described soft tissue tumor. Several additional case reports and small series published since their initial description further support that this lesion is a new and distinct entity.[5–8] Angiofibroma of soft tissue is a slow-growing tumor of the subcutis or deep soft tissue most commonly arising in the extremities (lower > upper) of adults, or, less frequently, children/adolescents. There is a roughly 2:1 female predominance. Most are well-circumscribed lesions with a median size of 3.5 cm (range: 1.2–12.0 cm). Although the histologic features of this tumor, particularly the prominent branching vessels, may lead to diagnostic confusion with several forms of sarcoma, angiofibroma of soft tissue is a benign neoplasm that may occasionally recur locally (14%) but does not metastasize.[4]

PATHOLOGIC FEATURES

Angiofibroma of soft tissue is composed of small spindle cells with bland uniform nuclei. These are set in a variably myxoid and collagenous background that displays numerous small branching blood vessels (**Fig.** 3A–C). The vascular pattern bears some resemblance to that of myxoid liposarcoma, except that in angiofibroma of soft tissue, the vessels are much more numerous and not as thin and delicate as in myxoid liposarcoma (see **Fig.** 3D, E). Lesser numbers of larger vessels are also present, often with ectatic, staghorn, hemangiopericytoma-like appearance. The tumor cells lack significant cytologic atypia, and mitoses are usually infrequent (<1 per 10 HPFs), although in a minority of cases may be more prominent (up to 4 per 10 HPFs); atypical mitoses are absent. Focal degenerative changes are occasionally seen, including ischemic necrosis, edema, or mild degenerative atypia.[4]

On immunohistochemistry, epithelial membrane antigen (EMA) is positive in nearly half of cases, usually only in scattered cells but rarely diffusely. Focal staining for desmin, smooth muscle actin (SMA), or CD34 may be seen in a subset of cases, but S100 protein is negative.[4] Angiofibroma of soft tissue has a unique molecular signature: t(5;8)

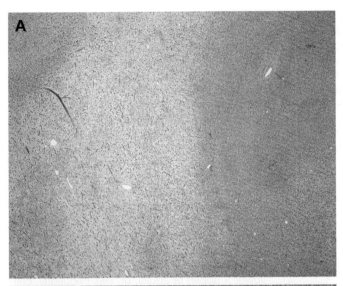

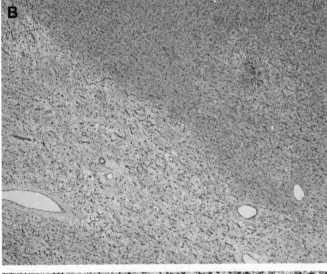

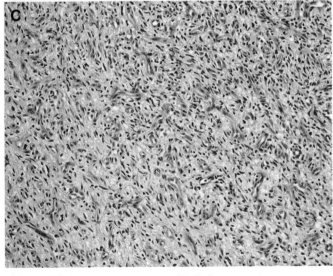

Fig. 3. (A) Angiofibroma of soft tissue displays a variably myxoid and collagenous background as well as variable cellularity. The numerous small branching vessels are visible even from low magnification. (B) More cellular collagenous areas are seen in the upper right of this image of angiofibroma of soft tissue, whereas the bottom left displays less cellularity and a more myxoid and edematous background. Most of the numerous vessels are small and plexiform, although occasional larger ectatic hemangiopericytoma-like vessels are also present. (C) The spindle cells in angiofibroma of soft tissue have small bland uniform nuclei. There is minimal cytologic atypia, and mitoses are usually infrequent.

Fig. 3. (continued). (*D*) The thin branching vessels, intervening small uniform spindle cells, and myxoid background in some areas of angiofibroma of soft tissue may bear some resemblance to myxoid liposarcoma. (*E*) Although their vascular patterns are similar, in angiofibroma of soft tissue the vessels are usually much more numerous and not quite as thin and delicate as in myxoid liposarcoma. (*Courtesy of* Dr Scott Lauer, Omaha, NE.)

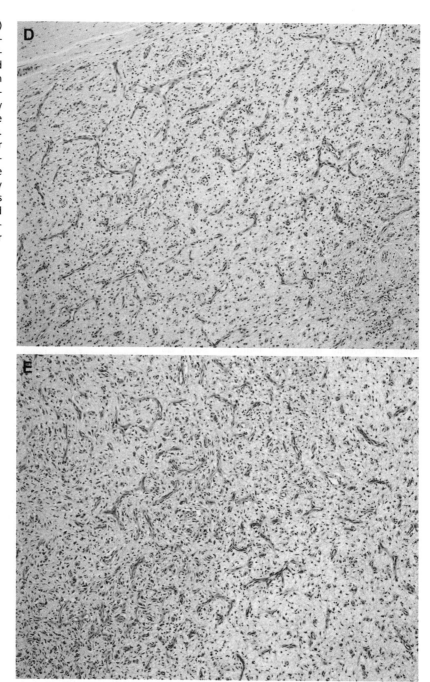

(p15;q13), resulting in fusion of the genes *AHRR* and *NCOA2*. This translocation can be detected by conventional cytogenetic karyotyping, reverse-transcriptase polymerase chain reaction (RT-PCR), or break-apart FISH.[4,5,8,9]

DIFFERENTIAL DIAGNOSIS

The differential diagnosis most notably includes myxoid liposarcoma, low-grade fibromyxoid sarcoma (LGFMS), solitary fibrous tumor (SFT), low-grade myxofibrosarcoma, and cellular angiofibroma. Myxoid liposarcoma is perhaps the most important of these in light of the relative similarity in the vascular pattern of both tumors and the vastly different treatment and prognosis. As mentioned previously, the vessels of myxoid liposarcoma are much more thin and delicate and fewer in number than those of angiofibroma of soft tissue. Furthermore, myxoid liposarcoma has characteristic translocations, resulting in rearrangement of *DDIT3*. LGFMS enters the differential because it also possesses bland spindle cells set in a variably myxoid and collagenous background, but LGFMS lacks the prominent plexiform vascular pattern seen in angiofibroma of soft tissue. Additionally, LGFMS usually expresses the relatively specific immunohistochemical marker MUC4 and also has characteristic translocations resulting in fusions of *FUS* and either *CREB3L1* or *CREB3L2*.[10] SFT has several overlapping histologic features with angiofibroma of soft tissue. Although both entities often possess ectatic staghorn vessels, these are more frequent in SFT and not typically accompanied by numerous thin branching vessels. SFT usually displays strong diffuse CD34 expression, nuclear STAT6 expression, and recurrent *NAB2-STAT6* gene fusions.[5,11] Low-grade myxofibrosarcoma has a myxoid background but usually with long curvilinear vessels rather than abundant plexiform vessels; it also differs from angiofibroma of soft tissue by the presence of overtly malignant features, such as prominent nuclear pleomorphism and mitotic activity. Cellular angiofibroma is similar in name, but unlike angiofibroma of soft tissue, it occurs mostly in the genital region, has thicker vessels with less branching, and has histologic and molecular features similar to spindle cell lipoma.[4,8]

Key Pathologic Features

1. Bland uniform spindle cells with minimal atypia
2. Variably myxoid and collagenous background
3. Numerous branching thin-walled blood vessels
4. t(5;8) *AHRR-NCOA2* gene fusion

Main Differential Diagnosis

1. Myxoid liposarcoma
2. Low-grade fibromyxoid sarcoma
3. Solitary fibrous tumor
4. Low-grade myxofibrosarcoma
5. Cellular angiofibroma

Pitfall

! Can be confused with several other more aggressive soft tissue neoplasms

LOW-GRADE SINONASAL SARCOMA WITH NEURAL AND MYOGENIC FEATURES

Low-grade sinonasal sarcoma with neural and myogenic features (LGSSNMF), also known as biphenotypic sinonasal sarcoma, is a recently described entity based on review of sinonasal sarcomas from several decades of cases and consults.[12,13] Sinonasal sarcomas in general are very rare and oftentimes these lesions were believed to be examples of known entities (fibrosarcoma, malignant peripheral nerve sheath tumor [MPNST], synovial sarcoma). However, these cases were found to all have similar characteristic histology, along with evidence of neural and myogenic differentiation.

The clinical presentation is similar to other sinonasal neoplasms and includes general features of sinusitis: difficulty breathing, facial pressure, congestion, and, rarely, facial pain. The age range is 24 to 85 years (mean: 52 years), and there is female predominance in the original series (21 women, 7 men). The lesion most commonly affects multiple sites, including the nasal cavity proper (54%) and ethmoid sinus (57%); extension into the orbit (25%) and cribriform plate (11%) were not uncommon. One tumor extended into the cranial vault. Local recurrence is common, but metastases or mortality from disease have not yet been reported.[12]

PATHOLOGIC FEATURES

Lewis and colleagues[12] defined the inclusion criteria as highly cellular, infiltrative spindle cell neoplasm with uniform, elongated nuclei and at least focal S100 positivity. Specimens are typically received as multiple polypoid tan/red fragments measuring up to 4 cm in greatest dimension, possibly more firm than the typical inflammatory nasal polyp, but otherwise with no distinctive features. The histologic features demonstrate a poorly circumscribed, infiltrative, cellular neoplasm composed of bland spindle cells often arranged in short fascicles reminiscent of a "herringbone" pattern (**Fig. 4**A–D). Wavy or buckled nuclei are often identified (see **Fig. 4**E). No significant atypia is present; however, a minority of tumors will show focal rhabdomyoblastic-type cells with larger hyperchromatic nuclei and abundant eosinophilic

Fig. 4. (*A*) LGSSNMF is a cellular spindle cell proliferation in the nasal submucosa. (*B*) LGSSNMF is composed of bland spindle cells arranged in hypercellular fascicles. (*C*) The hypercellular fascicles in LGSSNMF often display an intersecting herringbone pattern, a finding that may cause confusion with synovial sarcoma or malignant peripheral nerve sheath tumor.

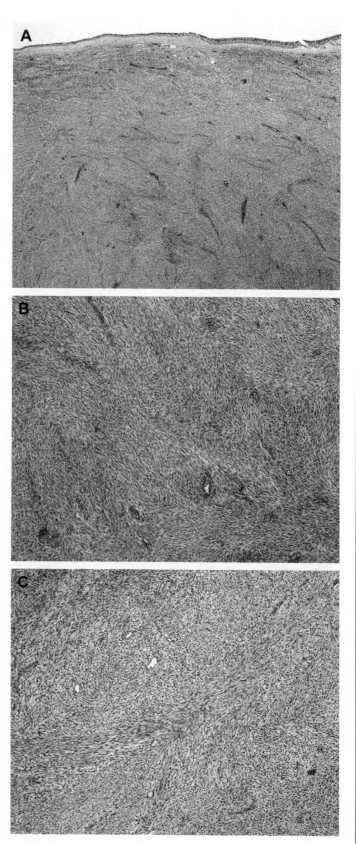

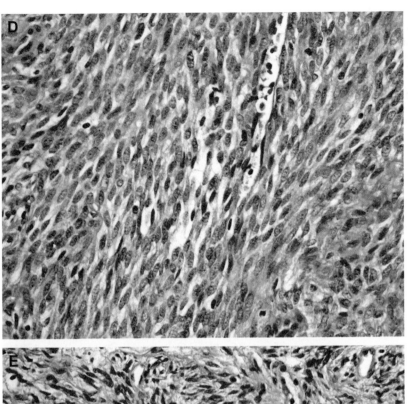

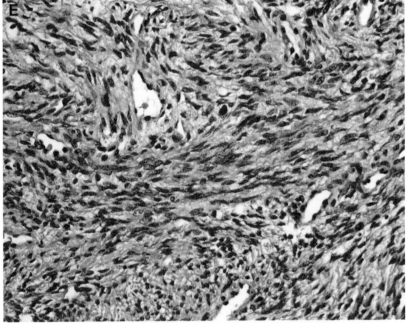

Fig. 4. (continued). (D) The spindle cells of LGSSNMF are bland and uniform with minimal atypia. Mitoses are infrequent. (E) Wavy or buckled nuclei are often identified in LGSSNMF, imparting a neural appearance. (Courtesy of [A–D] Dr Scott Lauer, Omaha, NE; and [E] Dr Raul Gonzalez, Rochester, NY.)

cytoplasm. Mitoses are infrequent. Vessels are typically not prominent; however, a minority of cases may show areas of hemangiopericytic-patterned vasculature. No dense or ropey collagen is present, with the intercellular collagen being scanty to moderate and arranged in delicate strands. A characteristic finding present in most cases is a benign proliferation of the surface respiratory epithelium leading to invaginations of small glands or cystic spaces. These glandular structures are often admixed among the tumor cells and impart a histologic image similar to adenosarcoma of the female genital tract. It is important to be aware of this associated proliferation, as shallow biopsies may be misdiagnosed as inverted papilloma.

The immunohistochemical features are characteristic in that they have S100 positivity in addition to SMA and/or muscle-specific actin (MSA). The staining of S100 and muscle markers is often diffuse, but sometime patchy or only in isolated tumor cells. Other stains that may be rarely focally positive are CD34, desmin, EMA, and cytokeratin AE1/3. No estrogen receptor (ER), progesterone receptor (PR), or myogenin staining is seen. A recent study by Wang and colleagues[13] found *PAX3* rearrangement by FISH in 96% of LGSSNMF (n = 25); 79% of these cases were positive for *PAX3-MAML3* fusion by RT-PCR.[12]

Of note, one recently reported case showed only focal SMA and MSA, but did have staining for caldesmon and β-catenin, and the electron microscopy findings were also different.[14] The investigators raised the possibility that maybe the tumor has fibroblastic differentiation instead of myogenic differentiation. Given that the first series did not perform β-catenin and the later series did not do molecular studies, it is possible that these represent tumors with variable myofibroblastic differentiation on a spectrum or possibly 2 different tumor types.

DIFFERENTIAL DIAGNOSIS

The histologic differential diagnosis for LGSSNMF includes mainly fibrosarcoma, MPNST, and monophasic synovial sarcoma, and possibly glomangiopericytoma, SFT, and cellular schwannoma. Indeed, many of these cases have probably been reported as such in the past. In general, immunohistochemistry should be helpful in distinguishing these lesions. However, given the potentially focal/patchy nature of both S100 and muscle markers, conceivably a small biopsy could lack one or both markers, leading to an incorrect diagnosis. The rare and focal cytokeratin staining may lead one to think of synovial sarcoma, but all LGSSNMF tested have been negative for *SS18 (SYT)* translocations, so FISH would prove helpful in this differential.[12]

Key Pathologic Features

1. Poorly circumscribed, infiltrative

2. Highly cellular, bland spindle cells, in vague "herringbone" pattern, without atypia or frequent mitoses

3. Positivity for S100 and muscle markers (SMA, MSA)

4. Benign proliferation of respiratory epithelium with variable admixture with tumor cells

5. Rarely: rhabdomyoblastic differentiation, hemangiopericytic vascular pattern

Main Differential Diagnosis

1. Fibrosarcoma

2. Malignant peripheral nerve sheath tumor

3. Synovial sarcoma, monophasic-type

Pitfalls

! Patchy immunohistochemical staining for S100 and actins, which may not be present on small biopsies

! Overlying epithelial proliferation may lead to misdiagnosis as inverted papilloma

! Focal cytokeratin expression may lead to misdiagnosis as monophasic synovial sarcoma

MALIGNANT GASTROINTESTINAL NEUROECTODERMAL TUMOR

Malignant gastrointestinal neuroectodermal tumor (GNET) is a rare, aggressive tumor of the gastrointestinal (GI) tract that has previously been referred to as "clear cell sarcoma-like tumor of the GI tract with osteoclast-like giant cells."[15–19] The name was proposed by Stockman and colleagues[15] after a review of 16 cases showed histologic features, immunohistochemical pattern, and molecular findings similar to clear cell sarcoma of soft tissue, but with distinct differences, including no evidence of melanocytic differentiation.[20]

GNET has an equal male/female distribution with an age range of 17 to 77 years (mean, 42 years). Patients often present with abdominal pain, intestinal obstruction, or an abdominal mass, with anorexia, anemia, weight loss, high-grade fever, and weakness also reported. Tumors are more common in the small bowel, but also may occur in the stomach and colon. If the tumor can be completely removed, the prognosis may be good; however, metastases are common (over 50%), often to liver and lymph nodes. In the Stockman and colleagues[15] series, 50% of patients died of disease (most within 2–3 years), and most remaining living patients had regional and liver metastasis.

PATHOLOGIC FEATURES

Grossly, the lesions range in size from 2 to 15 cm (mean, 5.2 cm; median, 3.8 cm) and are firm, solid, tan-white lobulated masses with focal areas of hemorrhage and necrosis. Lesions are based primarily in the submucosa and muscularis propria and may grow in an exophytic fashion protruding into the bowel lumen, circumferentially mimicking carcinoma, or transmurally with overlying mucosal ulceration (Fig. 5A).[15]

Histologically, the lesion consists of diffuse sheets or nests of uniform, predominately epithelioid/polygonal cells with variable amounts of eosinophilic to clear cytoplasm (see Fig. 5B–D). Scattered oval-to-spindle cells are variably seen. The nuclei are vesicular with marginated chromatin, indistinct to small nucleoli and scattered intranuclear cytoplasmic inclusions (see Fig. 5E). Mitoses vary from 0 to 20 per 10 HPFs (mean, 6 per 10 HPFs). Focal pseudoalveolar, pseudopapillary, microcystic, fascicular, or cord-like patterns may be seen.[15]

Immunohistochemically, the tumors appear to be uniformly positive for S100, SOX10, and vimentin. S100 positivity is typically strong and diffuse, although rarely may be focal. Neuroendocrine markers are variably present (CD56, 70%; synaptophysin, 56%; NB84, 50%; NSE, 45%; and neurofilament, 14%). Notably, the melanocytic markers (HMB-45, melan A, tyrosinase, and MiTF) and GI stromal tumor (GIST) markers (DOG1, CD34, and CD117) are all negative. Other negative markers are glial fibrillary acidic protein, desmin, SMA, CD99, and NeuN, and epithelial markers (very rare cases may show focal CAM5.2 positivity). Ki-67 is often 20% to 30%.[15]

FISH analysis will be positive for *EWSR1* break apart in 86% of cases. The fusion genes are typically *CREB1* or *ATF1*. These translocations are not unique and may be seen in clear cell sarcoma of soft tissue and angiomatoid fibrous histiocytoma. *FUS* rearrangements are not present in GNET.[15]

DIFFERENTIAL DIAGNOSIS

The histologic differential diagnosis for GNET includes GIST, monophasic synovial sarcoma, melanoma, soft tissue clear cell sarcoma involving the GI tract, and, rarely, variants of perivascular epithelioid cell tumor (PEComa) and epithelioid MPNST. It is important to distinguish GNET from these entities, as treatment and prognosis may be quite different. A thorough immunohistochemical and/or molecular workup can usually sort these out (see Main Differential Diagnosis box).

Key Pathologic Features

1. Epithelioid/polygonal cells with variable amount of eosinophilic cytoplasm

2. Vesicular nuclei with chromatin margination and scattered intranuclear cytoplasmic inclusions

3. S100, SOX10, and neuroendocrine markers positive, but specific melanocytic markers negative

4. *EWSR1* translocation

Main Differential Diagnosis

	S100	SOX10	MART1/HMB-45	Actin/Desmin	CK/EMA	CD117	DOG1	*EWSR1*[a]	*SS18*[a]
GNET	+	+	−	−	−	−	−	+	−
CCS	+	+	+	−	−	−	−	+	−
Melanoma	+	+	+	−	−	+/−	−	−	−
GIST	−	−	−	−	−	+	+	−	−
SS[21]	+/−	−	−	−	+	−	−	−	+
PEComa[22,23]	+/−	−	+	+	−	−	−	−	−
E-MPNST	+	+	−	−	−	−	−	−	−

Note: This table shows typical immunophenotype and molecular profile for these entities; exceptions exist.

Abbreviations: +, usually positive; −, usually negative; +/−, sometimes positive; CCS, soft tissue clear cell sarcoma involving GI tract; E-MPNST, epithelioid malignant peripheral nerve sheath tumor; GIST, gastrointestinal stromal tumor; GNET, gastrointestinal neuroectodermal tumor; PEComa, perivascular epithelioid cell tumor; SS, monophasic synovial sarcoma.

[a] By break-apart FISH.

Fig. 5. (*A*) Malignant GNET is usually based primarily in the submucosa and muscularis propria and may grow in an exophytic fashion with overlying mucosal ulceration, as seen in this case. (*B*) GNET is composed of tumor cells arranged in sheets or nests that are sometimes divided by dense fibrous bands. (*C*) This example of GNET displays trabeculae of uniform eosinophilic cells with intervening dense fibrosis. The pattern is similar to that of clear cell sarcoma of soft tissue.

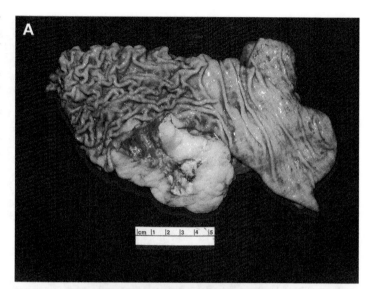

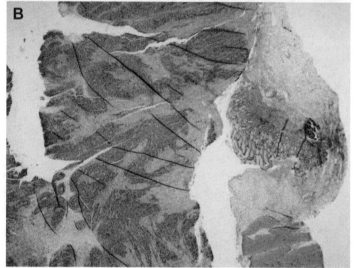

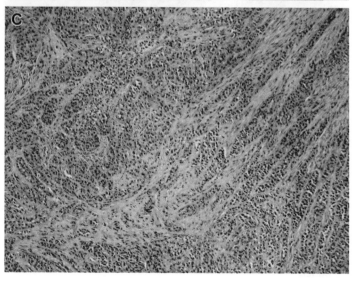

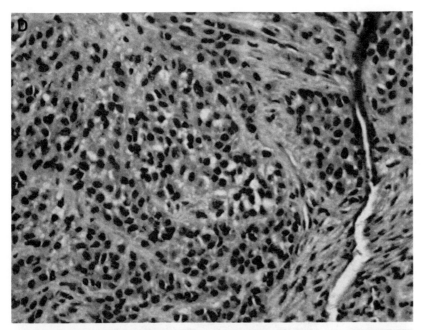

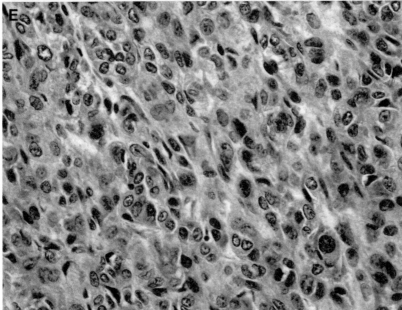

Fig. 5. (continued). (*D*) GNET is composed of uniform epithelioid cells with variable amounts of clear or eosinophilic cytoplasm. (*E*) Tumor nuclei in GNET are vesicular with marginated chromatin and indistinct to small nucleoli. (*Courtesy of* [*A, E*] Dr Rhonda Yantiss, New York, NY; and [*B–D*] Dr Raul Gonzalez, Rochester, NY.)

 Pitfalls

! Similar histology and chromosomal aberration as clear cell sarcoma of soft tissue; differs by absence of melanocytic marker expression, such as MART-1 and HMB-45 in GNET.

! GIST, a much more common GI tract tumor with more pathologist awareness, may have similar histologic appearance to GNET; misdiagnosis can be avoided by using a simple immunohistochemical panel.

HEMOSIDEROTIC FIBROLIPOMATOUS TUMOR

First described in 2000, hemosiderotic fibrolipomatous tumor (HFLT) was originally believed to be a reactive process.[24] However, recent studies have shown a consistent t(1;10) abnormality and reports have been made of cases transforming into myxoinflammatory fibroblastic sarcoma (MIFS), as well as PHAT,[25] thus confirming the neoplastic nature of this lesion.[2,26–28]

HFLT is a slow-growing, but locally aggressive lesion with a striking predilection for the foot/ankle region of middle-aged adults. However, reported ages range from 8 months to 74 years and locations have included the thigh, hand, and cheek. Local recurrence is common if HFLT is not fully removed. The initial series of patients had a high incidence of previous trauma leading to the belief that these were reactive lesions. But further reports have not shown a connection to previous trauma and indeed have supported occasional true malignant transformation.[25,28–31]

PATHOLOGIC FEATURES

HFLT is grossly fatty/gelatinous and ranges in size from 1 to 19 cm. Histologically, it is an unencapsulated lesion with varying proportions of mature adipocytes with admixed fibroblastic spindle cells (Fig. 6A). A consistent feature is variable amounts of hemosiderin deposition, predominantly within macrophages in the spindled component, but also in the spindled cells proper. The spindle cell component often has a streaming, swirling, or honeycomb pattern and scattered osteoclast-like giant cells are common (see Fig. 6B–D). A lymphoplasmacytic inflammatory component is scattered throughout the lesion with occasional mast cells or eosinophils. Mitoses, atypia, and necrosis are rarely seen. Immunohistochemistry is not specific and includes positivity for CD34 and calponin and negativity for SMA, desmin, CD68, S100, and keratins.[32]

As referenced previously, several studies have shown translocations involving *TGFBR3* and *MGEA5* genes, a molecular signature shared with some cases of both PHAT and MIFS.[2,25,27] HFLT appears to be a precursor lesion to PHAT, with many cases of PHAT having HFLT areas around the periphery.[25,28] However, these areas of HFLT are very infrequently seen in association with classic MIFS.[25,28] Rare cases of HFLT recurring as MIFS have been reported.[30,31] In light of these findings, one proposal is that these entities might be grouped into the "*TGFBR3-MGEA5* family of tumors."[25,28] Recent work by Zreik and colleagues[25] (presented at the United States and Canadian Academy of Pathology [USCAP] Annual Meeting 2015 but not yet published) suggests that hybrid HFLT/MIFS lesions do not actually show classic features of MIFS and thus might be better regarded as "HFLT showing progression to myxoid sarcoma" rather than progression to bona fide MIFS; thus, they suggest that MIFS is likely unrelated to HFLT and PHAT. As evidenced by multiple presentations on this topic at the recent USCAP 2015 annual meeting in Boston, the relationship between HFLT, PHAT, and MIFS is a clearly a matter of ongoing debate and investigation.

DIFFERENTIAL DIAGNOSIS

Based on the morphologic features and typical location, the differential for HFLT includes primarily plexiform fibrohistiocytic tumor, atypical lipomatous tumor, spindle cell lipoma, and giant cell tumor of soft tissue. In children, the differential would include lipofibromatosis and fibrous hamartoma of infancy, although this location would be uncommon for the latter. And in cases with minimal fat component, nodular fasciitis and fibrous histiocytoma may be a consideration. The presence of both hemosiderin deposition and admixed adipose tissue in HFLT would be unusual for most of these entities, but the distinction can sometimes be challenging, particularly on small biopsies.

Key Pathologic Features

1. Fascicles of fibroblastic spindle cells containing hemosiderin and hemosiderin-laden macrophages
2. Variable amounts of admixed adipose tissue
3. Osteoclast-like giant cells
4. No significant atypia, mitoses, or necrosis

Main Differential Diagnosis

1. Plexiform fibrohistiocytic tumor
2. Atypical lipomatous tumor
3. Spindle cell lipoma
4. Giant cell tumor of soft tissue
5. Children: lipofibromatosis, fibrous hamartoma of infancy
6. Minimal fatty component: nodular fasciitis, fibrous histiocytoma

Pitfalls

! No specific immunohistochemical pattern: CD34 and calponin positivity

! May be associated with pleomorphic hyalinizing angiectactic tumor or myxoinflammatory fibroblastic sarcoma.

EPITHELIOID INFLAMMATORY MYOFIBROBLASTIC SARCOMA

Inflammatory myofibroblastic tumor (IMT) is a mesenchymal tumor of intermediate malignant potential composed of spindled myofibroblasts with admixed inflammation. It often displays *ALK* rearrangements with a variety of partner genes and diffuse cytoplasmic staining for ALK by immunohistochemistry. A rare epithelioid variant of IMT

Fig. 6. (*A*) HFLT is an unencapsulated lesion with varying proportions of mature adipocytes with admixed fibroblastic spindle cells. (*B*) HFLT often has a honeycomb pattern with clusters of mature adipocytes surrounded by spindle cells. Hemosiderin deposition is a consistent finding.

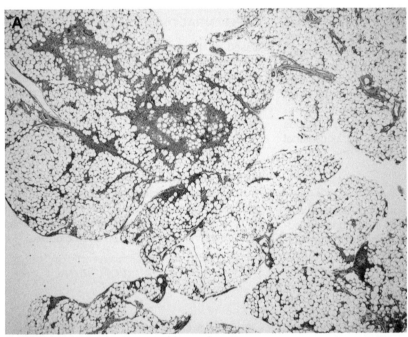

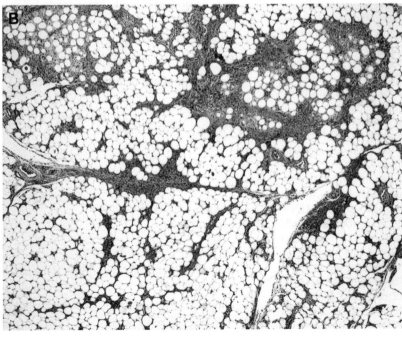

Fig. 6. (*continued*). (*C*) The spindle cells of HFLT swirl and stream between mature adipocytes. There is minimal atypia or mitotic activity. (*D*) Hemosiderin is present both in the neoplastic spindle cells of HFLT and in background siderophages. (*Courtesy of* Dr Scott Lauer, Omaha, NE.)

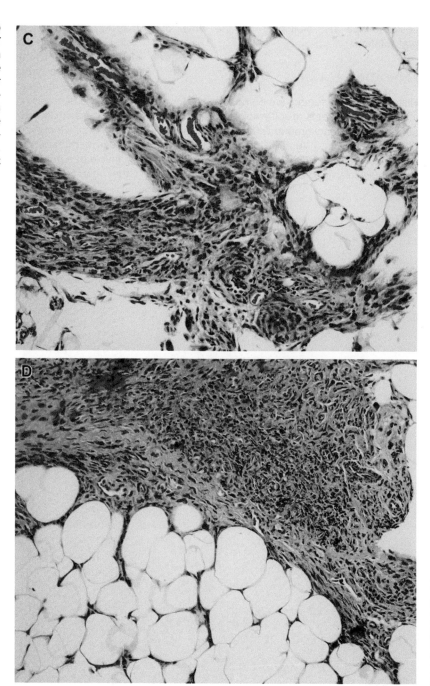

with distinctive nuclear membrane or perinuclear ALK staining was recently described and termed "epithelioid inflammatory myofibroblastic sarcoma" (EIMS) in light of its more aggressive behavior than conventional IMT. EIMS has a marked male predominance and wide age range (7 months–63 years, median 39 years).[33] They are almost exclusively found in the abdominal cavity with a single report in the pleural cavity.[34] The lesions range in size from 8 to 26 cm, and accordingly commonly present with abdominal pain and fullness and various gastrointestinal symptoms.[35]

Lesions may be multifocal at the time of presentation.

PATHOLOGIC FEATURES

Histologically, the tumors are composed predominantly of loose sheets of epithelioid-to-round cells set in a myxoid background with abundant mixed inflammation (Fig. 7A). The tumor cells have eosinophilic-to-amphophilic cytoplasm and large round vesicular nuclei with prominent nucleoli

(see Fig. 7B, C). Most cases have focal spindle cell areas. The inflammatory infiltrate may be neutrophilic or lymphocytic predominant, but plasma cells are typically conspicuously absent. Mitotic activity is variable (average rate: 4 per 10 HPFs), and necrosis may be present.[33]

EIMS essentially always displays ALK staining by immunohistochemistry, usually in a distinctive nuclear membrane pattern, or less commonly, a perinuclear cytoplasmic pattern (see Fig. 7D). Other commonly positive markers are CD30

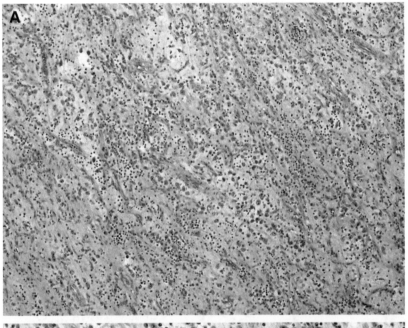

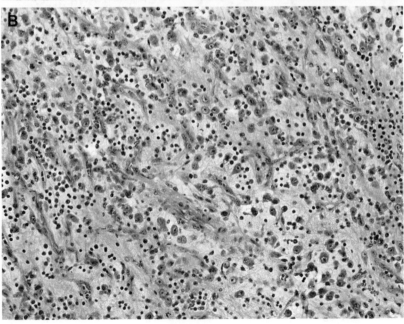

Fig. 7. (A) EIMS is composed predominantly of loose sheets of epithelioid-to-round cells set in a myxoid background with abundant mixed inflammation. (B) The tumor cells in EIMS have eosinophilic-to-amphophilic cytoplasm and large round vesicular nuclei with prominent nucleoli.

Fig. 7. (*continued*). (*C*) The background inflammatory cells are predominantly lymphocytes in this case of EIMS. The tumor cells have eosinophilic-to-amphophilic cytoplasm and large round vesicular nuclei with prominent nucleoli. Mitoses are present. (*D*) EIMS essentially always displays ALK staining by immunohistochemistry, usually in a distinctive *nuclear* membrane pattern. (*Courtesy of* Dr Karen Fritchie, Rochester, MN.)

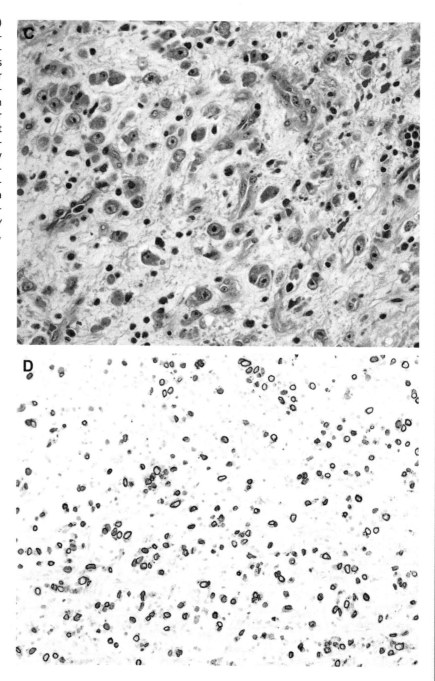

(100%), desmin (90%), and focal SMA (50%). S100, caldesmon, EMA, and keratins are uniformly negative.[33] *ALK* gene rearrangement with *RANBP2* has been reported in EIMS and this specific fusion appears to be related to the unique nuclear membrane ALK staining pattern and the more aggressive behavior seen in this rare epithelioid variant of IMT.[35] Importantly, there is new anecdotal evidence that these lesions may respond to ALK inhibitors.[36]

DIFFERENTIAL DIAGNOSIS

The diagnosis of EIMS may be very challenging given its rarity and lack of histologic similarity to typical IMT. The common differential includes anaplastic large cell lymphoma (ALCL), epithelioid leiomyosarcoma, rhabdomyosarcoma (RMS), and dedifferentiated liposarcoma (DDL), among others. The differential with ALCL may be especially difficult given the overlapping morphology and immunohistochemical pattern; however, desmin and nuclear membrane ALK staining are not present in ALCL. DDL may also mimic either IMT or EIMS, as it has vast histologic variations and may have associated inflammation; the presence of a well-differentiated liposarcoma component and MDM2 amplification by FISH can help confirm a diagnosis of DDL over EIMS. Alveolar rhabdomyosarcoma is desmin positive and often expresses ALK, but the cytologic features are that of a round blue cell neoplasm with relatively little cytoplasm, and myogenin, which is almost always strongly expressed in alveolar RMS, is negative in EIMS. For all of the entities in the differential, a full immunohistochemical workup is essential, and molecular studies for ALK rearrangements can be done in particularly difficult cases.

Key Pathologic Features

1. Epithelioid cells with vesicular nuclei and prominent nucleoli

2. Myxoid stroma

3. Inflammatory infiltrate of either predominantly neutrophils or lymphocytes

4. ALK positivity in unique nuclear membrane or perinuclear cytoplasmic pattern

5. ALK gene rearrangement, often fused with RANBP2

Table 1
Recent molecular findings in soft tissue tumors

Tumor Name	Molecular Findings
Angiofibroma of soft tissue	AHRR-NCOA2 fusion[4,5,9]
Angiomatoid fibrous histiocytoma	EWSR1-CREB1, EWSR1-ATF1, or FUS-ATF1 fusion[37]
Chondroid lipoma	C11orf95-MKL2 fusion[38]
EIMS and other IMT	ALK- RANBP2 fusion & other ALK rearrangements[35,39,40]
Ewing-like round cell sarcomas	CIC-DUX4 fusion[41–43] or BCOR-CCNB3 fusion[44,45]
Glomus tumors (benign and malignant)	MIR143-NOTCH fusions[46]
GNET	EWSR1-ATF1 or EWSR1-CREB1 fusion[15]
HFLT, MIFS, and PHAT[a]	TGFBR3 & MGEA5 rearrangments[2,25,27,28]
Intimal sarcoma of heart and great vessels	MDM2 & CDK4 amplification (12q13-14)[47–50]
Low-grade fibromyxoid sarcoma	FUS-CREB3L2, FUS-CREB3L1, or EWSR1-CREB3L1 fusion[51]
LGSSNMF	PAX3-MAML3 fusion[12,13]
Nodular fasciitis	MYH9-USP6 fusion[52]
Ossifying fibromyxoid tumor	PHF1 rearrangements[53–56]
Phosphaturic mesenchymal tumor	FN1-FGFR1 fusion[57]
Spindle cell hemangioma	IDH1 & IDH2 mutations[58,59]
Spindle cell rhabdomyosarcomas (adults)	MYOD1 mutation[60,61]
Spindle cell rhabdomyosarcoma (infants)	NCOA2 rearrangements with SRF or TEAD1[62]
Sclerosing epithelioid fibrosarcoma	EWSR1-CREB3L1 fusion, FUS rearrangements rare[63,64]
Solitary fibrous tumor	NAB2-STAT6 fusion[11]

Abbreviations: EIMS, epithelioid inflammatory myofibroblastic sarcoma; GNET, malignant gastrointestinal neuroectodermal tumor; HFLT, hemosiderotic fibrolipomatous tumor; IMT, inflammatory myofibroblastic tumor; LGSSNMF, low-grade sinonasal sarcoma with neural and myogenic features; MIFS, myxoinflammatory myofibroblastic sarcoma; PHAT, pleomorphic hyalinizing angiectactic tumor.
[a] The molecular findings and relationships among HFLT, MIFS, and PHAT are ongoing topics of debate and investigation.

Main Differential Diagnosis

1. ALCL
2. Epithelioid leiomyosarcoma
3. Rhabdomyosarcoma
4. Dedifferentiated liposarcoma

Pitfalls

! Epithelioid histology is not classically associated with IMT or related entities and may lead the pathologist away from recognition of this unique aggressive variant of IMT

! Similar histology and immunohistochemical staining to ALCL

RECENT MOLECULAR FINDINGS IN SOFT TISSUE TUMORS

In addition to the molecular findings associated with the novel entities discussed in this article, a variety of molecular alterations have been recently reported in many established soft tissue tumors, as well. Although space does not permit full discussion of each, we have attempted to summarize many of these in **Table 1**.

REFERENCES

1. Carter JM, Weiss SW, Linos K, et al. Superficial CD34-positive fibroblastic tumor: report of 18 cases of a distinctive low-grade mesenchymal neoplasm of intermediate (borderline) malignancy. Mod Pathol 2014;27:294–302.
2. Antonescu CR, Zhang L, Nielsen GP, et al. Consistent t(1;10) with rearrangements of TGFBR3 and MGEA5 in both myxoinflammatory fibroblastic sarcoma and hemosiderotic fibrolipomatous tumor. Genes Chromosomes Cancer 2011;50:757–64.
3. Deyrup AT, Chibon F, Guillou L, et al. Fibrosarcoma-like lipomatous neoplasm: a reappraisal of so-called spindle cell liposarcoma defining a unique lipomatous tumor unrelated to other liposarcomas. Am J Surg Pathol 2013;37:1373–8.
4. Mariño-Enríquez A, Fletcher CD. Angiofibroma of soft tissue: clinicopathologic characterization of a distinctive benign fibrovascular neoplasm in a series of 37 cases. Am J Surg Pathol 2012;36:500–8.
5. Sugita S, Aoyama T, Kondo K, et al. Diagnostic utility of NCOA2 fluorescence in situ hybridization and Stat6 immunohistochemistry staining for soft tissue angiofibroma and morphologically similar fibrovascular tumors. Hum Pathol 2014;45:1588–96.
6. Fukuda Y, Motoi T, Kato I, et al. Angiofibroma of soft tissue with fibrohistiocytic features and intratumor genetic heterogeneity of NCOA2 gene rearrangement revealed by chromogenic in situ hybridization: a case report. Pathol Int 2014;64:237–42.
7. Lee JJ, Bredella MA, Springfield DS, et al. Soft tissue angiofibroma: a case report. Skeletal Radiol 2014; 43:403–7.
8. Edgar MA, Lauer SR, Bridge JA, et al. Soft tissue angiofibroma: report of 2 cases of a recently described tumor. Hum Pathol 2013;44:438–41.
9. Jin Y, Moller E, Nord KH, et al. Fusion of the AHRR and NCOA2 genes through a recurrent translocation t(5;8)(p15;q13) in soft tissue angiofibroma results in upregulation of aryl hydrocarbon receptor target genes. Genes Chromosomes Cancer 2012;51:510–20.
10. Doyle LA, Moller E, Dal Cin P, et al. MUC4 is a highly sensitive and specific marker for low-grade fibromyxoid sarcoma. Am J Surg Pathol 2011;35:733–41.
11. Robinson DR, Wu YM, Kalyana-Sundaram S, et al. Identification of recurrent NAB2-STAT6 gene fusions in solitary fibrous tumor by integrative sequencing. Nat Genet 2013;45:180–5.
12. Lewis JT, Oliveira AM, Nascimento AG, et al. Low-grade sinonasal sarcoma with neural and myogenic features: a clinicopathologic analysis of 28 cases. Am J Surg Pathol 2012;36:517–25.
13. Wang X, Bledsoe KL, Graham RP, et al. Recurrent PAX3-MAML3 fusion in biphenotypic sinonasal sarcoma. Nat Genet 2014;46:666–8.
14. Powers KA, Han LM, Chiu AG, et al. Low-grade sinonasal sarcoma with neural and myogenic features—diagnostic challenge and pathogenic insight. Oral Surg Oral Med Oral Pathol Oral Radiol 2015; 119(5):e265–9.
15. Stockman DL, Miettinen M, Suster S, et al. Malignant gastrointestinal neuroectodermal tumor: clinicopathologic, immunohistochemical, ultrastructural, and molecular analysis of 16 cases with a reappraisal of clear cell sarcoma-like tumors of the gastrointestinal tract. Am J Surg Pathol 2012;36:857–68.
16. Kosemehmetoglu K, Folpe AL. Clear cell sarcoma of tendons and aponeuroses, and osteoclast-rich tumour of the gastrointestinal tract with features resembling clear cell sarcoma of soft parts: a review and update. J Clin Pathol 2010;63:416–23.
17. Friedrichs N, Testi MA, Moiraghi L, et al. Clear cell sarcoma-like tumor with osteoclast-like giant cells in the small bowel: further evidence for a new tumor entity. Int J Surg Pathol 2005;13:313–8.
18. Zambrano E, Reyes-Mugica M, Franchi A, et al. An osteoclast-rich tumor of the gastrointestinal tract

with features resembling clear cell sarcoma of soft parts: reports of 6 cases of a GIST simulator. Int J Surg Pathol 2003;11:75–81.

19. Huang W, Zhang X, Li D, et al. Osteoclast-rich tumor of the gastrointestinal tract with features resembling those of clear cell sarcoma of soft parts. Virchows Arch 2006;448:200–3.

20. Antonescu CR, Nafa K, Segal NH, et al. EWS-CREB1: a recurrent variant fusion in clear cell sarcoma–association with gastrointestinal location and absence of melanocytic differentiation. Clin Cancer Res 2006;12:5356–62.

21. Karamchandani JR, Nielsen TO, van de Rijn M, et al. Sox10 and S100 in the diagnosis of soft-tissue neoplasms. Appl Immunohistochem Mol Morphol 2012; 20:445–50.

22. Folpe AL, Mentzel T, Lehr HA, et al. Perivascular epithelioid cell neoplasms of soft tissue and gynecologic origin: a clinicopathologic study of 26 cases and review of the literature. Am J Surg Pathol 2005;29:1558–75.

23. Miettinen M, McCue PA, Sarlomo-Rikala M, et al. Sox10: a marker for not only schwannian and melanocytic neoplasms but also myoepithelial cell tumors of soft tissue: a systematic analysis of 5134 tumors. Am J Surg Pathol 2015;39(6):826–35.

24. Marshall-Taylor C, Fanburg-Smith JC. Hemosiderotic fibrohistiocytic lipomatous lesion: ten cases of a previously undescribed fatty lesion of the foot/ankle. Mod Pathol 2000;13:1192–9.

25. Zreik RT, Carter JM, Sukov WR, et al. Myxoinflammatory fibroblastic sarcoma and hybrid hemosiderotic fibrolipomatous tumor/myxoinflammatory fibroblastic sarcoma: related or not? United States and Canadian Academy of Pathology Annual Meeting (platform presentation). Boston, March 23, 2015.

26. Wettach GR, Boyd LJ, Lawce HJ, et al. Cytogenetic analysis of a hemosiderotic fibrolipomatous tumor. Cancer Genet Cytogenet 2008;182:140–3.

27. Hallor KH, Sciot R, Staaf J, et al. Two genetic pathways, t(1;10) and amplification of 3p11-12, in myxoinflammatory fibroblastic sarcoma, haemosiderotic fibrolipomatous tumour, and morphologically similar lesions. J Pathol 2009;217:716–27.

28. Carter JM, Sukov WR, Montgomery E, et al. TGFBR3 and MGEA5 rearrangements in pleomorphic hyalinizing angiectatic tumors and the spectrum of related neoplasms. Am J Surg Pathol 2014;38: 1182–992.

29. Browne TJ, Fletcher CD. Haemosiderotic fibrolipomatous tumour (so-called haemosiderotic fibrohistiocytic lipomatous tumour): analysis of 13 new cases in support of a distinct entity. Histopathology 2006; 48:453–61.

30. Solomon DA, Antonescu CR, Link TM, et al. Hemosiderotic fibrolipomatous tumor, not an entirely benign entity. Am J Surg Pathol 2013;37:1627–30.

31. Elco CP, Marino-Enriquez A, Abraham JA, et al. Hybrid myxoinflammatory fibroblastic sarcoma/hemosiderotic fibrolipomatous tumor: report of a case providing further evidence for a pathogenetic link. Am J Surg Pathol 2010;34:1723–7.

32. Fletcher CDM, Bridge JA, Hogendoorn PC, et al. WHO classification of tumours of soft tissue and bone. 4th edition. Lyon (France): World Health Organization; 2013.

33. Marino-Enriquez A, Wang WL, Roy A, et al. Epithelioid inflammatory myofibroblastic sarcoma: an aggressive intra-abdominal variant of inflammatory myofibroblastic tumor with nuclear membrane or perinuclear ALK. Am J Surg Pathol 2011;35:135–44.

34. Kozu Y, Isaka M, Ohde Y, et al. Epithelioid inflammatory myofibroblastic sarcoma arising in the pleural cavity. Gen Thorac Cardiovasc Surg 2014;62:191–4.

35. Li J, Yin WH, Takeuchi K, et al. Inflammatory myofibroblastic tumor with RANBP2 and ALK gene rearrangement: a report of two cases and literature review. Diagn Pathol 2013;8:147.

36. Kimbara S, Takeda K, Fukushima H, et al. A case report of epithelioid inflammatory myofibroblastic sarcoma with RANBP2-ALK fusion gene treated with the ALK inhibitor, crizotinib. Jpn J Clin Oncol 2014;44:868–71.

37. Antonescu CR, Dal Cin P, Nafa K, et al. EWSR1-CREB1 is the predominant gene fusion in angiomatoid fibrous histiocytoma. Genes Chromosomes Cancer 2007;46:1051–60.

38. Huang D, Sumegi J, Dal Cin P, et al. C11orf95-MKL2 is the resulting fusion oncogene of t(11;16)(q13;p13) in chondroid lipoma. Genes Chromosomes Cancer 2010;49:810–8.

39. Lovly CM, Gupta A, Lipson D, et al. Inflammatory myofibroblastic tumors harbor multiple potentially actionable kinase fusions. Cancer Discov 2014;4:889–95.

40. Takeuchi K, Soda M, Togashi Y, et al. Pulmonary inflammatory myofibroblastic tumor expressing a novel fusion, PPFIBP1-ALK: reappraisal of anti-ALK immunohistochemistry as a tool for novel ALK fusion identification. Clin Cancer Res 2011;17:3341–8.

41. Choi EY, Thomas DG, McHugh JB, et al. Undifferentiated small round cell sarcoma with t(4;19)(q35;q13.1) CIC-DUX4 fusion: a novel highly aggressive soft tissue tumor with distinctive histopathology. Am J Surg Pathol 2013;37:1379–86.

42. Graham C, Chilton-MacNeill S, Zielenska M, et al. The CIC-DUX4 fusion transcript is present in a subgroup of pediatric primitive round cell sarcomas. Hum Pathol 2012;43:180–9.

43. Specht K, Sung YS, Zhang L, et al. Distinct transcriptional signature and immunoprofile of CIC-DUX4 fusion-positive round cell tumors compared to EWSR1-rearranged Ewing sarcomas: further evidence toward distinct pathologic entities. Genes Chromosomes Cancer 2014;53:622–33.

44. Pierron G, Tirode F, Lucchesi C, et al. A new subtype of bone sarcoma defined by BCOR-CCNB3 gene fusion. Nat Genet 2012;44:461–6.

45. Puls F, Niblett A, Marland G, et al. BCOR-CCNB3 (Ewing-like) sarcoma: a clinicopathologic analysis of 10 cases, in comparison with conventional Ewing sarcoma. Am J Surg Pathol 2014;38:1307–18.

46. Mosquera JM, Sboner A, Zhang L, et al. Novel MIR143-NOTCH fusions in benign and malignant glomus tumors. Genes Chromosomes Cancer 2013;52:1075–87.

47. Bode-Lesniewska B, Zhao J, Speel EJ, et al. Gains of 12q13-14 and overexpression of mdm2 are frequent findings in intimal sarcomas of the pulmonary artery. Virchows Arch 2001;438:57–65.

48. Neuville A, Collin F, Bruneval P, et al. Intimal sarcoma is the most frequent primary cardiac sarcoma: clinicopathologic and molecular retrospective analysis of 100 primary cardiac sarcomas. Am J Surg Pathol 2014;38:461–9.

49. Zhang H, Macdonald WD, Erickson-Johnson M, et al. Cytogenetic and molecular cytogenetic findings of intimal sarcoma. Cancer Genet Cytogenet 2007;179:146–9.

50. Zhao J, Roth J, Bode-Lesniewska B, et al. Combined comparative genomic hybridization and genomic microarray for detection of gene amplifications in pulmonary artery intimal sarcomas and adrenocortical tumors. Genes Chromosomes Cancer 2002; 34:48–57.

51. Lau PP, Lui PC, Lau GT, et al. EWSR1-CREB3L1 gene fusion: a novel alternative molecular aberration of low-grade fibromyxoid sarcoma. Am J Surg Pathol 2013;37:734–8.

52. Erickson-Johnson MR, Chou MM, Evers BR, et al. Nodular fasciitis: a novel model of transient neoplasia induced by MYH9-USP6 gene fusion. Lab Invest 2011;91:1427–33.

53. Antonescu CR, Sung YS, Chen CL, et al. Novel ZC3H7B-BCOR, MEAF6-PHF1, and EPC1-PHF1 fusions in ossifying fibromyxoid tumors–molecular characterization shows genetic overlap with endometrial stromal sarcoma. Genes Chromosomes Cancer 2014;53:183–93.

54. Endo M, Kohashi K, Yamamoto H, et al. Ossifying fibromyxoid tumor presenting EP400-PHF1 fusion gene. Hum Pathol 2013;44:2603–8.

55. Gebre-Medhin S, Nord KH, Moller E, et al. Recurrent rearrangement of the PHF1 gene in ossifying fibromyxoid tumors. Am J Pathol 2012;181:1069–77.

56. Graham RP, Weiss SW, Sukov WR, et al. PHF1 rearrangements in ossifying fibromyxoid tumors of soft parts: a fluorescence in situ hybridization study of 41 cases with emphasis on the malignant variant. Am J Surg Pathol 2013;37:1751–5.

57. Lee JC, Jeng YM, Su SY, et al. Identification of a novel FN1-FGFR1 genetic fusion as a frequent event in phosphaturic mesenchymal tumour. J Pathol 2015;235:539–45.

58. Kurek KC, Pansuriya TC, van Ruler MA, et al. R132C IDH1 mutations are found in spindle cell hemangiomas and not in other vascular tumors or malformations. Am J Pathol 2013;182:1494–500.

59. Pansuriya TC, van Eijk R, d'Adamo P, et al. Somatic mosaic IDH1 and IDH2 mutations are associated with enchondroma and spindle cell hemangioma in Ollier disease and Maffucci syndrome. Nat Genet 2011;43:1256–61.

60. Agaram NP, Chen CL, Zhang L, et al. Recurrent MYOD1 mutations in pediatric and adult sclerosing and spindle cell rhabdomyosarcomas: evidence for a common pathogenesis. Genes Chromosomes Cancer 2014;53:779–87.

61. Szuhai K, de Jong D, Leung WY, et al. Transactivating mutation of the MYOD1 gene is a frequent event in adult spindle cell rhabdomyosarcoma. J Pathol 2014;232:300–7.

62. Mosquera JM, Sboner A, Zhang L, et al. Recurrent NCOA2 gene rearrangements in congenital/infantile spindle cell rhabdomyosarcoma. Genes Chromosomes Cancer 2013;52:538–50.

63. Arbajian E, Puls F, Magnusson L, et al. Recurrent EWSR1-CREB3L1 gene fusions in sclerosing epithelioid fibrosarcoma. Am J Surg Pathol 2014;38: 801–8.

64. Wang WL, Evans HL, Meis JM, et al. FUS rearrangements are rare in 'pure' sclerosing epithelioid fibrosarcoma. Mod Pathol 2012;25:846–53.

Non-mesenchymal Mimics of Sarcoma

Leona A. Doyle, MD

KEYWORDS

- Soft tissue • Tumor • Sarcoma • Melanoma • Sarcomatoid carcinoma • Immunohistochemistry
- Molecular genetics

ABSTRACT

A variety of different non-mesenchymal neoplasms may mimic sarcoma, in particular sarcomatoid carcinoma and melanoma, but also mesothelioma and rarely some lymphomas. This article reviews the key clinical and histologic features of such neoplasms in different settings, along with the use of ancillary studies to help identify the tumor types most frequently misdiagnosed as sarcoma.

OVERVIEW

Soft tissue tumors encompass a broad group of clinically, histologically, and molecularly diverse tumor types. Many soft tissue tumors show significant histologic overlap with one another (eg, spindle cell sarcomas, pleomorphic sarcomas), and distinguishing different sarcoma types often requires clinical correlation along with ancillary diagnostic tests, most often immunohistochemistry (IHC) and fluorescence in situ hybridization (FISH). However, many non-mesenchymal tumor types can also show significant histologic overlap with sarcomas, and should be considered in the differential diagnosis of many different soft tissue neoplasms. In most cases, distinction can be made with a combination of clinical correlation, identification of certain diagnostic histologic features, and a relatively limited panel of immunohistochemical stains. This article reviews some of the most commonly encountered situations in which non-mesenchymal neoplasms may show significant histologic overlap with sarcoma and provides a practical approach to such cases, incorporating the use of ancillary studies.

MALIGNANT MELANOMA

Malignant melanoma, both primary and metastatic, frequently mimics sarcoma. Most primary cutaneous melanomas are readily recognizable as such due to the presence of an in-situ component, with the exception of desmoplastic or spindle cell melanoma, which may be difficult to distinguish histologically from other intradermal spindle cell neoplasms, such as atypical fibroxanthoma/pleomorphic dermal sarcoma, and nerve sheath neoplasms. However, the diverse histologic features (epithelioid, spindled, round cell, pleomorphic, mixed) seen in metastatic melanoma accounts for the significant overlap with many different sarcoma types (Fig. 1). Although clinical history is clearly crucial, histologic clues to the diagnosis of metastatic melanoma include the presence of mixed architectural growth patterns, particularly a nested or theke-like growth pattern, cytologic pleomorphism, melanin pigmentation (often not present in metastatic tumors), and prominent "cherry-red" nucleoli. However, in many cases, and especially in small biopsy samples, IHC is needed to confirm the diagnosis and to exclude other entities. Most metastatic melanomas show at least focal nuclear and cytoplasmic S100 protein expression, but expression of secondary melanocytic markers, such as melan-A/MART-1, HMB45, tyrosinase, and MiTF is highly variable, and many metastatic tumors are negative for all these markers. In addition, melanomas with a spindled morphology, both primary and metastatic, are usually negative for secondary melanocytic markers. Quite recently, however, SOX10 has been described as a highly sensitive and relatively specific marker of neuroectodermal differentiation, and has proven to be very useful

Department of Pathology, Brigham and Women's Hospital, Harvard Medical School, 75 Francis Street, Boston, MA 02115, USA
E-mail address: ladoyle@partners.org

Surgical Pathology 8 (2015) 493–513
http://dx.doi.org/10.1016/j.path.2015.05.010
1875-9181/15/$ – see front matter © 2015 Elsevier Inc. All rights reserved.

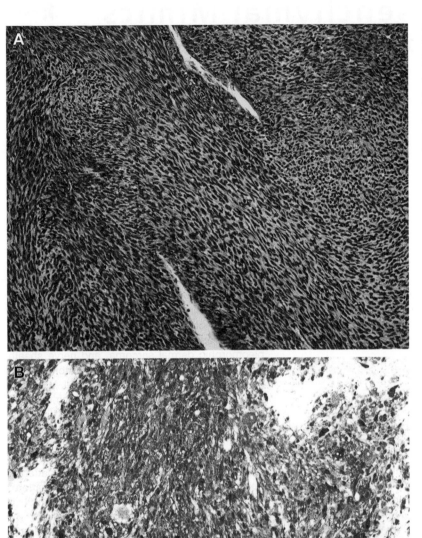

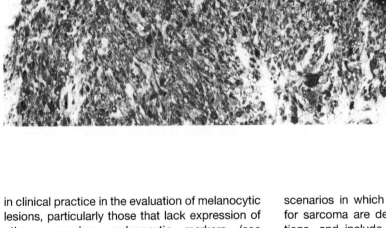

Fig. 1. Metastatic malignant melanoma involving bone and showing a fascicular growth pattern virtually indistinguishable from MPNST (*A*). The tumor cells show diffuse nuclear and cytoplasmic expression of S100 protein (*B*).

in clinical practice in the evaluation of melanocytic lesions, particularly those that lack expression of other secondary melanocytic markers (see **Fig.** 1D).[1] Expression of SOX10 is seen in more than 99% of melanocytic and nerve sheath neoplasms, as well as a subset of (usually benign) myoepithelial tumors.[2–4] Three relatively common

scenarios in which melanoma may be mistaken for sarcoma are described in the following sections, and include the distinction of melanoma from malignant peripheral nerve sheath tumor (MPNST) and clear cell sarcoma, as well as the occurrence of metastatic melanoma in the absence of a known primary tumor.

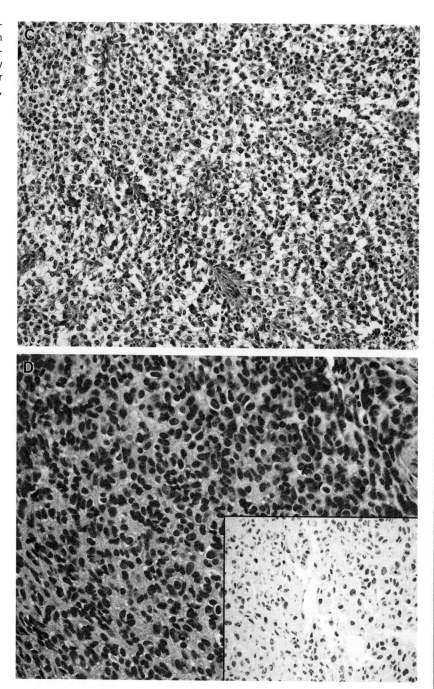

Fig. 1. (*continued*). Metastatic melanoma with round cell (*C*) and epithelioid (*D*) morphology showing diffuse nuclear positivity for SOX10 (*D*, inset).

MELANOMA AND MALIGNANT PERIPHERAL NERVE SHEATH TUMOR

Malignant melanoma is occasionally mistaken for MPNST, due to shared S100 expression in both tumors, in addition to overlapping histologic features (see **Fig. 1**A). MPNST is a variably cellular fascicular spindle cell neoplasm that shows S100 protein expression in approximately 50% of cases.[5,6] Importantly, however, the distribution of S100 expression in MPNST is usually focal or multifocal at most when present, and the presence of diffuse S100 expression is far more commonly seen in melanoma (see Fig. 1B). The presence of diffuse S100 positivity in MPNST is generally seen only in pediatric cases associated with neurofibromatosis.[5] Anatomic location is also important in this differential diagnosis: "conventional" MPNST arises in deep soft tissues and virtually never in skin, and therefore the presence of an S100-positive cytologically atypical dermal tumor is far more likely to represent melanoma, with the exception of the very rare variant of epithelioid MPNST. Epithelioid MPNST is a clinico-pathologically distinctive neoplasm characterized by a multinodular growth pattern and composed of a relatively monomorphic population of epithelioid cells with distinct nucleoli. In contrast to conventional MPNST, this variant arises in the dermis and shows diffuse S100 positivity. It is distinguished from melanoma by its multinodular growth pattern, relative cytologic monotony, loss of INI1 expression in 50% of cases, and absence of expression of secondary melanocytic markers, such as HMB-45 and melan-A.[7]

MELANOMA AND CLEAR CELL SARCOMA

Distinguishing malignant melanoma from clear cell sarcoma can be extremely difficult, particularly in core biopsy samples, again due to overlapping IHC features. Clear cell sarcoma classically involves tendons or aponeuroses of distal extremities, usually around the ankle, and is composed of nests of spindled or epithelioid cells with prominent nucleoli and usually mild cytologic pleomorphism. Similar to melanoma, the tumor cells show expression of S100, SOX10, and secondary melanocytic markers, but characteristically show more intense or diffuse staining for HMB-45 compared with S100, a finding that is uncommon in melanoma. However, this feature alone is generally not reliable enough in a given case to distinguish these tumor types, and distinction relies on a combination of clinicopathologic and molecular features. Clear cell sarcoma is a translocation-associated sarcoma that generally occurs in young to middle-aged adults, and is characterized by either a t(12;22)(q13;q12) resulting in EWSR1-ATF fusion gene, or less commonly t(2;22)(q34;q12) resulting in EWSR1-CREB1 fusion,[8–10] and identification of EWSR1 rearrangement by FISH is a reliable ancillary test to confirm this diagnosis. Histologic features that favor a diagnosis of clear cell sarcoma include lack of a superficial epidermal component, infiltration of

tendinous tissue by tumor in a nested pattern, multinucleate tumor cells, and the presence of only mild atypia and pleomorphism. However, in many cases, the histologic and immunohistochemical overlap is sufficient enough that FISH to identify the EWSR1 rearrangement of clear cell sarcoma is needed to exclude melanoma.

METASTATIC MELANOMA WITH NO KNOWN PRIMARY

In approximately 5% of cases of metastatic melanoma a primary site is not identified, and given the overall incidence of metastatic melanoma, this is not an uncommon scenario. Axillary lymph nodes are frequently involved, followed by inguinal lymph nodes, and tumors may show epithelioid, spindled, or mixed features, usually with moderate to severe cytologic atypia and pleomorphism. In such cases, the diagnosis is usually suggested by the finding of S100 or SOX10 positivity, with or without expression of other melanocytic markers. Metastatic melanoma may also involve subcutaneous soft tissue sites, where it is usually well circumscribed, and shows a nested or "theke-like" growth pattern. Circumscription and lack of an overlying epidermal component are features suggestive of metastatic disease rather than primary tumor site.

Key Features
METASTATIC MELANOMA

- For approximately 5% of metastatic melanomas, no primary site is identified

- Broad range of morphologies, including spindled, epithelioid, pleomorphic, or round cell; spindled or round cell morphologies commonly mimic sarcoma

- Clues to diagnosis include presence of nested growth pattern, which may be focal, cytologic and architectual pleomorphism

- Many metastatic melanomas, either primary or metastatic, and most with spindle cell morphology, lack expression of secondary melanocytic markers; however, SOX10 remains highly sensitive in this setting

- SOX10 expression is present in more than 95% of melanocytic neoplasms; expression is also seen in nerve sheath tumors and a subset of myoepithelial tumors

Pitfalls
METASTATIC MELANOMA

! Diffuse positivity for S100 protein or SOX10 in a spindle cell neoplasm is far more likely to represent melanoma than MPNST, which only very rarely shows diffuse expression of these two markers

! Distinction of malignant melanoma from clear cell sarcoma may be very difficult, especially in small biopsies: FISH to identify *EWSR1* rearrangement characteristic of clear cell sarcoma is often needed to resolve this differential

CARCINOMA TYPES THAT MAY MIMIC SARCOMA (AND VICE VERSA)

Sarcomatoid carcinoma, or spindle cell carcinoma, can be present as a major or minor component of carcinomas at virtually any site, but is most often associated with primary breast carcinoma, renal cell carcinoma, and mucosal or cutaneous squamous cell carcinoma. At these sites and other primary sites, pure sarcomatoid carcinoma may be difficult to recognize as an epithelial neoplasm (**Fig. 2**), and sarcomatoid carcinoma is even more difficult to recognize at metastatic sites, such as in bone or somatic soft tissue (**Fig. 3**), unless one has a high level of suspicion or can identify more epithelioid-appearing areas. In addition, sarcomatoid carcinoma may show heterologous differentiation in the form of chondro-osseous/osteosarcomatous or rhabdomyosarcomatous differentiation (**Fig. 4**A), which may result in an erroneous diagnosis of osteosarcoma or rhabdomyosarcoma: the presence of either of these tumor types at visceral sites, or even at soft tissue sites, in an adult should prompt consideration of the possibility of heterologous differentiation within a carcinoma (see **Fig. 4**B). A panel of immunohistochemical markers to include several cytokeratins (both low-molecular weight and high-molecular weight) is usually needed to confirm the diagnosis of metastatic sarcomatoid carcinoma, and with the exception of TTF-1 and PAX-8, most "lineage-specific" markers or keratin subtypes are of little use in determining primary site. Three settings in which carcinoma may mimic different mesenchymal tumors are considered in the following sections.

SARCOMATOID CARCINOMA OF BREAST

Sarcomatoid or spindle cell carcinoma of the breast is often cytologically bland and thereby resembles desmoid fibromatosis or Phyllodes tumor[11,12] (**Fig. 5**A), or may show significant cytologic atypia and pleomorphism and mimic high-grade sarcoma.[13] For this reason, most practitioners advocate the use of multiple cytokeratins to include broad-spectrum cytokeratins (AE1/AE3, pan-cytokeratin) and those associated with a "basal" or myoepithelial phenotype (CK5, CK14, 34βE12) along with p63,[14] in the evaluation of any spindle cell lesion in the breast to exclude the possibility of sarcomatoid carcinoma, and this approach is generally optimal when dealing with most such lesions (see **Fig. 5**B). In some cases, small foci of epithelioid cells, gland formation, or in situ carcinoma are present, and therefore thorough sampling to identify any conventional component of adenocarcinoma is warranted. Desmoid fibromatosis is distinguished from low-grade spindle cell carcinoma of breast by the presence of nuclear beta-catenin expression and lack of cytokeratin expression. Sarcomatoid carcinoma of breast is typically negative for estrogen and progesterone receptors, as well as Her2-neu.

Clinically, sarcomatoid carcinoma of breast shows a wide spectrum of biologic behavior, with histologically low-grade fibromatosis-like cases having a relatively indolent clinical course with local recurrences and infrequent lymph node spread, similar to low-grade sarcomas,[12,15] whereas higher-grade lesions show a clinical course more analogous to conventional adenocarcinoma of breast.[13]

Key Features
SARCOMATOID CARCINOMA

• For any spindle cell neoplasm in the breast, consider a broad panel of keratins, as well as thorough sampling, to exclude possibility of sarcomatoid carcinoma

• The differential diagnosis of an atypical intradermal spindle cell neoplasm includes sarcomatoid carcinoma, melanoma, smooth muscle neoplasm, and spindle cell angiosarcoma; these tumors should be excluded before a diagnosis of atypical fibroxanthoma or pleomorphic dermal sarcoma is made

Pitfalls
SARCOMATOID CARCINOMA

! Sarcomatoid spindle cell carcinoma of breast can be morphologically low grade, resembling desmoid fibromatosis

! Keratin expression can be seen in many different soft tissue tumors, including leiomyosarcoma, inflammatory myofibroblastic tumor, schwannoma arising in the mediastinum, epithelioid sarcoma, and epithelioid vascular tumors

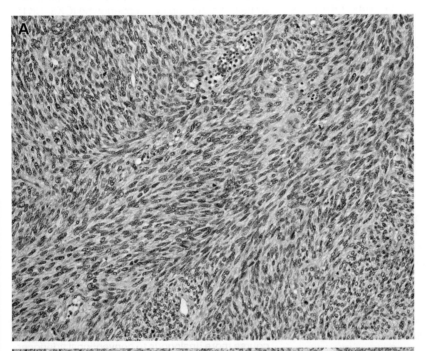

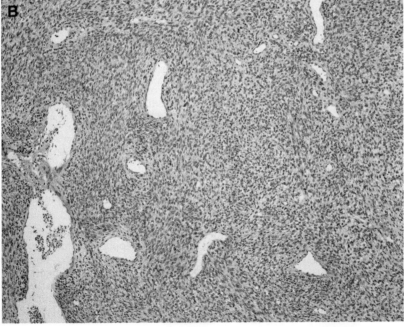

Fig. 2. Sarcomatoid carcinoma arising in the stomach and showing a fascicular spindle cell appearance more reminiscent of high-grade spindle cell sarcoma such as synovial sarcoma, (A) with areas of hemangiopericytomalike blood vessels (B). Other areas had a more round cell appearance (C), and just focally areas of epithelioid cytomorphology with gland formation were present (D): tumor cells in glandular areas were positive for CDX2 and pankeratin, whereas the spindle cell component was negative for keratins and showed only rare EMA-positive cells.

Fig. 2. (continued).

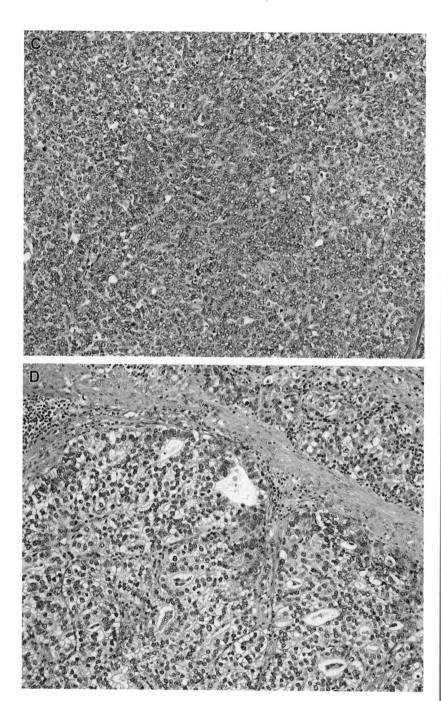

SARCOMATOID SQUAMOUS CELL CARCINOMA OF SKIN

Spindle cell/sarcomatoid squamous cell carcinoma falls into the differential diagnosis of virtually any atypical intradermal spindle cell neoplasm, commonly encountered in superficial skin biopsies or shaves. In addition to carcinoma, diagnostic considerations for such specimens include spindle cell melanoma, atypical fibroxanthoma, pleomorphic dermal sarcoma, and less often, atypical intradermal smooth muscle neoplasm (cutaneous leiomyosarcoma) or spindle cell angiosarcoma. The overlying epithelium should be evaluated

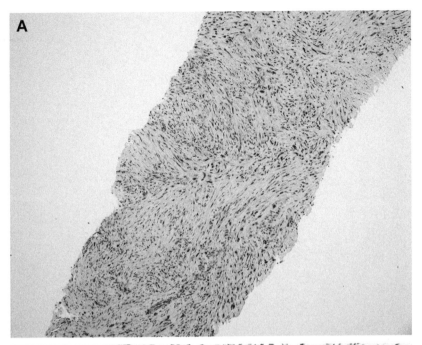

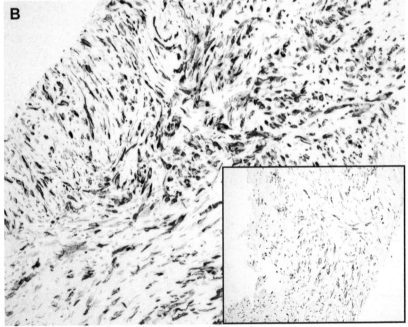

Fig. 3. Biopsy of a mass in the deep soft tissue of the leg of an 83-year-old man. The tumor is composed of fascicles of spindle cells with cytologic atypia and pleomorphism (*A*). The tumor cells were positive for CAM5.2 (*B*), whereas pancytokeratin (*B*, inset) showed positivity in just scattered cells. Based on the presence of keratin expression (and negativity for other markers including S100 and MDM2), the possibility of metastatic sarcomatoid carcinoma was raised: subsequently, a lung mass was identified and the resection showed a poorly differentiated adenosquamous carcinoma with sarcomatoid features.

for either squamous dysplasia to support a diagnosis of sarcomatoid squamous cell carcinoma or atypical melanocytic proliferation for melanoma. A useful initial IHC panel to evaluate such lesions therefore includes CK5, p63, S100, and SOX10. Sarcomatoid squamous cell carcinoma is typically positive for CK5 and p63. Spindle cell melanoma shows variable expression of S100 and is usually negative for HMB-45 and melan-A/MART-1, but SOX10 shows a higher sensitivity than all of these markers in this setting.[1] For smooth muscle neoplasms, expression of smooth muscle actin and desmin helps confirm the diagnosis, and for angiosarcoma, expression of

Fig. 4. Rhabdomyosarcomatous component of a sarcomatoid renal cell carcinoma, composed of dyshesive tumor cells with brightly eosinophilic cytoplasm (*A*) and desmin positivity (*A*, inset). Other areas of the tumor showed chondrosarcomatous components, within which conventional clear-cell renal cell carcinoma can be seen intermingled with the chondrosarcomatous elements (*B*).

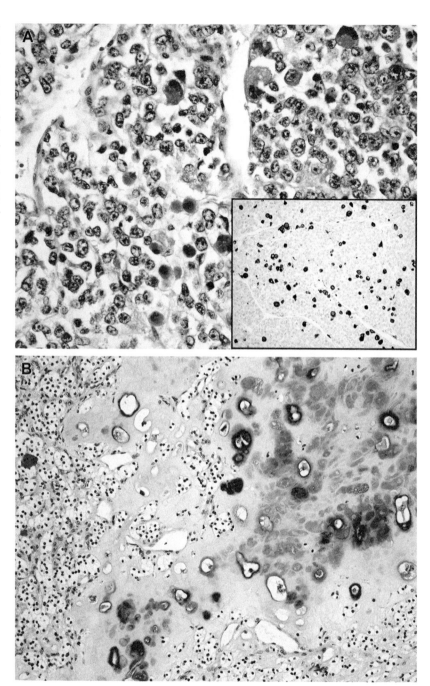

endothelial markers CD31 and ERG is diagnostic. For those tumors that fail to show a line of differentiation, either morphologically or immunohistochemically, the differential diagnosis usually lies between atypical fibroxanthoma and pleomorphic dermal sarcoma[16]; distinction between these two tumors requires complete excision to evaluate the depth of tumor involvement and determine whether invasion into subcutaneous tissue has occurred: atypical fibroxanthoma should be confined to the dermis or show only minimal extension into subcutaneous tissue.

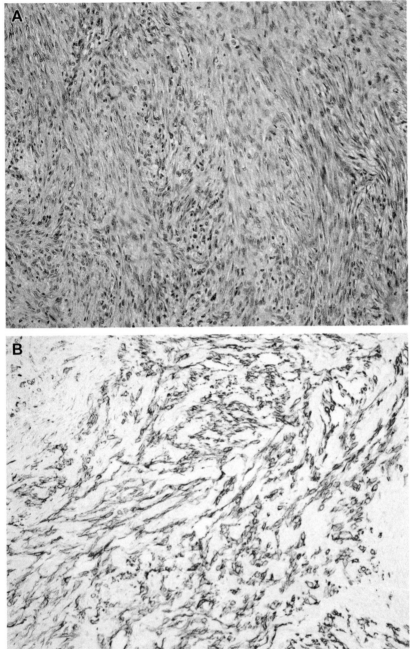

Fig. 5. Sarcomatoid carcinoma of breast showing a fascicular growth pattern of bland uniform spindle cells, resembling desmoid fibromatosis (*A*). The tumor cells show diffuse expression of the high-molecular-weight cytokeratin 34 betaE12 (*B*).

RENAL CELL CARCINOMA, ADRENOCORTICAL CARCINOMA, AND MESENCHYMAL MIMICS

Renal cell carcinoma may mimic several soft tissue tumors; in the kidney, anastomosing hemangioma may be difficult to distinguish from renal cell carcinoma, and outside the kidney renal cell carcinoma most often resembles perivascular epithelioid cell tumor (PEComa), chordoma, and epithelioid variant of pleomorphic liposarcoma.

Anastomosing hemangioma is composed of small capillaries lined by bland endothelial cells, which may have an epithelioid appearance or clear cytoplasm.[17] The capillaries are often compressed, resulting in a solid appearance and in combination with clear cell cytomorphology may mimic renal cell carcinoma.[18] Histologic clues that suggest the diagnosis of anastomosing hemangioma include a lobular growth pattern (may not be apparent on core biopsies), eosinophilic intracytoplasmic globules, stromal fibrosis, and hemorrhage. Expression of ERG and CD31 confirms the endothelial nature of the lesion, and PAX8 is negative, thereby distinguishing it from renal cell carcinoma.

Epithelioid variant of pleomorphic liposarcoma is composed of sheets, nests, or trabeculae of large epithelioid cells with variably clear, granular, or palely eosinophilic cytoplasm, thereby mimicking metastatic adrenocortical carcinoma or renal cell carcinoma (Fig. 6). Clinically, pleomorphic liposarcoma usually arises on the extremities, but occasionally can occur in the retroperitoneum.[19,20] Most adrenocortical carcinomas present with a large adrenal mass, and unlike renal cell carcinoma, occult adrenal cell carcinoma presenting with metastasis is exceptional, and therefore knowledge of the presence of an adrenal mass or history of renal cell carcinoma is helpful. The histologic clue to the diagnosis of pleomorphic liposarcoma is the presence of true lipoblasts (ie, univacuolated or multivacuolated cells with indented or scalloped nuclei); these cells may be numerous or present only focally within a given tumor (see inset in Fig. 6). Although there are no specific IHC markers to confirm the diagnosis of pleomorphic liposarcoma, IHC for inhibin and melan-A/mart1, or PAX8 and EMA, can help exclude adrenocortical carcinoma or renal cell carcinoma, respectively. Epithelioid variant of pleomorphic liposarcoma shows focal expression of broad-spectrum cytokeratins (usually high-molecular weight) in 20% of cases.[19,20]

Finally, it is important to remember that keratin expression can be seen in many different soft tissue tumors. Of those with spindle cell morphology, leiomyosarcoma[21] and schwannoma arising in the mediastinum or retroperitoneum[22] can show expression of cytokeratins, which is usually at most multifocal in distribution. In addition, keratin expression is characteristic of some epithelioid soft tissue tumors, most notably epithelioid sarcoma[23] and synovial sarcoma (biphasic and monophasic types), and also may be present in any epithelioid vascular tumor.[24] Of round cell sarcomas, Ewing sarcoma can show focal expression of cytokeratin as well as neuroendocrine markers, which may lead to an erroneous diagnosis of neuroendocrine tumor.

HEMATOLYMPHOID NEOPLASMS

Although lymphoma is generally readily distinguishable from sarcoma, several hematolymphoid neoplasms may mimic sarcoma and are discussed in the following sections.

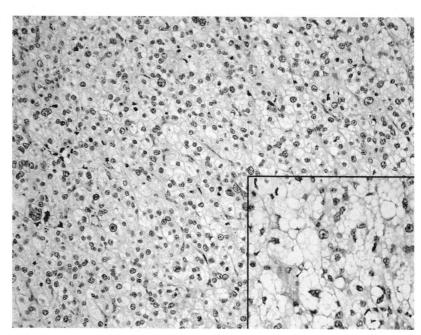

Fig. 6. Epithelioid variant of pleomorphic liposarcoma showing a trabecular growth pattern and composed of cells with abundant palely eosinophilic or clear cytoplasm, resembling adrenal cortical or renal cell carcinoma. The histologic clue to the diagnosis is identification of true lipoblasts, that is, cells with vacuolated cytoplasm and indented or scalloped hyperchromatic nuclei (inset).

ACUTE LYMPHOBLASTIC LYMPHOMA VERSUS ROUND CELL SARCOMA

Lymphoblastic lymphoma, both T-cell and B-cell types, is composed of sheets of relatively monotonous-appearing small to medium-sized lymphocytes with minimal cytoplasm, finely dispersed nuclear chromatin, irregular nuclear contours, and frequent mitoses, and may mimic round cell sarcoma (Fig. 7A). These tumors usually arise in children, and may form tumors in bone but also frequently occur in somatic soft tissue and skin

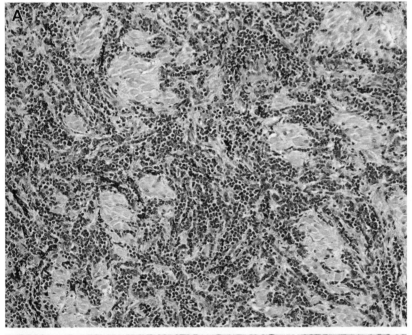

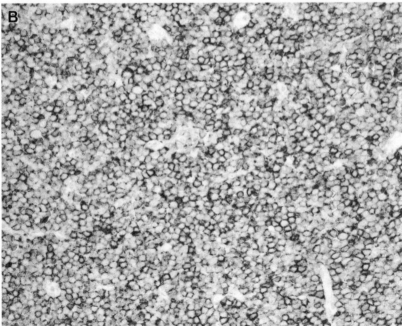

Fig. 7. Lymphoblastic lymphoma may mimic Ewing sarcoma due to both overlapping morphologic and immunohistochemical features. Lymphoblastic lymphoma is composed of sheets of round cells with minimal or small amounts of clear cytoplasm, and may have an associated sclerotic stroma (A). Diffuse membranous CD99 expression is seen in many cases (B), and is a major pitfall in the differential with Ewing sarcoma. Nuclear expression of TdT in lymphoblastic lymphoma (C) distinguishes it from Ewing sarcoma, which is negative for TdT, and subclassification by more specific B-cell and T-cell markers. This case showed expression of CD19 (D), consistent with early precursor B-lymphoblastic lymphoma.

Fig. 7. (continued).

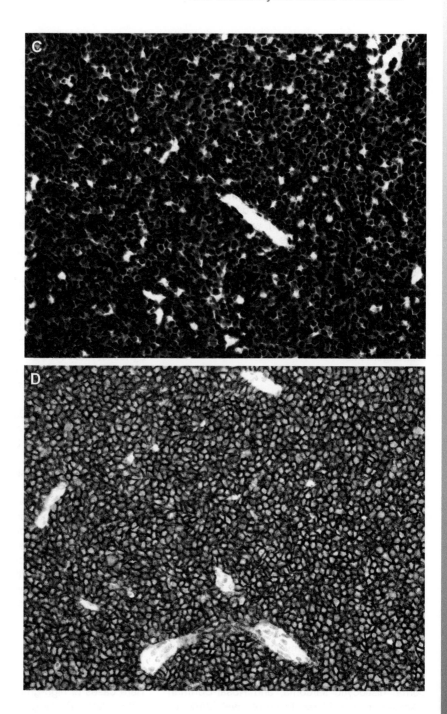

(and mediastinum for T lymphoblastic lymphoma), where they most frequently mimic Ewing sarcoma.[25–27] This is not only because of their shared morphologic features, but also because up to 80% of cases show diffuse membranous expression of CD99, the pattern usually appreciated in Ewing sarcoma (see **Fig. 7**B). Because of this, a high index of suspicion for the diagnosis of lymphoblastic lymphoma should be maintained when faced with any round cell sarcoma. This is particularly important from a prognostic and predictive standpoint, as the chemotherapeutic regimens and prognosis for Ewing sarcoma and lymphoblastic lymphoma differ greatly. Histologic features that favor a diagnosis of Ewing sarcoma include nested growth pattern, rosette formation, and clear cytoplasm, whereas the presence of irregular nuclear membranes is more characteristic of lymphoblastic lymphoma. However, in a given case or in small biopsies, these features may not be identifiable. Fortunately, immunohistochemistry readily distinguishes lymphoblastic lymphoma from its mimics: lymphoblastic lymphoma shows diffuse nuclear positivity for TdT (see Fig. 7C), which is not seen in Ewing sarcoma and is highly specific for lymphoid differentiation in this setting.[28] Further subclassification is afforded by more specific IHC to identify T-cell and B-cell lineage (see Fig. 7D). Other round cell sarcomas that also may mimic lymphoblastic lymphoma include solid variant of alveolar rhabdomyosarcoma, and round cell sarcomas with CIC-DUX4 and BC0R-CCNB3 rearrangements.[29–31]

HISTIOCYTIC SARCOMA

The classification of histiocytic sarcoma as a sarcoma rather than a hematolymphoid neoplasm is somewhat controversial; in fact, many of these tumors were previously classified as lymphoma and they are currently classified in the World Health Organization Classification of Tumors of Hematopoietic and Lymphoid Tissues. However, these tumors tend to show little response to conventional chemotherapeutic agents used in the treatment of lymphoma, and also show a broader range of anatomic sites of involvement, features that in part explain the shift in nomenclature. However, regardless of nosology, because of their rarity and potential to mimic other tumor types (in particular sarcoma), recognition of these neoplasms is often difficult. Histiocytes are phagocytic cells that are derived from myeloid/monocytic cells, and correspondingly histiocytic tumors (including Langerhans cell histiocytosis, Langerhans cell sarcoma, histiocytic sarcoma, and Rosai-Dorfman disease) are considered to be of myeloid/monocyte lineage.

Histiocytic sarcoma is an aggressive malignant neoplasm composed of large pleomorphic cells that show morphologic and immunohistochemical features of mature histiocytes. Patients are usually middle-aged adults, but there is a wide age range. Most tumors arise in extranodal sites, including somatic soft tissue, gastrointestinal tract, and skin, and present with solitary or multiple masses.[32,33] A subset of cases arises in association with

lymphoma (usually non-Hodgkin) or leukemia.[34–36] Histiocytic sarcoma consists of sheets of large round to oval (Fig. 8A, B), and occasionally spindled cells (see Fig. 8C, D), with abundant eosinophilic cytoplasm that may be vacuolated.[32,33] Nuclei are also large and round with irregular nuclear membranes, vesicular chromatin, and variable atypia (see Fig. 8; Fig. 9). The tumor cells are usually pleomorphic, but in some cases may be monomorphic. A prominent inflammatory infiltrate is generally seen, comprising lymphocytes, plasma cells, non-neoplastic histiocytes, and neutrophils. Histiocytic sarcoma therefore may mimic many different tumor types (melanoma, carcinoma, lymphoma), but of mesenchymal neoplasms the main diagnostic considerations include pleomorphic sarcomas, such as undifferentiated/unclassified type, pleomorphic liposarcoma or malignant PEComa, as well as other sarcomas that show a prominent inflammatory infiltrate such as dedifferentiated liposarcoma. Immunohistochemistry is extremely helpful in resolving these differential diagnoses. Histiocytic sarcoma shows membranous and/or cytoplasmic expression of CD163, LCA, and CD45RO, and cytoplasmic expression of CD68 and lysozyme.[32,33] In addition, positivity for CD4, lysozyme, and CD31 is common (see Figs. 8 and 9). S100 protein positivity is found in 50% of cases.[33] Markers of Langerhans cells, B-cells and T-cells are negative, as are CD21, CD35, keratins, and EMA. When arising in the retroperitoneum, the principal differential diagnosis is dedifferentiated liposarcoma; however, in addition to the above immunophenotypic findings, histiocytic sarcoma lacks coexpression of MDM2 and CDK4. At present, relatively little is known about the genetic pathogenesis of histiocytic sarcoma; for cases arising in association with lymphoma or leukemia, similar genetic changes can be seen in both components, but otherwise histiocytic sarcoma lacks clonal IgH or T-cell receptor gene rearrangements.[32]

LYMPHOMA WITH SPINDLE CELL FEATURES

Rare cases of high-grade lymphoma, particularly diffuse large B-cell lymphoma, show a spindled morphology and may have a sclerotic stroma (see Fig. 9A). Recognition of such cases as lymphoma can be extremely difficult, and is usually helped by knowledge of a preceding history of lymphoma or the presence of more conventional-appearing lymphoma within the tumor. Other histologic clues include a somewhat dyshesive growth pattern, convoluted nuclear membranes, and admixed small lymphocytes or other inflammatory cells. Expression of LCA, CD20, and

Fig. 8. Histiocytic sarcoma is typically composed of large polygonal cells with abundant palely eosinophilic cytoplasm and variable amounts of nuclear atypia and pleomorphism with an admixed inflammatory infiltrate (*A, B*). Convoluted nuclear membranes, and somewhat spindled, ovoid or "footprint" nuclear shape may suggest histiocytic lineage (*B*). In some cases, tumor cells have a spindled morphology and are difficult to recognize as histiocytic (*C*).

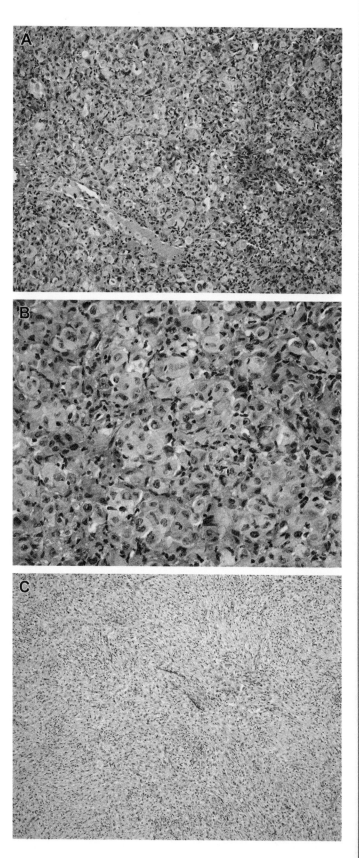

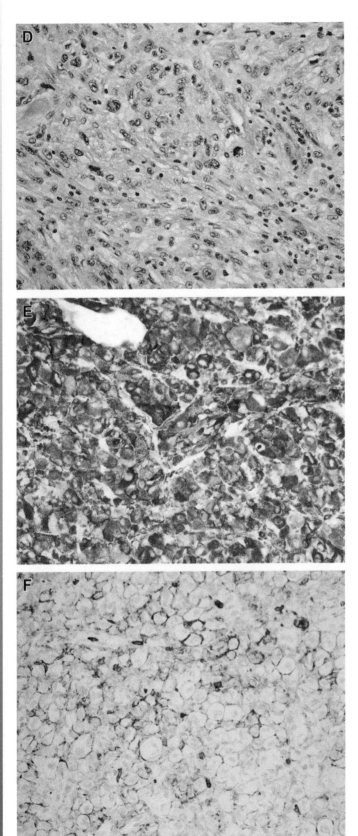

Fig. 8. (continued). The presence of pale eosinophilic and somewhat granular cytoplasm along with nuclear morphology aid recognition (D), but IHC is typically needed to confirm this diagnosis. Tumor cells show variable expression of CD163 (E) and LCA (F). (Cases courtesy of Dr Christopher Fletcher, Brigham and Women's Hospital, Boston, MA.)

Fig. 9. Diffuse large B-cell lymphoma with spindle cell morphology (*A*). The tumor cells show diffuse expression of LCA (*B*) and CD20 (*B,* inset). (*Case courtesy of* Dr Christopher Fletcher, Brigham and Women's Hospital, Boston, MA.)

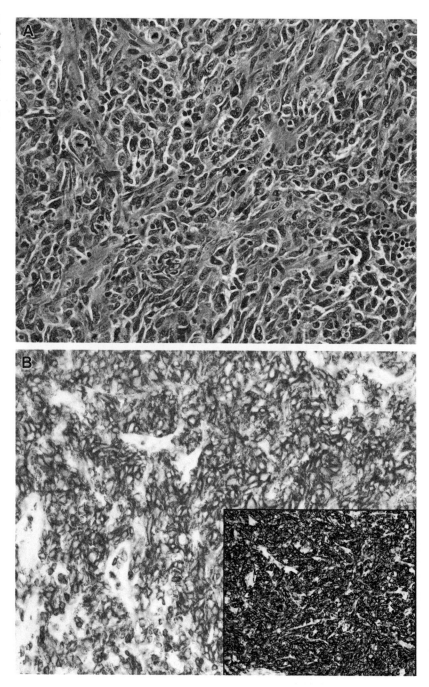

BSAP/PAX5 confirms B-lymphocytic differentiation (see Fig. 9B). The presence of PAX8 expression in lymphoma, due to cross-reactivity with PAX5, should be kept in mind to avoid an erroneous diagnosis of sarcomatoid renal cell carcinoma. Other lymphomas that may show a spindled morphology include anaplastic lymphoma kinase (ALK)-positive anaplastic large-cell lymphoma and primary cutaneous follicle center lymphoma.[37–39]

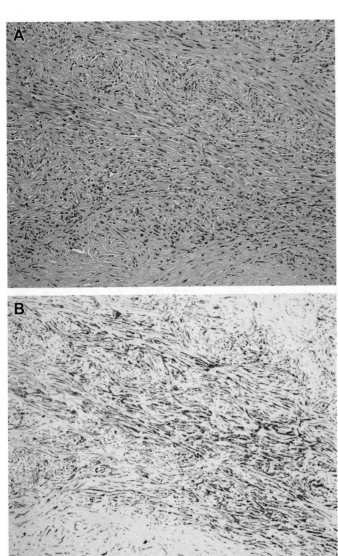

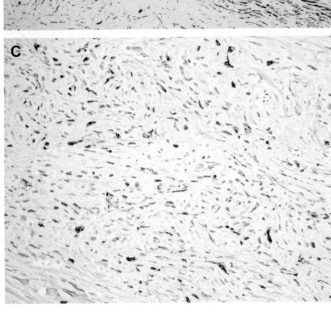

Fig. 10. Sarcomatoid malignant mesothelioma may resemble many different
sarcoma types or sarcomatoid carcinoma
(*A*). The tumor cells show variable
expression of keratins, in this case AE1/
AE3 (*B*). Nuclear WT-1 expression is
only occasionally seen in sarcomatoid
malignant mesothelioma, and in this
case is multifocal (*C*).

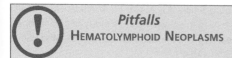

Pitfalls
HEMATOLYMPHOID NEOPLASMS

! Lymphoblastic lymphoma may mimic round-cell sarcomas, in particular Ewing sarcoma due to the presence of diffuse membranous CD99 expression in both tumor types, and should be distinguished if any uncertainty remains, either by IHC for TdT or FISH/reverse-transcriptase polymerase cell reaction to identify fusion genes of Ewing sarcoma

! Rarely, diffuse large B-cell lymphoma has a spindled morphology and may mimic sarcoma

! Expression of PAX8 can be seen in lymphoid neoplasms due to cross reactivity for PAX5

! Histiocytic sarcoma may mimic high-grade pleomorphic sarcomas or spindle cell sarcomas, and should be considered in tumors that show a prominent admixed inflammatory infiltrate

MALIGNANT MESOTHELIOMA

Within the pleura and less commonly the abdominal cavity, malignant mesothelioma may mimic several different sarcoma types, most often when it shows spindled or sarcomatoid morphology. Most primary peritoneal mesotheliomas are epithelioid, and the main differential diagnosis is with papillary serous carcinoma of gynecologic origin or other carcinomas. Although epithelioid mesothelioma is usually readily recognizable, sarcomatoid mesothelioma is more difficult to recognize, and is less likely to be considered as a diagnostic possibility within the abdominal cavity. Sarcomatoid variants may mimic dedifferentiated liposarcoma, inflammatory myofibroblastic tumor (IMT), sclerosing mesenteritis, or sarcomatoid carcinoma when occurring in the abdominal cavity (**Fig. 10A**).

Features suggestive of sarcomatoid mesothelioma include diffuse growth throughout the abdomen and keratin positivity in an otherwise nondescript spindle cell neoplasm without features of dedifferentiated liposarcoma, IMT, or other spindle cell mesenchymal neoplasms that occur in the retroperitoneum. Although mesothelioma generally shows consistent expression of cytokeratins, such as pancytokeratin or AE1/AE3, more specific "mesothelioma" markers (ie, CK5/6 and WT1) are usually negative in sarcomatoid variants (see **Fig. 10B, C**).[40] Calretinin is expressed in 70% of sarcomatoid mesotheliomas, but expression also is seen in 60% of sarcomatoid

carcinomas and up to 20% of sarcomas.[40,41] Due to the variability of staining between different tumors, a panel of stains is usually needed. IHC for MDM2/CDK4 and ALK should distinguish mesothelioma from dedifferentiated liposarcoma and IMT, respectively. The rare "deciduoid" variant of mesothelioma that arises within pleural or peritoneal cavities is composed of sheets of large cells with abundant eosinophilic cytoplasm and prominent nucleoli, resembling ectopic decidua.[42,43] This variant of mesothelioma may mimic histiocytic neoplasms, germ cell tumors, or carcinoma, and has an aggressive clinical course.

SUMMARY

Knowledge of the histologic overlap between non-mesenchymal neoplasms (melanoma, sarcomatoid carcinoma, mesothelioma, and some hematolymphoid neoplasms) and different sarcoma types is essential in all areas of pathology to avoid erroneous diagnoses, which may have significant clinical implications. This article has reviewed the most commonly encountered settings in which such differential diagnoses are encountered, along with clinical and histologic clues to distinguish these different tumor types and to guide the appropriate use of ancillary tests.

REFERENCES

1. Nonaka D, Chiriboga L, Rubin BP. Sox10: a pan-schwannian and melanocytic marker. Am J Surg Pathol 2008;32:1291–8.

2. Karamchandani JR, Nielsen TO, van de Rijn M, et al. Sox10 and S100 in the diagnosis of soft-tissue neoplasms. Appl Immunohistochem Mol Morphol 2012; 20:445–50.

3. Naujokas A, Charli-Joseph Y, Ruben BS, et al. SOX-10 expression in cutaneous myoepitheliomas and mixed tumors. J Cutan Pathol 2014;41:353–63.

4. Mohamed A, Gonzalez RS, Lawson D, et al. SOX10 expression in malignant melanoma, carcinoma, and normal tissues. Appl Immunohistochem Mol Morphol 2013;21:506–10.

5. Zhou H, Coffin CM, Perkins SL, et al. Malignant peripheral nerve sheath tumor: a comparison of grade, immunophenotype, and cell cycle/growth activation marker expression in sporadic and neurofibromatosis 1-related lesions. Am J Surg Pathol 2003;27:1337–45.

6. Wick MR, Swanson PE, Scheithauer BW, et al. Malignant peripheral nerve sheath tumor. An immunohistochemical study of 62 cases. Am J Clin Pathol 1987;87:425–33.

7. Jo VY, Fletcher CD. Epithelioid malignant peripheral nerve sheath tumor: clinicopathologic analysis of 63 cases. Am J Surg Pathol 2015;39(5):673–82.

8. Hiraga H, Nojima T, Abe S, et al. Establishment of a new continuous clear cell sarcoma cell line: morphological and cytogenetic characterization and detection of chimaeric EWS/ATF-1 transcripts. Virchows Arch 1997;431:45–51.

9. Stenman G, Kindblom LG, Angervall L. Reciprocal translocation t(12;22)(q13;q13) in clear-cell sarcoma of tendons and aponeuroses. Genes Chromosomes Cancer 1992;4:122–7.

10. Antonescu CR, Nafa K, Segal NH, et al. EWS-CREB1: a recurrent variant fusion in clear cell sarcoma–association with gastrointestinal location and absence of melanocytic differentiation. Clin Cancer Res 2006;12:5356–62.

11. Dwyer JB, Clark BZ. Low-grade fibromatosis-like spindle cell carcinoma of the breast. Arch Pathol Lab Med 2015;139:552–7.

12. Gobbi H, Simpson JF, Borowsky A, et al. Metaplastic breast tumors with a dominant fibromatosis-like phenotype have a high risk of local recurrence. Cancer 1999;85:2170–82.

13. Tse GM, Tan PH, Putti TC, et al. Metaplastic carcinoma of the breast: a clinicopathological review. J Clin Pathol 2006;59:1079–83.

14. Carter MR, Hornick JL, Lester S, et al. Spindle cell (sarcomatoid) carcinoma of the breast: a clinicopathologic and immunohistochemical analysis of 29 cases. Am J Surg Pathol 2006;30:300–9.

15. Davis WG, Hennessy B, Babiera G, et al. Metaplastic sarcomatoid carcinoma of the breast with absent or minimal overt invasive carcinomatous component: a misnomer. Am J Surg Pathol 2005;29:1456–63.

16. Miller K, Goodlad JR, Brenn T. Pleomorphic dermal sarcoma: adverse histologic features predict aggressive behavior and allow distinction from atypical fibroxanthoma. Am J Surg Pathol 2012;36(9):1317–26.

17. Montgomery E, Epstein JI. Anastomosing hemangioma of the genitourinary tract: a lesion mimicking angiosarcoma. Am J Surg Pathol 2009;33:1364–9.

18. Kryvenko ON, Roquero L, Gupta NS, et al. Low-grade clear cell renal cell carcinoma mimicking hemangioma of the kidney: a series of 4 cases. Arch Pathol Lab Med 2013;137:251–4.

19. Hornick JL, Bosenberg MW, Mentzel T, et al. Pleomorphic liposarcoma: clinicopathologic analysis of 57 cases. Am J Surg Pathol 2004;28:1257–67.

20. Huang HY, Antonescu CR. Epithelioid variant of pleomorphic liposarcoma: a comparative immunohistochemical and ultrastructural analysis of six cases with emphasis on overlapping features with epithelial malignancies. Ultrastruct Pathol 2002;26:299–308.

21. Iwata J, Fletcher CD. Immunohistochemical detection of cytokeratin and epithelial membrane antigen in leiomyosarcoma: a systematic study of 100 cases. Pathol Int 2000;50:7–14.

22. Fanburg-Smith JC, Majidi M, Miettinen M. Keratin expression in schwannoma; a study of 115 retroperitoneal and 22 peripheral schwannomas. Mod Pathol 2006;19:115–21.

23. Miettinen M, Fanburg-Smith JC, Virolainen M, et al. Epithelioid sarcoma: an immunohistochemical analysis of 112 classical and variant cases and a discussion of the differential diagnosis. Hum Pathol 1999;30:934–42.

24. McCluggage WG, Clarke R, Toner PG. Cutaneous epithelioid angiosarcoma exhibiting cytokeratin positivity. Histopathology 1995;27:291–4.

25. Maitra A, McKenna RW, Weinberg AG, et al. Precursor B-cell lymphoblastic lymphoma. A study of nine cases lacking blood and bone marrow involvement and review of the literature. Am J Clin Pathol 2001;115:868–75.

26. Lin P, Jones D, Dorfman DM, et al. Precursor B-cell lymphoblastic lymphoma: a predominantly extranodal tumor with low propensity for leukemic involvement. Am J Surg Pathol 2000;24:1480–90.

27. Sheibani K, Nathwani BN, Winberg CD, et al. Antigenically defined subgroups of lymphoblastic lymphoma. Relationship to clinical presentation and biologic behavior. Cancer 1987;60:183–90.

28. Kung PC, Long JC, McCaffrey RP, et al. Terminal deoxynucleotidyl transferase in the diagnosis of leukemia and malignant lymphoma. Am J Med 1978;64:788–94.

29. Choi EY, Thomas DG, McHugh JB, et al. Undifferentiated small round cell sarcoma with t(4;19)(q35;q13.1) CIC-DUX4 fusion: a novel highly aggressive soft tissue tumor with distinctive histopathology. Am J Surg Pathol 2013;37:1379–86.

30. Italiano A, Sung YS, Zhang L, et al. High prevalence of CIC fusion with double-homeobox (DUX4) transcription factors in EWSR1-negative undifferentiated small blue round cell sarcomas. Genes Chromosomes Cancer 2012;51:207–18.

31. Pierron G, Tirode F, Lucchesi C, et al. A new subtype of bone sarcoma defined by BCOR-CCNB3 gene fusion. Nat Genet 2012;44:461–6.

32. Copie-Bergman C, Wotherspoon AC, Norton AJ, et al. True histiocytic lymphoma: a morphologic, immunohistochemical, and molecular genetic study of 13 cases. Am J Surg Pathol 1998;22:1386–92.

33. Hornick JL, Jaffe ES, Fletcher CD. Extranodal histiocytic sarcoma: clinicopathologic analysis of 14 cases of a rare epithelioid malignancy. Am J Surg Pathol 2004;28:1133–44.

34. Feldman AL, Minniti C, Santi M, et al. Histiocytic sarcoma after acute lymphoblastic leukaemia: a common clonal origin. Lancet Oncol 2004;5:248–50.

35. Feldman AL, Arber DA, Pittaluga S, et al. Clonally related follicular lymphomas and histiocytic/dendritic cell sarcomas: evidence for transdifferentiation of the follicular lymphoma clone. Blood 2008;111:5433–9.

36. Shao H, Xi L, Raffeld M, et al. Clonally related histio-cytic/dendritic cell sarcoma and chronic lympho-cytic leukemia/small lymphocytic lymphoma: a study of seven cases. Mod Pathol 2011;24:1421–32.
37. Charli-Joseph Y, Cerroni L, LeBoit PE. Cutaneous spindle-cell B-cell lymphomas: most are neoplasms of follicular center cell origin. Am J Surg Pathol 2015; 39:737–43.
38. Jghaimi F, Hocar O, Akhdari N, et al. Primary cuta-neous spindle-cell B-cell lymphoma of follicle center cell origin. Am J Dermatopathol 2013;35:871–3.
39. Wang L, Lv Y, Wang X, et al. Giant primary cuta-neous spindle cell B-cell lymphoma of follicle center cell origin. Am J Dermatopathol 2010;32:628–32.
40. Lucas DR, Pass HI, Madan SK, et al. Sarcomatoid mesothelioma and its histological mimics: a compar-ative immunohistochemical study. Histopathology 2003;42:270–9.
41. Zhang K, Deng H, Cagle PT. Utility of immunohisto-chemistry in the diagnosis of pleuropulmonary and mediastinal cancers: a review and update. Arch Pathol Lab Med 2014;138:1611–28.
42. Shia J, Erlandson RA, Klimstra DS. Deciduoid meso-thelioma: a report of 5 cases and literature review. Ultrastruct Pathol 2002;26:355–63.
43. Ordonez NG. Deciduoid mesothelioma: report of 21 cases with review of the literature. Mod Pathol 2012; 25:1481–95.

Genetics of Gastrointestinal Stromal Tumors
A Heterogeneous Family of Tumors?

Deepa T. Patil, MD[a],*, Brian P. Rubin, MD, PhD[a,b]

KEYWORDS

• GIST • KIT • PDGFRA • Succinate dehydrogenase • BRAF

ABSTRACT

pproximately 85–90% of adult gastrointestinal stromal tumors (GISTs) harbor *KIT* and *PDGFRA* mutations. The remaining cases, including the majority of pediatric GISTs, lack these mutations, and have been designated as *KIT/PDGFRA* wild-type (WT) GISTs. Nearly 15% of WT GISTs harbor *BRAF* mutations, while others arise in patients with type I neurofibromatosis. Recent work has confirmed that 20–40% of *KIT/PDGFRA* WT GISTs show loss of function of succinate dehydrogenase complex. Less than 5% of GISTs lack known molecular alterations ("quadruple-negative" GISTs). Thus, it is important to consider genotyping these tumors to help better define their clinical behavior and therapy.

OVERVIEW

Gastrointestinal stromal tumors (GIST) are the most common mesenchymal tumors of the gastrointestinal tract. Since the first report of gain-of-function *KIT* mutations by Hirota and colleagues,[1] our understanding regarding the genetic alterations in GISTs has significantly evolved to a point that GISTs are now best considered as tumors with heterogeneous disease-initiating molecular events. The goal of this review is to elaborate on the latest molecular underpinnings of GISTs and to discuss their implications on clinical management.

GENOTYPES OF GASTROINTESTINAL STROMAL TUMOR

It is now widely accepted that GISTs arise from interstitial cells of Cajal (ICC) or from an ICC precursor.[2,3] Because it was noted that KIT deficiency causes loss of ICC in mouse models, Hirota and colleagues[1] decided to examine GISTs, and found that they showed strong KIT expression, and had activating *KIT* mutations. This seminal study was followed by many subsequent studies that confirmed and expanded this finding.[4] Nearly 75% to 80% of GISTs harbor *KIT* mutations, whereas 10% demonstrate gain-of-function mutations in platelet-derived growth factor receptor alpha (*PDGFRA*). The remaining 10% to 15% of GISTs lack *KIT* and *PDGFRA* mutations, and have previously been designated as wild-type (WT) GISTs. Several studies have now shown that the subgroup of WT-GISTs consists of GISTs that harbor molecular abnormalities in genes encoding succinate dehydrogenase (SDH)-ubiquinone complex II,[5–10] as well as those that carry mutations in *BRAF*[11–14] and *NF-1*.[15] The frequency of these genotypes has been summarized in **Table 1**.

KIT MUTATIONS

KIT mutations found in GIST result in constitutive activation of the receptor tyrosine kinase pathway in the absence of KIT ligand. Exons 9, 11, 13, and

Disclaimers: B.P. Rubin is a member of the Novartis Speakers Bureau and has served on Advisory Boards for Novartis.
[a] Department of Pathology, Robert J. Tomsich Pathology and Laboratory Medicine Institute, Cleveland Clinic, 9500 Euclid Avenue, L-25, Cleveland, OH 44195, USA; [b] Department of Molecular Genetics, Cleveland Clinic and Lerner Research Institute, 9500 Euclid Avenue, L-25, Cleveland, OH 44195, USA
* Corresponding author. Department of Pathology, Cleveland Clinic Lerner College of Medicine, Cleveland Clinic, 9500 Euclid Avenue, L-25, Cleveland, OH 44195.
E-mail address: patild@ccf.org

surgpath.theclinics.com

Table 1
GIST genotypes

Genotype	Relative Frequency	Germline Examples
KIT mutation (relative frequency 70%–80%)		
Exon 8	Rare	Yes
Exon 9 insertion AY502–503	10%	None
Exon 11 (deletions, single nucleotide substitutions and insertions)	67%	Yes
Exon 13 K642E	1%	Yes
Exon 17 D820Y, N822K, and Y823D	1%	Yes
PDGFRA mutation (relative frequency 5%–15%)		
Exon 12	1%	Yes
Exon 14	<1%	None
Exon 18 D842V	5%	None
Exon 18 (such as deletion of amino acids IMHD 842–846)	1%	Yes
KIT and *PDGFRA* wild-type (relative frequency 12%–15%)		
BRAF V600E	3%	None
SDHA, SDHB, SDHC, and *SDHD* mutations	3%	Yes, including Carney-Stratakis
SDHC hypermethylation – Carney Triad	Rare	No
NF1-related	Rare	Yes
Quadruple wild-type	Rare	No

Abbreviations: GIST, gastrointestinal stromal tumor; NF1, neurofibromatosis type 1; *PDGFRA*, platelet-derived growth factor receptor a; SDH, succinate dehydrogenase.

17 are most often mutated in sporadic GISTs. The vast majority of *KIT* mutations (nearly 65%) involve the juxtamembrane domain (exon 11), followed by extracellular domain (exon 9, 9%), tyrosine kinase I: ATP binding pocket (exon 13; 1%) and tyrosine kinase II: kinase activation loop (exon 17; 1%; **Fig. 1**).[16,17] Very rarely, mutations in exons 8, 12, 14, and 18, have been found in primary GISTs.

Exon 11 mutations include missense mutations, in-frame deletions, insertions, or a combination of these alterations. Oncogenic exon 11 mutations are most commonly composed of in-frame deletions of one or more codons; some of these (codons 557–558) are typically associated with poor clinical outcome.[18] Missense point mutations are the next most common type of mutations. Stomach is the most common site of involvement, and these tumors often show a spindled morphology (**Fig. 2A–C**). In gastric GISTs, exon 11 mutations are associated with a better prognosis, and a more reliable response to imatinib therapy.[19] However, no such correlation has been documented with exon 11–mutated small intestinal GISTs.[20,21]

Virtually all exon 9 mutations are characterized by a 6-nucleotide duplication encoding Ala and Tyr at amino acid residues 502 and 503.[22] These mutations are usually associated with small or large intestinal GISTs (especially rectum).[21,23] A meta-analysis of randomized phase 3 clinical trials has shown that patients with *KIT* exon-9 mutant GISTs have a median progression-free survival that is 1 year longer in those treated with 800 mg imatinib versus those treated with a 400-mg dose.[24] More recently, it was shown that in itself, the presence of this mutation does not have any prognostic relevance.[23]

Exon 13 and 17 mutations are very rare (<1%–2%). Exon 13 mutations are almost always a substitution of aspartate for lysine at residue 642, and most commonly arise in the stomach. Exon 17 mutations are mostly substitutions and occur predominantly in small intestinal GISTs.[4] Although in vitro studies have indicated that they may be less sensitive to imatinib, there are reports of clinical responses with imatinib in primary exon 17–mutant GISTs.[4,16]

PLATELET-DERIVED GROWTH FACTOR RECEPTOR ALPHA MUTATIONS

Like KIT, PDGFRA is a type III receptor tyrosine kinase and similar to KIT, activating mutations result in downstream activation of multiple

Fig. 1. Schematic diagram showing the locations and frequency of activating KIT and PDGFRA mutations in gastrointestinal stromal tumor. [a] Refers to exons most commonly involved by secondary/acquired mutations. (*From* Patil DT, Rubin BP. Gastrointestinal stromal tumor: advances in diagnosis and management. Arch Path Lab Med 2011;135:1303; with permission from College of American Pathologists.)

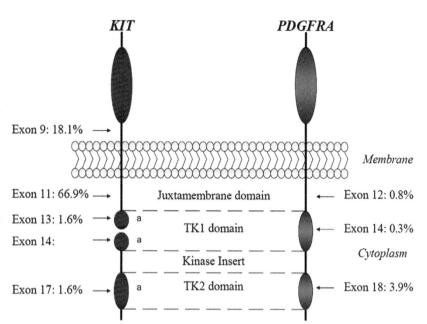

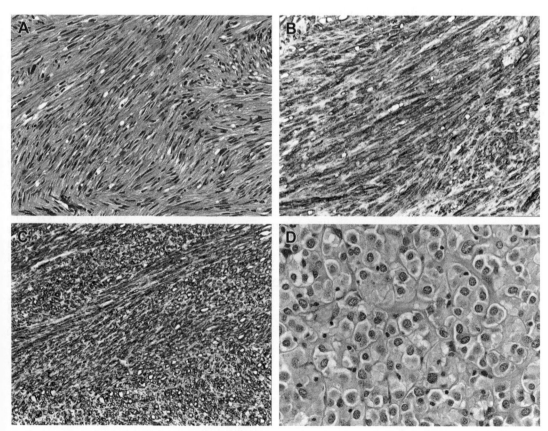

Fig. 2. Gastrointestinal stromal tumor with *KIT* exon 11 mutation showing spindle-cell phenotype (*A*). The tumor showed diffuse expression of CD117 (*B*) and DOG1 (*C*). Part (*D*) shows an example of an epithelioid GIST with *PDGFRA* mutation ([A, D] Hematoxylin-eosin, original magnification [A] ×100; [B] ×100; [C] ×100; [D] ×400).

cell-signaling cascades that control vital cellular functions. Both *KIT* and *PDGFRA* are located on the long arm of chromosome 4.[25] Exon 18, exon 12, and exon 14 are the 3 *PDGFRA* regions that are mutated in GISTs. They correspond to the exon 17, exon 11, and exon 13 *KIT* mutations (see **Fig. 1**). Overall, nearly 7% of GISTs harbor *PDGFRA* mutations and more than 80% are missense D842V mutations in exon 18. They have a strong predilection for stomach, mesentery, and omentum. Histologically, they exhibit an epithelioid phenotype accompanied by myxoid stroma and multinucleated and rhabdoid cells (see **Fig. 2D**). *KIT* and *PDGFRA* mutations are mutually exclusive.[26] *PDGFRA*-mutant GISTs tend to be faintly positive or completely negative for KIT by immunohistochemistry. In general, this subset of GISTs has a lower risk of recurrence compared with *KIT*-mutant GISTs.

FAMILIAL GASTROINTESTINAL STROMAL TUMOR SYNDROME

Although quite rare, some individuals carry germline mutations in *KIT* or *PDGFRA* that result in an inherited predisposition to developing multiple GISTs.[27,28] Since their original description by Nishida and colleagues,[29] an additional 27 families with familial GIST have been identified.[27,30] These mutations are identical to those found in sporadic tumors, and are inherited in an autosomal dominant pattern.[29,31–33] Every family member who harbors a germline *KIT* mutation will develop Cajal

cell hyperplasia and eventually, one or more GISTs, usually at a much younger age when compared with sporadic tumors. Clinically, many members of familial GIST syndrome kindreds manifest with cutaneous findings that include hyperpigmentation (especially perineal), increased numbers of nevi, and mast cell disease in the form of urticaria pigmentosa or even systemic mastocytosis.[33,34] Morphologically, these tumors are indistinguishable from sporadic GISTs.

SO-CALLED *KIT*/PLATELET-DERIVED GROWTH FACTOR RECEPTOR ALPHA–WILD-TYPE GASTROINTESTINAL STROMAL TUMORS

Tumors that do not harbor either the *KIT* or *PDGFRA* mutations account for approximately 15% of GISTs. Based on recent studies, we now know that other molecular alterations account for this subset of tumors. These include SDHB-deficient GISTs, *BRAF*-mutated GISTs, and those that contain *NF-1* mutations.

SUCCINATE DEHYDROGENASE B–DEFICIENT GASTROINTESTINAL STROMAL TUMORS

SDH is an enzyme complex located within the inner mitochondrial membrane that participates in the citric acid cycle and the electron transport chain (**Fig. 3**). This complex consists of SDHA, SDHB, SDHC, and SDHD subunits, and is normally present in mitochondria of all nucleated eukaryotic cells. Inactivation of any one of these

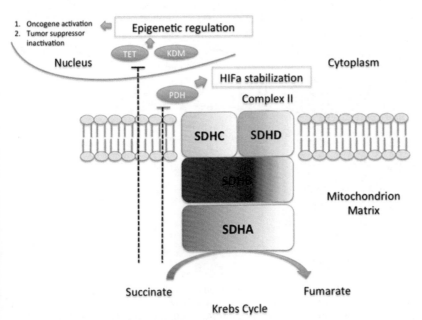

Fig. 3. SDH complex and epigenetic regulation. PHD, prolyl hydroxylase. (*Adapted from* Boikos SA, Stratakis CA. The genetic landscape of gastrointestinal stromal tumor lacking KIT and PDGFRA mutations. Endocrine 2014;47:402; with permission; and *Courtesy of* Springer Science and Business Media ©2014; with permission.)

SDH subunits results in loss of enzymatic function. Between 20% and 40% of KIT/PDGFRA wild-type GISTs show loss of function of SDH. In general, these tumors have been variably designated as SDH-deficient GISTs, "Type 2" GISTs, "pediatric-type" GISTs, or SDHB-negative GISTs, because they show loss of SDHB expression by immunohistochemistry.

Much of the recent effort has been geared toward understanding the oncogenic effect of the SDH enzyme complex dysfunction. The most frequent molecular events include germline mutations in SDH in at least half of the patients with SDH-deficient GISTs, complemented by somatic mutations in the second SDH allele in these tumors. SDH deficiency leads to accumulation of succinate, which inhibits dioxygenases ten-eleven translocation (TET) and histone lysine (K) demethylases (KDM).[35] In addition, succinate inhibits hypoxia-inducible factor 1 alpha (HIF-1α)-prolyl hydroxylases in the cytosol, leading to stabilization and activation of HIF-1α.[36] More recently, it was shown that SDH-deficient GISTs arise as a result of a failure in TET2 maintenance demethylation.[37] Elevated levels of intracellular succinate are toxic for the dioxygenase TET2, an enzyme required to catalyze DNA demethylation by conversion of 5-methylcytosine to 5-hydroxymethyl-cytosine, which is the initial step in the DNA demethylation pathway.

In patients who lack SDH-germline mutations, activation of the HIF signaling pathway was shown to be one of the mechanisms driving tumorigenesis. In another study, overexpression of type 1 insulin-like growth factor receptor (IGF1R) was found to be associated with SDH-deficient GISTs.[38] In this study, 89% of gastric SDH-deficient GISTs expressed IGF1R by immunohistochemistry, compared with 1% of gastric GISTs with intact SDHB expression. The exact molecular mechanism for IGF1R expression is yet to be determined; although phase 1b trials using R1507, a monoclonal antibody to IGF1R,[39] appear promising, and results from another phase 2 clinical trial using Linsitinib (NCT01560260) for WT-GISTs are pending. More recently, in an attempt to further understand the mechanism of SDH deactivation, Killian and colleagues[40] performed genome-wide DNA methylation and expression profiling on 59 SDH-deficient GISTs. SDHC promoter-specific CpG island hypermethylation and resultant gene silencing was observed in 15 of 16 (94%) of SDH-deficient GISTs that lacked actual SDH mutations. These results indicate that SDHC epimutation is the molecular basis for dysfunction of the SDH complex in most SDH-deficient GISTs that lack SDH mutations. In addition, SDHC epimutation appears to be the basis for the Carney triad (see later in this article).

SDH-deficient GISTs can be subdivided into syndromic (associated with Carney-Stratakis syndrome and Carney triad) versus nonsyndromic GISTs. SDH-deficient GISTs share some distinctive clinicopathologic features. The tumors commonly arise in the stomach, especially distal stomach and antrum. Histologically, they have a characteristic multinodular/plexiform growth pattern, with nodules that are separated by smooth muscle fibers of muscularis propria (Fig. 4). The individual cells show a predominantly epithelioid morphology with variably eosinophilic cytoplasm. Lymphovascular invasion can be seen in up to 50% of cases, and lymph node metastasis appears to be a characteristic feature of this group of GISTs.[41,42]

Immunohistochemically, the tumors are diffusely positive for KIT and DOG1. Regardless of the subtype of the deficient subunit (A, B, C, or D), SDH-deficient GISTs lack granular cytoplasmic staining with anti-SDHB antibody. Presence of intact staining within the adjacent stromal and vascular endothelial cells serves as a useful internal control when interpreting this stain (see Fig. 4).

Despite demonstrating aggressive features, such as lymphovascular invasion, lymph node metastasis, and liver and/or peritoneal involvement, most SDH-deficient GISTs follow an indolent clinical course. These tumors do not follow the risk assessment prediction model of conventional KIT/PDGFRA-mutated GISTs, and often show limited (if any) response to imatinib therapy.[43,44]

CARNEY-STRATAKIS SYNDROME–RELATED GASTROINTESTINAL STROMAL TUMORS

Carney-Stratakis syndrome (CSS)-related GISTs occur as a result of germline mutation in the SDH enzyme subunits.[45] CSS shows an autosomal dominant mode of inheritance with incomplete penetrance. Clinically, patients with CSS present with multifocal GISTs, paragangliomas, and pheochromocytomas. CSS-related GISTs also lack SDHB staining by immunohistochemistry.[6,7] Patients are usually older than those with Carney triad and the male-to-female ratio is 1:1.

CARNEY TRIAD–RELATED GASTROINTESTINAL STROMAL TUMORS

Carney triad usually occurs in young women who present with a combination of gastric GIST, para-ganglioma, and pulmonary chondroma.[46–48] The etiology of Carney triad continues to remain

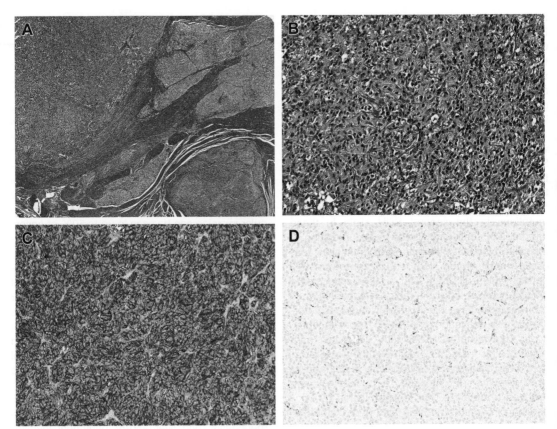

Fig. 4. SDH-deficient GIST. This gastric tumor shows a characteristic multinodular/plexiform growth pattern separated by fibers of muscularis propria (*A*). The individual cells show an epithelioid morphology with abundant eosinophilic cytoplasm (*B*). The cells are diffusely positive for DOG1 (*C*) and show loss of SDHB protein expression (*D*). Note that the stromal and endothelial cells retain granular immunoreactivity with SDHB and serve as a positive internal control ([A, B] Hematoxylin-eosin, original magnification [A] ×20; [B] x100; [C] ×100; [D] ×100).

elusive. Comparative genomic hybridization study by Matyakhina and colleagues[48] have shown genetic alterations in the 1q, 1p, 14q, and 22q chromosomal loci. Although *SDHB* and *SDHC* are localized to 1p and 1q regions, sequencing studies have not identified any of these mutations in patients with Carney triad.[45] In an attempt to further investigate the molecular events in Carney triad, Haller and colleagues[49] performed a broad, high-resolution, and quantitative assessment of DNA methylation in the proximity of transcriptional initiation sites of all 4 genes encoding the SDH subunits in tumors from 4 patients with Carney triad who did not have any SDH-coding sequence abnormalities. They found a novel recurrent aberrant dense DNA methylation at the gene locus of *SDHC* in tumors of patients with Carney triad, which was not present in tumors of patients with Carney-Stratakis syndrome or paragangliomas, or in sporadic GISTs with *KIT* mutations. This DNA methylation pattern was found to result in reduced mRNA expression of SDHC, and

concurrent loss of SDHC protein expression. In the study by Killian and colleagues,[40] 6 of 8 patients with Carney triad showed *SDHC* promoter methylation (5-homozygous, 1-hemimethylated). The other 2 patients who lacked *SDHC* promoter methylation in their tumors were found to harbor *SDHA* mutations. These data highlight epigenetic inactivation of *SDHC* as a common tumorigenic event in GISTs in patients with Carney triad; however, there appears to be a small subset of Carney triad GISTs that may have mutations in other SDH subunits, and still maintain *SDHC* transcription.

SPORADIC SUCCINATE DEHYDROGENASE–DEFICIENT GASTROINTESTINAL STROMAL TUMORS

In a recent study, it was observed that patients with WT-GISTs, with or without *SDH* mutations, can lack SDHB expression.[8] Based on cumulative data, it appears that approximately one-fourth of GISTs that lack SDHB expression by immunohistochemistry

(IHC) show mutations in *SDHA*.[50–52] These patients lack SDHA expression by IHC, and compared with tumors with intact SDHA expression, they tend to have an older median age at presentation, a lower female-to-male ratio, and are associated with *SDHA* germline mutations.[52]

BRAF-MUTATED GASTROINTESTINAL STROMAL TUMORS

Recently, nearly 7% to 13% of adult WT-GISTs have been shown to harbor *BRAF* V600E mutations at exon 15.[11–13] BRAF belongs to the RAF family of serine/threonine protein kinases that is involved in cell-cycle regulation and growth signaling via the MAP kinase pathway. Located downstream of KIT, BRAF is activated by the V600E mutation and supports KIT-independent growth of GIST cells.

Historically, these mutations have been detected using sequencing-based techniques. More recently, the *BRAF* V600E mutant-specific antibody VE1 became available for detecting *BRAF* mutations via IHC.[53]

In a recent study performed at the Cleveland Clinic, we found strong and diffuse BRAF expression in 2 of 38 (5.2%) consecutive cases of GISTs.[54] Sequencing analysis confirmed the presence of *BRAF* V600E mutation in both these cases, thus documenting 100% specificity and 100% sensitivity in detecting *BRAF* V600E mutation using the VE1 antibody. Both these tumors were incidentally found within the stomach, and measured 0.8 cm and 1.0 cm in greatest dimension (**Fig. 5**). Based on previous studies that have examined *BRAF* mutations in GISTs,[11–13,55] most *BRAF*-mutated tumors appear to originate within the small bowel and demonstrate spindle-cell morphology. Stomach is an uncommon site of origin, and only 4 examples of gastric *BRAF*-mutated GISTs have been described thus far.[11–13,55] Similar to our cases, all 4 cases of gastric *BRAF*-mutated GISTs reported in the literature demonstrated spindle-cell morphology. The tumor sizes (documented in 3 cases) and risk of

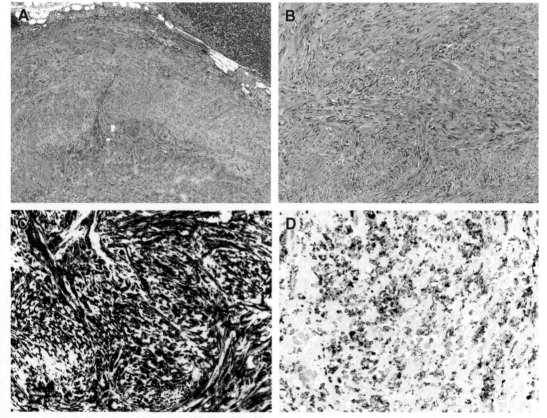

Fig. 5. BRAF V600E allele-specific antibody-positive GIST. This example was a 0.8-cm gastric GIST from a 42-year-old woman. The tumors were composed of spindle cells (*A, B*) and were diffusely positive for CD117 and DOG1 (*C*). Note the diffuse and strong granular cytoplasmic BRAF V600E expression (*D*). This lesion was confirmed to have heterozygous *BRAF* V600E mutation ([A, B] Hematoxylin-eosin, original magnification [A] ×20; [B] ×100; [C] ×100; [D] ×100).

progressive disease were 3 cm (very low), 4 cm (very low), and 10.5 cm (intermediate). Thus far, it appears that there are no histologic features that are distinctive of *BRAF*-mutated GISTs. Based on the results of our study, we believe that VE1 antibody can be used as a reflex test in routine practice, specifically in unresectable/metastatic GISTs that are found to be negative for *KIT/PDGFRA* mutation and that would benefit from targeted therapy using BRAF-inhibitors.

NEUROFIBROMATOSIS TYPE 1-ASSOCIATED GASTROINTESTINAL STROMAL TUMORS

Multiple GISTs also arise in the setting of neurofibromatosis type 1 (NF1). This syndrome results from germline mutation of the *NF1* gene, which encodes for a GTPase-activating protein, neurofibromin. Approximately 7% of patients with NF1 have GISTs.[56] NF1-related GISTs most commonly occur as multiple small tumors in the small bowel and exhibit spindle-cell morphology. They are replete with skenoid fibers. These tumors do not harbor *KIT* or *PDGFRA* mutations. They do, however, express KIT; a subset of them also shows S-100 protein immunoreactivity.[21,34,57]

"QUADRUPLE WILD-TYPE" GASTROINTESTINAL STROMAL TUMORS

Pantaleo and colleagues[58] recently proposed that approximately 5% of all GISTs that lack mutations in KIT exons 8, 9, 11, 13, 14, 17/PDFRA exons 12, 14, 18, or RAS pathways (BRAF exons 11, 15/RAS exons 2, 3, or NF1), and still retain SDH complex function (intact SDHB staining and no SDHA/B/C/D mutations) should be designated as quadruple WT-GISTs. Needless to say, this group of tumors deserves additional studies to better characterize their clinicopathologic features, molecular abnormalities, and potential medical trials for targeted therapy.

SUMMARY

GISTs demonstrate diverse clinical profiles in that they can arise in any part of the gastrointestinal tract, and can present as tumors ranging from incidental microscopic tumors to those that follow a malignant and life-threatening course by virtue of widespread metastasis. This diversity is also reflected in the oncogenetic events that lead to their development. Although most GISTs can be risk-stratified using conventional parameters of size, location, and mitotic activity,[59] the current knowledge about molecular alterations in these tumors

suggests that perhaps incorporating mutational status is even more important for providing accurate information regarding prognosis and treating advanced tumors using pathway-specific inhibitors.

REFERENCES

1. Hirota S, Isozaki K, Moriyama Y, et al. Gain-of-function mutations of c-kit in human gastrointestinal stromal tumors. Science 1998;279:577–80.
2. Sommer G, Agosti V, Ehlers I, et al. Gastrointestinal stromal tumors in a mouse model by targeted mutation of the Kit receptor tyrosine kinase. Proc Natl Acad Sci U S A 2003;100:6706–11.
3. Rubin BP, Antonescu CR, Scott-Browne JP, et al. A knock-in mouse model of gastrointestinal stromal tumor harboring kit K641E. Cancer Res 2005;65:6631–9.
4. Lasota J, Corless CL, Heinrich MC, et al. Clinicopathologic profile of gastrointestinal stromal tumors (GISTs) with primary KIT exon 13 or exon 17 mutations: a multicenter study on 54 cases. Mod Pathol 2008;21:476–84.
5. van Nederveen FH, Gaal J, Favier J, et al. An immunohistochemical procedure to detect patients with paraganglioma and phaeochromocytoma with germline SDHB, SDHC, or SDHD gene mutations: a retrospective and prospective analysis. Lancet Oncol 2009;10:764–71.
6. Gill AJ, Chou A, Vilain RE, et al. "Pediatric-type" gastrointestinal stromal tumors are SDHB negative ("type 2") GISTs. Am J Surg Pathol 2011;35:1245–7 [author reply: 1247–8].
7. Gaal J, Stratakis CA, Carney JA, et al. SDHB immunohistochemistry: a useful tool in the diagnosis of Carney-Stratakis and Carney triad gastrointestinal stromal tumors. Mod Pathol 2011;24:147–51.
8. Janeway KA, Kim SY, Lodish M, et al. Defects in succinate dehydrogenase in gastrointestinal stromal tumors lacking KIT and PDGFRA mutations. Proc Natl Acad Sci U S A 2011;108:314–8.
9. Miettinen M, Wang ZF, Sarlomo-Rikala M, et al. Succinate dehydrogenase-deficient GISTs: a clinicopathologic, immunohistochemical, and molecular genetic study of 66 gastric GISTs with predilection to young age. Am J Surg Pathol 2011;35:1712–21.
10. Doyle LA, Nelson D, Heinrich MC, et al. Loss of succinate dehydrogenase subunit B (SDHB) expression is limited to a distinctive subset of gastric wild-type gastrointestinal stromal tumours: a comprehensive genotype-phenotype correlation study. Histopathology 2012;61:801–9.
11. Agaram NP, Wong GC, Guo T, et al. Novel V600E BRAF mutations in imatinib-naive and imatinib-resistant gastrointestinal stromal tumors. Genes Chromosomes Cancer 2008;47:853–9.

12. Agaimy A, Terracciano LM, Dirnhofer S, et al. V600E BRAF mutations are alternative early molecular events in a subset of KIT/PDGFRA wild-type gastrointestinal stromal tumours. J Clin Pathol 2009;62: 613–6.

13. Hostein I, Faur N, Primois C, et al. BRAF mutation status in gastrointestinal stromal tumors. Am J Clin Pathol 2010;133:141–8.

14. Miranda C, Nucifora M, Molinari F, et al. KRAS and BRAF mutations predict primary resistance to imatinib in gastrointestinal stromal tumors. Clin Cancer Res 2012;18:1769–76.

15. Maertens O, Prenen H, Debiec-Rychter M, et al. Molecular pathogenesis of multiple gastrointestinal stromal tumors in NF1 patients. Hum Mol Genet 2006;15:1015–23.

16. Heinrich MC, Corless CL, Demetri GD, et al. Kinase mutations and imatinib response in patients with metastatic gastrointestinal stromal tumor. J Clin Oncol 2003;21:4342–9.

17. Corless CL, Fletcher JA, Heinrich MC. Biology of gastrointestinal stromal tumors. J Clin Oncol 2004; 22:3813–25.

18. Martin J, Poveda A, Llombart-Bosch A, et al. Deletions affecting codons 557-558 of the c-KIT gene indicate a poor prognosis in patients with completely resected gastrointestinal stromal tumors: a study by the Spanish Group for Sarcoma Research (GEIS). J Clin Oncol 2005;23:6190–8.

19. Heinrich MC, Maki RG, Corless CL, et al. Primary and secondary kinase genotypes correlate with the biological and clinical activity of sunitinib in imatinib-resistant gastrointestinal stromal tumor. J Clin Oncol 2008;26:5352–9.

20. Miettinen M, Sobin LH, Lasota J. Gastrointestinal stromal tumors of the stomach: a clinicopathologic, immunohistochemical, and molecular genetic study of 1765 cases with long-term follow-up. Am J Surg Pathol 2005;29:52–68.

21. Miettinen M, Makhlouf H, Sobin LH, et al. Gastrointestinal stromal tumors of the jejunum and ileum: a clinicopathologic, immunohistochemical, and molecular genetic study of 906 cases before imatinib with long-term follow-up. Am J Surg Pathol 2006; 30:477–89.

22. Lux ML, Rubin BP, Biase TL, et al. KIT extracellular and kinase domain mutations in gastrointestinal stromal tumors. Am J Surg Pathol 2000;156:791–5.

23. Kunstlinger H, Huss S, Merkelbach-Bruse S, et al. Gastrointestinal stromal tumors with KIT exon 9 mutations: Update on genotype-phenotype correlation and validation of a high-resolution melting assay for mutational testing. Am J Surg Pathol 2013;37: 1648–59.

24. Gastrointestinal stromal tumor meta-analysis group (metaGIST). Comparison of two doses of imatinib for the treatment of unresectable or metastatic gastrointestinal stromal tumors: a meta-analysis of 1,640 patients. J Clin Oncol 2010;28:1247–53.

25. Stenman G, Eriksson A, Claesson-Welsh L. Human PDGFA receptor gene maps to the same region on chromosome 4 as the KIT oncogene. Genes Chromosomes Cancer 1989;1:155–8.

26. Heinrich MC, Corless CL, Duensing A, et al. PDGFRA activating mutations in gastrointestinal stromal tumors. Science 2003;299:708–10.

27. Neuhann TM, Mansmann V, Merkelbach-Bruse S, et al. A novel germline KIT mutation (p.L576P) in a family presenting with juvenile onset of multiple gastrointestinal stromal tumors, skin hyperpigmentations, and esophageal stenosis. Am J Surg Pathol 2013;37:898–905.

28. Ponti G, Luppi G, Martorana D, et al. Gastrointestinal stromal tumor and other primary metachronous or synchronous neoplasms as a suspicion criterion for syndromic setting. Oncol Rep 2010;23:437–44.

29. Nishida T, Hirota S, Taniguchi M, et al. Familial gastrointestinal stromal tumours with germline mutation of the KIT gene. Nat Genet 1998;19:323–4.

30. Burgoyne AM, Somaiah N, Sicklick JK. Gastrointestinal stromal tumors in the setting of multiple tumor syndromes. Curr Opin Oncol 2014;26:408–14.

31. O'Riain C, Corless CL, Heinrich MC, et al. Gastrointestinal stromal tumors: insights from a new familial GIST kindred with unusual genetic and pathologic features. Am J Surg Pathol 2005;29:1680–3.

32. Kleinbaum EP, Lazar AJ, Tamborini E, et al. Clinical, histopathologic, molecular and therapeutic findings in a large kindred with gastrointestinal stromal tumor. Int J Cancer 2008;122:711–8.

33. Li FP, Fletcher JA, Heinrich MC, et al. Familial gastrointestinal stromal tumor syndrome: phenotypic and molecular features in a kindred. J Clin Oncol 2005; 23:2735–43.

34. Agarwal R, Robson M. Inherited predisposition to gastrointestinal stromal tumor. Hematol Oncol Clin North Am 2009;23:1–13, vii.

35. Boikos SA, Stratakis CA. The genetic landscape of gastrointestinal stromal tumor lacking KIT and PDGFRA mutations. Endocrine 2014;47:401–8.

36. Selak MA, Armour SM, MacKenzie ED, et al. Succinate links TCA cycle dysfunction to oncogenesis by inhibiting HIF-alpha prolyl hydroxylase. Cancer Cell 2005;7:77–85.

37. Killian JK, Kim SY, Miettinen M, et al. Succinate dehydrogenase mutation underlies global epigenomic divergence in gastrointestinal stromal tumor. Cancer Discov 2013;3:648–57.

38. Lasota J, Wang Z, Kim SY, et al. Expression of the receptor for type i insulin-like growth factor (IGF1R) in gastrointestinal stromal tumors: an immunohistochemical study of 1078 cases with diagnostic and therapeutic implications. Am J Surg Pathol 2013; 37:114–9.

39. Mahadevan D, Theiss N, Morales C, et al. Novel receptor tyrosine kinase targeted combination therapies for imatinib-resistant gastrointestinal stromal tumors (GIST). Oncotarget 2015;6(4):1954–66.

40. Killian JK, Miettinen M, Walker RL, et al. Recurrent epimutation of SDHC in gastrointestinal stromal tumors. Sci Transl Med 2014;6:268ra177.

41. Miettinen M, Lasota J. Histopathology of gastrointestinal stromal tumor. J Surg Oncol 2011;104:865–73.

42. Doyle LA, Hornick JL. Gastrointestinal stromal tumours: from KIT to succinate dehydrogenase. Histopathology 2014;64:53–67.

43. Pappo AS, Janeway K, Laquaglia M, et al. Special considerations in pediatric gastrointestinal tumors. J Surg Oncol 2011;104:928–32.

44. Janeway KA, Pappo A. Treatment guidelines for gastrointestinal stromal tumors in children and young adults. J Pediatr Hematol Oncol 2012;34(Suppl 2):S69–72.

45. Pasini B, McWhinney SR, Bei T, et al. Clinical and molecular genetics of patients with the Carney-Stratakis syndrome and germline mutations of the genes coding for the succinate dehydrogenase subunits SDHB, SDHC, and SDHD. Eur J Hum Genet 2008;16:79–88.

46. Carney JA. Gastric stromal sarcoma, pulmonary chondroma, and extra-adrenal paraganglioma (Carney Triad): natural history, adrenocortical component, and possible familial occurrence. Mayo Clin Proc 1999;74:543–52.

47. Carney JA, Stratakis CA. Familial paraganglioma and gastric stromal sarcoma: a new syndrome distinct from the Carney triad. Am J Med Genet 2002;108:132–9.

48. Matyakhina L, Bei TA, McWhinney SR, et al. Genetics of Carney triad: recurrent losses at chromosome 1 but lack of germline mutations in genes associated with paragangliomas and gastrointestinal stromal tumors. J Clin Endocrinol Metab 2007;92:2938–43.

49. Haller F, Moskalev EA, Faucz FR, et al. Aberrant DNA hypermethylation of SDHC: a novel mechanism of tumor development in Carney triad. Endocr Relat Cancer 2014;21:567–77.

50. Oudijk L, Gaal J, Korpershoek E, et al. SDHA mutations in adult and pediatric wild-type gastrointestinal stromal tumors. Mod Pathol 2013;26:456–63.

51. Wagner AJ, Remillard SP, Zhang YX, et al. Loss of expression of SDHA predicts SDHA mutations in gastrointestinal stromal tumors. Mod Pathol 2013;26:289–94.

52. Miettinen M, Killian JK, Wang ZF, et al. Immunohistochemical loss of succinate dehydrogenase subunit A (SDHA) in gastrointestinal stromal tumors (GISTs) signals SDHA germline mutation. Am J Surg Pathol 2013;37:234–40.

53. Capper D, Preusser M, Habel A, et al. Assessment of BRAF V600E mutation status by immunohistochemistry with a mutation-specific monoclonal antibody. Acta Neuropathol 2011;122:11–9.

54. Patil D, Shuang M, Konishi M, et al. Utility of BRAF V600E mutation-specific immunohistochemistry in detecting BRAF V600E-mutated gastrointestinal stromal tumors. American Journal of Clinical Pathology; 2015, in press.

55. Daniels M, Lurkin I, Pauli R, et al. Spectrum of KIT/PDGFRA/BRAF mutations and Phosphatidylinositol-3-Kinase pathway gene alterations in gastrointestinal stromal tumors (GIST). Cancer Lett 2011;312:43–54.

56. Rubin BP, Heinrich MC, Corless CL. Gastrointestinal stromal tumour. Lancet 2007;369:1731–41.

57. Takazawa Y, Sakurai S, Sakuma Y, et al. Gastrointestinal stromal tumors of neurofibromatosis type I (von Recklinghausen's disease). Am J Surg Pathol 2005;29:755–63.

58. Pantaleo MA, Nannini M, Corless CL, et al. Quadruple wild-type (WT) GIST: defining the subset of GIST that lacks abnormalities of KIT, PDGFRA, SDH, or RAS signaling pathways. Cancer Med 2015;4:101–3.

59. Miettinen M, Lasota J. Gastrointestinal stromal tumors: pathology and prognosis at different sites. Semin Diagn Pathol 2006;23:70–83.

Advances in the Molecular Analysis of Soft Tissue Tumors and Clinical Implications

Adrian Marino-Enriquez, MD

KEYWORDS

- Molecular diagnostics • Targeted therapy • Soft tissue tumor • Sarcoma

ABSTRACT

The emergence of high-throughput molecular technologies has accelerated the discovery of novel diagnostic, prognostic and predictive molecular markers. Clinical implementation of these technologies is expected to transform the practice of surgical pathology. In soft tissue tumor pathology, accurate interpretation of comprehensive genomic data provides useful diagnostic and prognostic information, and informs therapeutic decisions. This article reviews recently developed molecular technologies, focusing on their application to the study of soft tissue tumors. Emphasis is made on practical issues relevant to the surgical pathologist. The concept of genomically-informed therapies is presented as an essential motivation to identify targetable molecular alterations in sarcoma.

OVERVIEW

Recent technological advances have dramatically changed the molecular analysis of tumor samples. The development of high throughput genome-wide analytical methods, notably massively parallel sequencing (MPS) technologies and associated computational algorithms, provides the ability to generate comprehensive profiles from tumor cells and tissues at several biological levels – such as genome, epigenome, or transcriptome. Such an abundance of data is transforming molecular pathology and oncology into data-intensive sciences, a transformation that is expected to have a tremendous impact on many aspects of clinical practice. From a scientific and research perspective, these technologies are perceived as disruptive, revolutionary,[1] or paradigm changing[2] and have generated an impressive body of knowledge, contributing to a much improved understanding of tumor biology. In the field of diagnostic pathology of soft tissue tumors, however, the overall impact has been rather incremental, and represents the natural continuation of pioneer molecular genetic studies evolving over the past 40 years from classical cytogenetics,[3] DNA hybridization techniques and FISH,[4] and PCR-based single gene assays.[5] Arguably, the biggest innovation is the accelerated pace of advances and the large volume of novel information, both truly unprecedented.

The purpose of this review is to introduce recently developed molecular technologies and to briefly discuss their potential for clinical implementation (Table 1), focusing on their various applications to the evaluation of soft tissue tumors. A special emphasis is made on practical diagnostic uses relevant to the surgical pathologist, with illustrative examples of how these newer technologies have helped characterize and diagnose soft tissue lesions. Finally, the concept of genomically informed therapies in sarcoma is presented as an essential motivation to implement molecular tests to identify potentially targetable alterations. An orientative glossary of terms widely used in this field is provided in Box 1.

Financial Support: A. Marino-Enriquez is supported by a Career Development Award from The Sarcoma Alliance for Research through Collaboration.
Conflict of Interest: The author has nothing to disclose.
Department of Pathology, Brigham and Women's Hospital, Harvard Medical School, 75 Francis Street, Boston, MA 02115, USA
E-mail address: admarino@partners.org

Surgical Pathology 8 (2015) 525–537
http://dx.doi.org/10.1016/j.path.2015.06.001

Table 1
Molecular techniques discussed in this review

Technique	Alterations Detected	Limitations	Research Contributions	Clinical Implementation
MPS technologies (next-generation sequencing)				
Genome sequencing				
Targeted sequencing (cancer gene panels and exome sequencing)	SNV, CNA	Not comprehensive, transl detection	Mutational landscape	+
WGS	SNV, CNA, transl	Cost/depth		±
Transcriptome sequencing (RNA-seq)	Transl	RNA workflow	Gene fusions	−
Non–sequencing-based high-throughput molecular techniques				
Array CGH	CNA	No detection of transl or SNVs	Somatic CNA landscape	+
SNP arrays	CNA			+
Low-throughput technologies				
Single gene sequencing assays	Hotspot SNV	Low throughput, not scalable	Historical landmark discoveries	++
FISH	Transl, CNA	Fluorescence, cost, low throughput, not scalable	Translocation mapping	++
Immunohistochemistry as a surrogate for molecular alterations	Protein expression	Low throughput	(Many)	+++

Abbreviation: Transl, translocation and rearrangements.

Box1
Glossary of terms commonly used in cancer genomics

Shotgun sequencing	Sequencing strategy in which the DNA/RNA is sheared, generating numerous random short fragments to create a sequencing library
Alignment or mapping	Matching sequence reads to a reference
Paired-end sequencing	Sequencing linear DNA fragments from both ends
Mate pairs	Sequence reads corresponding to both ends of a unique DNA fragment
Hybrid capture	Enrichment method to select target sequences from a pool, by tagging them with oligos or capture probes
Read	String of text that corresponds to a single DNA fragment (data output from the sequencer)
Coverage/depth	Often used interchangeably to refer to the number of individual reads for each specific position on a target sequence
Reference genome	Fully assembled version of a genome that can be used as a map to locate new sequences (current human version is GRCh38.p3, released by the Genome Reference Consortium in April 2015)
Variants	Differences at specific positions between 2 aligned sequences
Variant calling	Process of detecting sequence variants, which is variably automated through computational algorithms
SNV	Single nucleotide variant: a single base difference between a fragment and the reference
SNP	Single nucleotide polymorphism: an SNV that is frequent in the population (present in at least 1% of individuals)
VUS	Variant of unknown significance: variants for which the functional effect is unknown
Indel	Structural aberration of the DNA in which a segment is either deleted or inserted (usually applied to small deletions or insertions)
CNA	Copy number alteration: numeric alteration of the DNA by which the number of copies of a segment is increased (copy number gain) or reduced (copy number loss)
Allelic fraction	The proportion of a specific variant (allele) among all variants observed for that locus
Actionable mutation	A sequence variant that provides clinically useful diagnostic, prognostic, or therapeutic information
Targetable mutation	A sequence variant that confers sensitivity to a specific therapy
Driver mutation	A mutation that provides selective advantage to a clone and hence contributes significantly to cancer initiation and/or progression (in contrast with passenger mutations, which provide no significant fitness improvement)
Precision medicine	Emerging approach for disease treatment and prevention that takes into account individual variability in genes, environment, and lifestyle for each person using high-density data sets; in oncology, often used as synonymous of genomics-driven patient care

APPLICATIONS OF MASSIVELY PARALLEL SEQUENCING TECHNOLOGIES

MASSIVELY PARALLEL SEQUENCING (SO-CALLED NEXT-GENERATION SEQUENCING OR NGS)

MPS technologies allow for high throughput multiplex detection of a wide range of genetic aberrations, including single nucleotide variants (SNVs), copy number alterations (CNAs), insertions and deletions (*indels*), and chromosomal rearrangements.[6] Different sequencing platforms vary in their enzymology, chemistry, signal detection, instrument, and software, variables that determine their relative strengths and limitations for each application (the specifics are beyond the scope of this article and have been described extensively in several excellent reviews[7,8]). For all platforms, the initial step is to extract DNA or RNA molecules from the sample, break them down to fragments of a relatively homogeneous size (usually 100–300 bp long), and ligate molecular adaptors to each end to produce a library that contains the nucleic acid fragments of interest (library preparation). The fragments are then separated and immobilized on a glass surface or on synthetic beads, which permits the use of PCR amplification to create spatially distinct clusters with many identical copies of each fragment (although not all technologies use amplification steps). Multiple sequencing-by-synthesis reactions occur simultaneously, in parallel, on each of these clusters, in a cyclic process that is closely monitored by a detection system able to identify the nucleotides that are incorporated to the template, recording their sequence as individual reads.[9] Frequently, sequencing starts inbound from both ends of the linear target molecules, which generates *paired-end* sequencing reads that provide advantages over *single end* reads for mapping fragments to the reference. To maximize the mapping benefits of paired-end sequencing, input DNA may be fragmented into larger, 2- to 5-kb segments and then circularized to generate rearranged DNA stretches consisting of fragments originally distant (mate pairs), which provide increased ability to discover structural variation.[10] Differences between platforms on each of these steps determine their performance characteristics in terms of sensitivity, accuracy, read length, throughput, run time, coverage, error modes, and cost.[11,12] In all cases, several critical steps of computational processing, data analysis, and automated variant calling[13] are required to generate a clinically relevant report that may be useful for patient management.

MPS technologies can probe different input nucleic acid molecules extracting information from the genome (DNA), transcriptome (RNA, including large and small, and coding and noncoding), epigenome (methyl-Seq), or chromatin (ChIP-Seq), all widely used in research settings but at different levels of implementation in clinical laboratories. The amount of input material required for successful analysis is remarkably low, in the 0.1- to 1-μg range for most platforms and applications, which can be obtained from a few formalin-fixed, paraffin-embedded (FFPE) tissue sections (one 20–50 um thick tissue section, with >20% of tumor cells). The degradation resulting from routine FFPE tissue processing is not a significant problem for DNA-based applications; using RNA is more demanding, but continuous improvements in reagents chemistry and extraction protocols generate good quality libraries with appropriate representation in most instances.

CANCER GENOME SEQUENCING

In molecular pathology laboratories, the prevailing application of MPS technologies is sequencing different extensions of tumor genomic DNA to identify somatic aberrations. The potential advantages of a genome-wide comprehensive approach, *whole genome sequencing* (WGS), are outweighed thus far by the challenges regarding data analysis and storage and clinical interpretation. Similarly, capturing and sequencing all protein-coding DNA segments, *exome sequencing*, is thought to generate an excess of information of questionable clinical significance, at the expense of increased analytical challenges. Hence, most clinical cancer sequencing tests involve a panel of selected cancer-related genes (*targeted cancer gene panels*), of which every exon and some introns are covered at high reading depth (usually several hundred reads), which ensures robust detection of sequence changes and manageable data analysis. It is worth noting that any alterations present in the sequence are detected, not just a predefined set, in contrast with so-called genotyping technologies (*allelic-specific assays*).

The output of MPS-based cancer genome sequencing tests is a multipart, usually complex report, listing at least 3 types of somatic alterations: (1) nucleotide variants (SNVs) and their allelic frequency, usually classified according to the predicted biological effects on the protein (missense, nonsense, or silent); (2) copy number changes, an estimate of the copy number status of the locus of each gene, based on the number of reads of each position and the local and overall coverage; and (3) chromosomal rearrangements, by virtue of paired-end sequencing and the inclusion of intronic regions, which allow some fragments to be mapped to distant regions of the genome predicting a rearrangement. All these alterations are reported using a tier-based classification system that groups them according to the level of evidence supporting their clinical relevance.[14] Positive or pertinent negative findings that may affect patient management are emphasized, whereas changes of unknown significance are merely recorded. In this setting, the concept of *actionable mutation* has been defined as an alteration that has diagnostic, prognostic, or therapeutic implications in a given clinical context.[15] A *PDGFRA* exon 12 mutation detected in a gastric epithelioid mesenchymal tumor biopsy, for example, is an actionable mutation supporting a diagnosis of gastrointestinal stromal tumor (GIST), with a relatively good prognosis, predicting moderate sensitivity to imatinib. As the biological understanding of cancer pathogenesis progresses and novel targeted therapies are developed, the classification of each mutation will vary, with more variants increasingly considered clinically actionable.

TARGETED SEQUENCING (CANCER GENE PANELS AND EXOME SEQUENCING)

Different techniques, such as hybrid capture or selective circularization, allow for target enrichment during library preparation,[16] so only portions of the genome are sequenced. The selection of targets can range from tens or hundreds of genes to whole exome, resulting in the exclusion of more than 98% of the genomic DNA. This allows for much greater depth of sequence coverage, providing excellent sensitivity for detection of even low-abundance SNVs. Also, amplifications and small *indels* can be accurately estimated with targeted approaches. The sensitivity for detection of medium to large-sized deletions and importantly, chromosomal rearrangements, is much lower despite continuous improvements in bioinformatic algorithms.[17]

The difficulty in detecting chromosomal rearrangements by sequencing targeted cancer gene panels is particularly inconvenient for the field of soft tissue tumor pathology; the inclusion of intronic sequences, as well as specific computational approaches, may improve the detection of select rearrangements,[18–20] but the sensitivity is still low. This technical feature is, arguably, the main limitation of current DNA-based targeted sequencing approaches, severely reducing its diagnostic value for soft tissue tumors. Despite these limitations, anecdotal evidence indicates that identification of diagnostic gene fusions is possible using targeted cancer panels, as dramatically illustrated by the recently published case of a 42-year-old patient treated at the author's institution with a pulmonary lesion showing clinical and morphologic features consistent with an atypical carcinoid tumor, correctly diagnosed as Ewing sarcoma by targeted MPS.[21]

Several institutions have developed customized gene panels for targeted sequencing, which are rapidly evolving as new knowledge becomes available.[22] Some panels are organ or system-specific, whereas others are *pan-cancer* tests (**Table 2**). The largest in-house pan-cancer panels typically involve 100 to 300 genes, including known oncogenes and tumor suppressors. The overlap between the gene sets covered by each panel is remarkably limited (ie, different panels interrogate different genes),[23] which reflects the lack of standardization in these early days and speaks to the difficulty of defining a clinically relevant cancer gene census.

Exome sequencing (often designated *whole exome sequencing* or WES, to emphasize its comprehensive nature) has the obvious advantage of probing a much larger portion of the genome, its approximately 300,000 exons, including all the cancer-related genes present in focused panels. The reduced coverage that results may be problematic but only in limited samples with very low tumor content. The technique is becoming increasingly facile and cost effective, and some groups have demonstrated its feasibility in a

Table 2
Representative cancer gene panel tests for targeted sequencing at several US academic laboratories

Institution	Test Name	Number of Genes Sequenced (Introns)	Reference
Brigham and Women's Hospital/Dana-Farber Cancer Institute (Boston, Massachusetts)	OncoPanel	275 (91)	21
Memorial Sloan Kettering Cancer Center (New York, New York)	MSK-IMPACT	341 (33)	79
Washington University (St Louis, Missouri)	Comprehensive Cancer Gene Set v2	48 (6)	80
The Jackson Laboratory for Genomic Medicine (Bar Harbor, Maine)	JAX Cancer Treatment Profile	190 (0)	81
University of Washington (Seattle, Washington)	UW-OncoPlex	194 (15)	82
University of Pittsburgh (Pennsylvania)	ThyroSeq v2 (thyroid)	13 (42)	83
Knight Diagnostic Laboratories (Portland, Oregon)	GeneTrails genotyping panels (organ specific)	23–43 (0)	84

clinical environment in terms of turnaround time and other performance metrics.[24] In the research setting, exome sequencing has led to the identification of gene fusions, such as NAB2-STAT6 in solitary fibrous tumor.[25] The large volume of information generated by exome sequencing, however, and the computational and analytical challenges associated with the interpretation of the results have limited its clinical implementation thus far. Efforts to simplify and facilitate the clinical implementation of exome sequencing include interesting analytical algorithms and clinical decision support tools that harness the potential of publicly available knowledge bases using user-friendly interfaces and generating interactive reports.[24,26]

For soft tissue tumors, point mutations and indels detectable by targeted MPS involve an increasing number of relevant genes (Table 3), such as KIT/PDGFRA and SDHA/B in GIST, CTNNB1 in desmoid tumors, IDH1 or IDH2 in enchodroma/chondrosarcoma, COL2A1 in chondrosarcoma, the polycomb repressive complex components SUZ12 or EED in malignant peripheral nerve sheath tumor (MPNST), PIK3CA in myxoid liposarcoma, KDR in angiosarcomas,

STAG2 in Ewing sarcoma, N/K/HRAS and FGFR4 in embryonal rhabdomyosarcoma, MYOD1 in spindle cell rhabdomyosarcoma, MED12 in leiomyomas and a very small subset of leiomyosarcomas, and NF1 in MPNSTs and in an increasing number of other tumor types. SMARCB1 is rarely genomically inactivated in epithelioid sarcoma. The various amplicons characteristic of well-differentiated/dedifferentiated liposarcoma are also readily detected as copy number gains of MDM2 and CDK4, whereas MYC amplification is present in radiation-associated angiosarcoma. Mutations in TP53 are often identified in some sarcomas (osteosarcoma and leiomyosarcoma) as well as occasional PTEN loses, although with little value for diagnosis or patient management at this time. CDKN2A inactivating events are common (MPNSTs, fibrosarcomatous dermatofibrosarcoma protuberans, and advanced GISTs).

WHOLE GENOME SEQUENCING (WGS)

Sequencing the entire genome is still far from clinical application, due to logistic challenges that include high costs in a CLIA environment. The

---

Table 3
Clinically actionable genetic alterations commonly encountered in soft tissue tumors

Type of Alteration (Main Clinical Use)	Genes	Entities
Point mutation/small indels (potential therapeutic targets)	KIT/PDGFRA, SDHA/B	GIST
	CTNNB1	Desmoid tumor
	IDH1, IDH2	Enchondroma/chondrosarcoma
	COL2A1	Chondrosarcoma
	SUZ12, EED	MPNST
	PIK3CA	Myxoid liposarcoma
	KDR	Angiosarcoma
	STAG2	Ewing sarcoma
	N/K/HRAS, FGFR4	Embryonal rhabdomyosarcoma
	MYOD1	Spindle cell rhabdomyosarcoma
	MED12	Leiomyoma (and small subset of leiomyosarcoma)
	NF1	MPNST and others
Amplification (diagnostic markers)	MDM2, CDK4	Dedifferentiated liposarcoma
	MYC	Postradiation sarcoma
	MYOCD	Leiomyosarcoma
Deletion (diagnostic markers)	NF1	MPNST and others
	TP53	Osteosarcoma, leiomyosarcoma, and others
	CDKN2A	MPNST, fibrosarcomatous DFSP, advanced GIST
	RB1	Spindle cell lipoma, mammary-type myofibroblastoma, and others
Rearrangement (diagnostic markers)	Fusion oncogenes (constitutively active chimeric kinases, transcription factors)	Tumor-type specific (reviewed by Mertens and Tayebwa[35])

mean sequencing depth is approximately 30 to 60 reads, and the high number of sequence variants requires paired tumor and normal samples to filter out the germline variants from the tumor genome calls. Even then, the functional relevance of most genetic variants detected by WGS is unknown. The clinical implementation of WGS is further hampered by the need for fresh or frozen tissue, because FFPE tissues remain problematic for WGS, and the sequencing depth required for robust mutation detection from poor-quality DNA at this coverage is not yet cost effective. As a discovery tool, WGS has led to the discovery of *STAG2* mutations in Ewing sarcoma[27,28] and H3.3 mutations in chondroblastoma and giant cell tumor of bone.[29] Because these genes can be incorporated into cancer gene panels or sampled by exome sequencing, the use of WGS in clinical samples is generally considered overkill at the present time, but it may become more relevant in the future.[30]

An advantage of WGS is higher sensitivity for the detection of chromosomal rearrangements using specific algorithms to map paired-end reads[31]; this application has been widely validated in research settings, as for the discovery of *ALK* and *RET* gene fusions in lung adenocarcinoma.[32,33] For soft tissue tumors, most groups have favored the use of RNA-seq approaches for gene fusion detection. An additional feature of WGS is the ability to detect alterations in noncoding, gene regulatory regions, such as *TERT* promoter mutations first described in melanoma.[34] There is little information available for this type of genetic alterations in sarcoma.

TRANSCRIPTOME SEQUENCING (RNA-seq)

The use of RNA-seq is particularly attractive for the study of soft tissue tumors, given its ability to detect structural rearrangements.[35] The relevance of chromosomal rearrangements in soft tissue tumor pathogenesis and their diagnostic utility is well documented,[36,37] to a point that recurrent rearrangements have been used as a dichotomous classifier to define a whole category of translocation-associated soft tissue tumors. Most genomic breakpoints occur at variable locations within introns, which can be large, so the resulting chimeric RNA transcripts are usually smaller than the corresponding rearranged genomic DNA segments. The analysis of RNA also provides information about expression levels and transcript variants (expression profiling), which contributes to a better understanding of tumor biology and has prognostic implications in certain tumor types.

The usual workflow starts with RNA extraction and enrichment for protein-coding RNA molecules, by capturing the poly-A tails. Several approaches may be used to enrich for certain types of noncoding RNAs, such as micro-RNAs, and to deplete others (such as ribosomal RNA) to increase the desired signal. The quality of RNA from old FFPE tissue blocks may be suboptimal for some applications, but some technologies are specifically designed to extract information from substantially degraded RNA molecules using very short reads[38,39]; in addition, extraction protocols continue to improve and there are examples of successful RNA-seq application to archival material up to 10 years old.[40] Once the library is prepared and converted to cDNA, sequencing takes place by MPS as for genome-based approaches. The length of the reads (ultimately depending on the quality of the starting RNA) is a big determinant of the analytical sensitivity and the quality of the results. Several computational algorithms are available to detect fusion transcripts in RNA-seq data, such as deFuse, FusionSeq, or FusionHunter (reviewed by Carrara and colleagues[41]); in general, the algorithms work by iteratively mapping initially discarded reads, allowing for an increasing number of mismatches to the reference. The progress in this area is remarkable: recent RNA-seq studies managed to characterize the entire spectrum of kinase fusions in cancer, with direct therapeutic implications.[42]

Applied to the study of soft tissue tumors, RNA-seq has become the most popular mode of discovery for novel fusion genes. Notable examples of fusion genes detected by RNA-seq include *YWHAE-NUTM2A/B* in high-grade endometrial stromal sarcoma,[43] *WWTR1-CAMTA1* in epithelioid hemangioendothelioma,[44] and *BCOR-CCNB3* in undifferentiated round cell sarcoma.[45] A slightly different RNA-based detection approach was used to identify the *HEY1-NCOA2* in mesenchymal chondrosarcoma,[46] in which the data showed variable levels of expression of different exons from both genes, leading the investigators to identify the rearrangement (similar data were observed at the RNA level on the *NAB2-STAT6* study by Robinson and colleagues[25]). At present, RNA-seq is not used for clinical applications in soft tissue tumors, although suitable methods have been described.[47]

Gene expression profiling deserves a particular mention, because it has evolved almost completely to RNA-seq–based methods. Despite the initial good results of microarray-based assays in research settings,[48,49] attempts to clinically utilize gene expression profiling for sarcoma diagnosis or prognostication have generally failed, due to poor reproducibility and poor performance.[50] This may change with the increased sensitivity of sequencing technologies and algorithms, which could contribute to improved subclassification of currently heterogeneous categories of sarcoma. Paradigmatic examples are leiomyosarcoma and MPNSTs, both heterogeneous groups of sarcoma lacking subgroup-specific molecular markers to accurately predict clinical behavior.[51,52]

NON–SEQUENCING-BASED HIGH-THROUGHPUT MOLECULAR TECHNIQUES

ARRAY-BASED TECHNOLOGIES

The technological revolution undergone by sequencing technologies over the past 5 years has essentially eclipsed any other molecular genetic techniques. Array-based technologies, however, are also able to provide high-resolution analysis of tumor genomes and transcriptomes.[53] Current array comparative genomic hybridization (CGH) and single nucleotide polymorphism (SNP) array platforms are particularly suited to detect somatic copy number changes (deletions and amplifications) at a resolution much greater than sequencing techniques at the usual coverage. Copy number changes are common in cancer and induce significant functional changes that drive oncogenesis in proportions comparable to sequence variations.[54] In sarcoma, several oncogenic events are engaged by copy number changes, such as amplification of oncogenes (*MDM2* and *CDK4* in dedifferentiated liposarcoma and parosteal osteosarcoma) and deletion of critical tumor suppressors (*NF1* in MPNST and *DMD* in myogenic sarcomas[55]).

The use of array-based techniques is the natural evolution of karyotyping for genome-wide analysis, providing much richer information regarding gains and losses of genetic material, at higher resolution. In addition, these techniques can use interphase DNA, thus obviating culturing living cells to establish metaphase spreads (which, for cell culture enthusiasts, represents a painful loss!). The detection of balanced translocations, however, is not possible with high-resolution arrays and requires complementary technologies. Ideally, array-based techniques should be integrated into comprehensive, integrative genotyping approaches that include orthogonal assays based on sequencing. Such approaches have been successfully applied in soft tissue tumors for discovery purposes (leading to the identification of *GRM1* fusions in chondromyxoid fibroma).[56]

Pioneer experiences in the study of glioblastoma have shown promising results in terms of feasibility and clinical implementation.[57]

LOW-THROUGHPUT TECHNOLOGIES

SINGLE GENE SEQUENCING ASSAYS

Sanger sequencing (capillary electrophoresis, dye-terminator method) is still considered the gold standard for diagnostic detection of point mutations and *indels* in specific gene regions. For hotspot analysis and validation purposes, Sanger sequencing provides a convenient, inexpensive, and universally available method. The main limitation is its low sensitivity, with a detection threshold of approximately 30% allelic frequency (problematic in cases of low tumor content or in the detection of subclonal/heterogeneous genetic changes). In addition, the technique remains artisanal and laborious in terms of primer design and electropherogram interpretation, which leads to limited scalability. RT-PCR followed by sequencing is still widely used as validation method for gene fusion detection (although the extreme sensitivity of PCR amplification implies a high risk of carryover contamination, hence requiring stringent conditions and appropriate controls to avoid false-positive results).[58]

FLUORESCENCE IN SITU HYBRIDIZATION

FISH is a well-established approach to interrogate known chromosomal rearrangements and is still the preferred technique for the cytogenetic diagnosis of soft tissue tumors.[59,60] Copy number gains and deletions can also be readily detected. During clinical work-up, morphologic evaluation combined with pertinent immunohistochemical stains usually narrows down the differential diagnosis to a limited number of entities that occasionally can be confirmed by FISH. In this usual workflow, FISH mainly has a role in validating or confirming a suspected diagnosis. In research, FISH has been an essential technique as part of the classical route to discover new fusion genes: after identification of recurrent rearrangements by chromosome banding techniques, FISH mapping allows delineating breakpoints that can then be defined by RT-PCR–based techniques.[35] Technically, FISH consists of the hybridization of fluorescently labeled probes to specific nucleotide sequences (usually genomic DNA). The size of FISH probes is in the hundreds of kilobases range, and the resolution to detect rearrangements is limited by the fluorescence microscope used for evaluation (small insertions or complex rearrangements may be missed). At present, approximately 30 recurrent chromosomal rearrangements are known to be involved in soft tissue tumors and can be used for diagnostic purposes (reviewed by Mertens and Tayebwa[35] and Al-Zaid and collaegues[61]). An added value of FISH, when performed in tissue sections, is the preservation of tissue architecture and the ability to evaluate regional heterogeneity or specific cellular populations within the tumor.

IMMUNOHISTOCHEMISTRY AS A SURROGATE FOR MOLECULAR ALTERATIONS

Although immunohistochemistry is formally not considered a molecular technique, the remarkable impact of recent molecular genetic discoveries in the development of useful immunohistochemical markers deserves consideration. Since immunohistochemistry is fully integrated in the surgical pathology workflow, the greatest clinical impact of molecular discoveries is achieved when a corresponding immunohistochemical assay is developed. For soft tissue tumors, this rapid translation has successfully occurred in multiple instances in recent years.[62] The usual course of events is the discovery of a molecular alteration in a given soft tissue tumor type by gene expression profiling or MPS technologies, followed by the development and validation of antibodies with appropriate specificity and sensitivity to be used for immunohistochemistry. Following this paradigm, gene expression profiling has led to the discovery of DOG1 as a diagnostic marker for GIST,[63] TLE1 for synovial sarcoma,[64] and MUC4 for low-grade fibromyxoid sarcoma.[65] Overexpression of STAT6, TFE3, or ALK as a result of chromosomal rearrangements in solitary fibrous tumor, alveolar soft part sarcoma, and inflammatory myofibroblastic tumors, respectively, can also be detected by robust immunohistochemical techniques. Gene amplifications (*MDM2*, *CDK4*, and *MYC*) and deletions (*RB1* and *SMARCB1*) also correlate with protein expression and can be used for diagnostic purposes. Anecdotally, some experts have referred to the development of these markers as next-generation immunohistochemistry, which reflects how significant a change is perceived in the field (of note, the same designation has been proposed for mass spectrometry–based methods for protein identification in tissues[66]). It should be highlighted that immunohistochemistry is susceptible to preanalytical variables, requires intensive quality controls to

be performed routinely, and requires expert interpretation, similarly to molecular techniques.

DRUG TARGET IDENTIFICATION

One of the main forces driving the clinical implementation of high-throughput molecular techniques is the perception that high-density genetic information will enable better discrimination of patients with similar phenotypic and clinical presentations, ultimately allowing for a refined selection of the most appropriate treatment. Different variations on this theme are currently encompassed under the concept of *precision medicine*, the most recent designation for what has also been called personalized medicine or individualized medicine.[67] The emergence of the designation precision medicine is more than a terminological issue, and its rapid adoption reflects the widespread acceptance of its main principle, that the disruptive nature of high-throughput molecular technologies will fundamentally transform patient care. The tremendous excitement surrounding precision medicine is exemplified by ambitious academic endeavors (such as a report from the Committee on a Framework for Developing a New Taxonomy of Disease[68]), the deployment of large-scale research initiatives (such as the Presidential Precision Medicine Initiative[69]), and the considerable revenue of specialized biotechnology companies,[70] all of which are taking place amid great enthusiasm in the academic medical community.[71] In oncology, the prevailing opinion is that genomic information, layered on top of "traditional" clinicopathologic variables, will inform therapeutic selection and improve patient outcomes.[72] This genomics-driven paradigm in oncology will require validation in clinical trials with innovative designs (involving molecularly stratified groups matched to their drugs in umbrella protocol, and likely requiring serial biopsies, for example),[73] but anecdotal evidence and extraordinary responses observed in multiple instances contribute to a general sense of optimism.[74]

Successful clinical implementation of genomics-driven oncology will depend on the development of effective targeted agents. It is estimated that 550 genes encode drug targets used by currently established pharmaceuticals, only a small fraction of which corresponds to cancer targets, whereas the druggable genome is predicted to comprise approximately 1000 genes (2%–5% of the genome).[75] At present, many potentially druggable mutations are identified for which there are no effective inhibitors. Conversely, most tumors harbor at least 1 targetable genomic alteration.[76] In soft tissue tumors, several clinically relevant drug targets have been identified through improved understanding of tumor genomics,[77] but thus far only 5 targeted agents are approved by the FDA for sarcoma patient treatment in the United States: the RANK ligand inhibitor denosumab for the treatment of giant cell tumor; the multikinase inhibitor pazopanib for several soft tissue sarcomas; and the receptor tyrosine kinase inhibitors imatinib, sunitinib, and regorafenib for the treatment of GIST. A series of up to 20 additional compounds are at different stages of clinical development, including the ALK inhibitor crizotinib, the mTOR inhibitor sirolimus, and the CDK4 inhibitor palbociclib (reviewed elsewhere[61,78]). The molecular abnormalities underlying activation of these oncogenes can be readily detected by MPS technologies.

CONCLUDING REMARKS

The extraordinary development of high-throughput molecular technologies has the potential to transform the practice of surgical pathology. At present, appreciable changes are restricted to large academic centers and oncology institutes in which research and patient care–related activities are closely intertwined; but with continuously declining costs and increasing accessibility, it is fair to assume that some form of variably comprehensive genetic data will be available for most cancer samples. Accurate interpretation of these data may support the diagnostic process and inform therapeutic decisions. In soft tissue tumor pathology, integration of genetic information, specifically chromosomal rearrangements, has been part of the diagnostic process over the past 2 decades. Novel diagnostic, prognostic, and predictive markers will be described and incorporated into clinical practice. In upcoming years, most molecular data will be generated by MPS technologies and, possibly, high-density arrays, both of which will likely replace FISH for most clinical applications. Recording clinically actionable somatic mutations and pertinent negatives will be part of the routine pathology report and will inform therapeutic decisions from the medical oncology team. In the immediate future, the biggest contributions of high-throughput genetic technologies will have an impact on the research arena, generating knowledge and increasing understanding of the molecular pathogenetic basis of soft tissue tumors. Once knowledge bases are saturated, a huge impact in patient care is expected, with the ultimate result of improved outcomes for sarcoma patients.

REFERENCES

1. Garraway LA, Verweij J, Ballman KV. Precision oncology: an overview. J Clin Oncol 2013;31: 1803–5.
2. Dienstmann R, Rodon J, Barretina J, et al. Genomic medicine frontier in human solid tumors: prospects and challenges. J Clin Oncol 2013;31:1874–84.
3. Turc-Carel C, Philip I, Berger MP, et al. Chromosome study of Ewing's sarcoma (ES) cell lines. Consistency of a reciprocal translocation t(11;22)(q24;q12). Cancer Genet Cytogenet 1984;12:1–19.
4. Guan XY, Zhang H, Bittner M, et al. Chromosome arm painting probes. Nat Genet 1996;12:10–1.
5. Sorensen PH, Liu XF, Delattre O, et al. Reverse transcriptase PCR amplification of EWS/FLI-1 fusion transcripts as a diagnostic test for peripheral primitive neuroectodermal tumors of childhood. Diagn Mol Pathol 1993;2:147–57.
6. MacConaill LE, Van Hummelen P, Meyerson M, et al. Clinical implementation of comprehensive strategies to characterize cancer genomes: opportunities and challenges. Cancer Discov 2011;1:297–311.
7. Mardis ER. Next-generation DNA sequencing methods. Annu Rev Genomics Hum Genet 2008;9: 387–402.
8. Ross JS, Cronin M. Whole cancer genome sequencing by next-generation methods. Am J Clin Pathol 2011;136:527–39.
9. MacConaill LE. Existing and emerging technologies for tumor genomic profiling. J Clin Oncol 2013;31: 1815–24.
10. Korbel JO, Urban AE, Affourtit JP, et al. Paired-end mapping reveals extensive structural variation in the human genome. Science 2007;318:420–6.
11. Lam HY, Clark MJ, Chen R, et al. Performance comparison of whole-genome sequencing platforms. Nat Biotechnol 2011;30:78–82.
12. Loman NJ, Misra RV, Dallman TJ, et al. Performance comparison of benchtop high-throughput sequencing platforms. Nat Biotechnol 2012;30:434–9.
13. Ramos AH, Lichtenstein L, Gupta M, et al. Oncotator: cancer variant annotation tool. Hum Mutat 2015;36:E2423–9.
14. Van Allen EM, Wagle N, Levy MA. Clinical analysis and interpretation of cancer genome data. J Clin Oncol 2013;31:1825–33.
15. MacConaill LE, Campbell CD, Kehoe SM, et al. Profiling critical cancer gene mutations in clinical tumor samples. PLoS One 2009;4:e7887.
16. Mertes F, Elsharawy A, Sauer S, et al. Targeted enrichment of genomic DNA regions for next-generation sequencing. Brief Funct Genomics 2011;10:374–86.
17. Ulahannan D, Kovac MB, Mulholland PJ, et al. Technical and implementation issues in using

next-generation sequencing of cancers in clinical practice. Br J Cancer 2013;109:827–35.

18. Abel HJ, Duncavage EJ, Becker N, et al. SLOPE: a quick and accurate method for locating non-SNP structural variation from targeted next-generation sequence data. Bioinformatics 2010;26:2684–8.

19. Duncavage EJ, Abel HJ, Szankasi P, et al. Targeted next generation sequencing of clinically significant gene mutations and translocations in leukemia. Mod Pathol 2012;25:795–804.

20. Abo RP, Ducar M, Garcia EP, et al. BreaKmer: detection of structural variation in targeted massively parallel sequencing data using kmers. Nucleic Acids Res 2015;43:e19.

21. Doyle LA, Wong KK, Bueno R, et al. Ewing sarcoma mimicking atypical carcinoid tumor: detection of unexpected genomic alterations demonstrates the use of next generation sequencing as a diagnostic tool. Cancer Genet 2014;207:335–9.

22. MacConaill LE, Garcia E, Shivdasani P, et al. Prospective enterprise-level molecular genotyping of a cohort of cancer patients. J Mol Diagn 2014;16:660–72.

23. Zutter MM, Bloom KJ, Cheng L, et al. The Cancer Genomics Resource List 2014. Arch Pathol Lab Med 2014. [Epub ahead of print].

24. Van Allen EM, Wagle N, Stojanov P, et al. Whole-exome sequencing and clinical interpretation of formalin-fixed, paraffin-embedded tumor samples to guide precision cancer medicine. Nat Med 2014;20:682–8.

25. Robinson DR, Wu YM, Kalyana-Sundaram S, et al. Identification of recurrent NAB2-STAT6 gene fusions in solitary fibrous tumor by integrative sequencing. Nat Genet 2013;45:180–5.

26. Aronson SJ, Clark EH, Babb LJ, et al. The GeneInsight Suite: a platform to support laboratory and provider use of DNA-based genetic testing. Hum Mutat 2011;32:532–6.

27. Tirode F, Surdez D, Ma X, et al. Genomic landscape of Ewing sarcoma defines an aggressive subtype with co-association of STAG2 and TP53 mutations. Cancer Discov 2014;4:1342–53.

28. Crompton BD, Stewart C, Taylor-Weiner A, et al. The genomic landscape of pediatric Ewing sarcoma. Cancer Discov 2014;4:1326–41.

29. Behjati S, Tarpey PS, Presneau N, et al. Distinct H3F3A and H3F3B driver mutations define chondroblastoma and giant cell tumor of bone. Nat Genet 2013;45:1479–82.

30. Garraway LA, Baselga J. Whole-genome sequencing and cancer therapy: is too much ever enough? Cancer Discov 2012;2:766–8.

31. Campbell PJ, Stephens PJ, Pleasance ED, et al. Identification of somatically acquired rearrangements in cancer using genome-wide massively parallel paired-end sequencing. Nat Genet 2008; 40:722–9.

32. Soda M, Choi YL, Enomoto M, et al. Identification of the transforming EML4-ALK fusion gene in non-small-cell lung cancer. Nature 2007;448:561–6.

33. Takeuchi K, Soda M, Togashi Y, et al. RET, ROS1 and ALK fusions in lung cancer. Nat Med 2012;18:378–81.

34. Huang FW, Hodis E, Xu MJ, et al. Highly recurrent TERT promoter mutations in human melanoma. Science 2013;339:957–9.

35. Mertens F, Tayebwa J. Evolving techniques for gene fusion detection in soft tissue tumours. Histopathology 2014;64:151–62.

36. Fletcher JA, Kozakewich HP, Hoffer FA, et al. Diagnostic relevance of clonal cytogenetic aberrations in malignant soft-tissue tumors. N Engl J Med 1991;324:436–42.

37. Mertens F, Johansson B, Fioretos T, et al. The emerging complexity of gene fusions in cancer. Nat Rev Cancer 2015;15:371–81.

38. Beck AH, Weng Z, Witten DM, et al. 3'-end sequencing for expression quantification (3SEQ) from archival tumor samples. PLoS One 2010;5:e8768.

39. Sweeney RT, Zhang B, Zhu SX, et al. Desktop transcriptome sequencing from archival tissue to identify clinically relevant translocations. Am J Surg Pathol 2013;37:796–803.

40. Huang W, Goldfischer M, Babyeva S, et al. Identification of a novel PARP14-TFE3 gene fusion from 10-year-old FFPE tissue by RNA-seq. Genes Chromosomes Cancer 2015. [Epub ahead of print].

41. Carrara M, Beccuti M, Cavallo F, et al. State of art fusion-finder algorithms are suitable to detect transcription-induced chimeras in normal tissues? BMC Bioinformatics 2013;14(Suppl 7):S2.

42. Stransky N, Cerami E, Schalm S, et al. The landscape of kinase fusions in cancer. Nat Commun 2014;5:4846.

43. Lee CH, Ou WB, Marino-Enriquez A, et al. 14-3-3 fusion oncogenes in high-grade endometrial stromal sarcoma. Proc Natl Acad Sci U S A 2012;109:929–34.

44. Tanas MR, Sboner A, Oliveira AM, et al. Identification of a disease-defining gene fusion in epithelioid hemangioendothelioma. Sci Transl Med 2011;3:98ra82.

45. Pierron G, Tirode F, Lucchesi C, et al. A new subtype of bone sarcoma defined by BCOR-CCNB3 gene fusion. Nat Genet 2012;44:461–6.

46. Wang L, Motoi T, Khanin R, et al. Identification of a novel, recurrent HEY1-NCOA2 fusion in mesenchymal chondrosarcoma based on a genome-wide screen of exon-level expression data. Genes Chromosomes Cancer 2012;51:127–39.

47. van de Rijn M, Guo X, Sweeney RT, et al. Molecular pathological analysis of sarcomas using paraffin-embedded tissue: current limitations and future possibilities. Histopathology 2014;64:163–70.

48. Subramanian S, West RB, Marinelli RJ, et al. The gene expression profile of extraskeletal myxoid chondrosarcoma. J Pathol 2005;206:433–44.

49. Nakayama R, Nemoto T, Takahashi H, et al. Gene expression analysis of soft tissue sarcomas: characterization and reclassification of malignant fibrous histiocytoma. Mod Pathol 2007;20:749–59.

50. West RB. Expression profiling in soft tissue sarcomas with emphasis on synovial sarcoma, gastrointestinal stromal tumor, and leiomyosarcoma. Adv Anat Pathol 2010;17:366–73.

51. Subramanian S, Thayanithy V, West RB, et al. Genome-wide transcriptome analyses reveal p53 inactivation mediated loss of miR-34a expression in malignant peripheral nerve sheath tumours. J Pathol 2010;220:58–70.

52. Guo X, Jo VY, Mills A, et al. Clinically relevant molecular subtypes in leiomyosarcoma. Clin Cancer Res 2015. [Epub ahead of print].

53. Beroukhim R, Mermel CH, Porter D, et al. The landscape of somatic copy-number alteration across human cancers. Nature 2010;463:899–905.

54. Zack TI, Schumacher SE, Carter SL, et al. Pan-cancer patterns of somatic copy number alteration. Nat Genet 2013;45:1134–40.

55. Wang Y, Marino-Enriquez A, Bennett RR, et al. Dystrophin is a tumor suppressor in human cancers with myogenic programs. Nat Genet 2014;46:601–6.

56. Nord KH, Lilljebjorn H, Vezzi F, et al. GRM1 is upregulated through gene fusion and promoter swapping in chondromyxoid fibroma. Nat Genet 2014; 46:474–7.

57. Ramkissoon SH, Bi WL, Schumacher SE, et al. Clinical implementation of integrated whole-genome copy number and mutation profiling for glioblastoma. Neuro Oncol 2015. [Epub ahead of print].

58. Fletcher CD, Fletcher JA, Dal Cin P, et al. Diagnostic gold standard for soft tissue tumours: morphology or molecular genetics? Histopathology 2001;39:100–3.

59. Lazar A, Abruzzo LV, Pollock RE, et al. Molecular diagnosis of sarcomas: chromosomal translocations in sarcomas. Arch Pathol Lab Med 2006;130: 1199–207.

60. Tanas MR, Goldblum JR. Fluorescence in situ hybridization in the diagnosis of soft tissue neoplasms: a review. Adv Anat Pathol 2009;16:383–91.

61. Al-Zaid T, Somaiah N, Lazar AJ. Targeted therapies for sarcomas: new roles for the pathologist. Histopathology 2014;64:119–33.

62. Doyle LA. Soft tissue tumor pathology: new diagnostic immunohistochemical markers. Semin Diagn Pathol 2015. [Epub ahead of print].

63. Espinosa I, Lee CH, Kim MK, et al. A novel monoclonal antibody against DOG1 is a sensitive and specific marker for gastrointestinal stromal tumors. Am J Surg Pathol 2008;32:210–8.

64. Terry J, Saito T, Subramanian S, et al. TLE1 as a diagnostic immunohistochemical marker for synovial sarcoma emerging from gene expression profiling studies. Am J Surg Pathol 2007;31:240–6.

65. Doyle LA, Moller E, Dal Cin P, et al. MUC4 is a highly sensitive and specific marker for low-grade fibromyxoid sarcoma. Am J Surg Pathol 2011;35:733–41.

66. Rimm DL. Next-gen immunohistochemistry. Nat Methods 2014;11:381–3.

67. Katsnelson A. Momentum grows to make 'personalized' medicine more 'precise'. Nat Med 2013;19: 249.

68. National Research Council (U.S.). Committee on a framework for developing a new taxonomy of disease. Toward precision medicine: building a knowledge network for biomedical research and a new taxonomy of disease. Washington, DC: National Academies Press; 2011.

69. Collins FS, Varmus H. A new initiative on precision medicine. N Engl J Med 2015;372:793–5.

70. Eisenstein M. Foundation medicine. Nat Biotechnol 2012;30:14.

71. Jameson JL, Longo DL. Precision medicine - personalized, problematic, and promising. N Engl J Med 2015;372:2229–34.

72. Macconaill LE, Garraway LA. Clinical implications of the cancer genome. J Clin Oncol 2010;28:5219–28.

73. Garraway LA. Genomics-driven oncology: framework for an emerging paradigm. J Clin Oncol 2013;31:1806–14.

74. Iyer G, Hanrahan AJ, Milowsky MI, et al. Genome sequencing identifies a basis for everolimus sensitivity. Science 2012;338:221.

75. Rask-Andersen M, Masuram S, Schioth HB. The druggable genome: evaluation of drug targets in clinical trials suggests major shifts in molecular class and indication. Annu Rev Pharmacol Toxicol 2014;54:9–26.

76. Dienstmann R, Jang IS, Bot B, et al. Database of genomic biomarkers for cancer drugs and clinical targetability in solid tumors. Cancer Discov 2015;5: 118–23.

77. Barretina J, Taylor BS, Banerji S, et al. Subtype-specific genomic alterations define new targets for soft-tissue sarcoma therapy. Nat Genet 2010;42:715–21.

78. Taylor BS, Barretina J, Maki RG, et al. Advances in sarcoma genomics and new therapeutic targets. Nat Rev Cancer 2011;11:541–57.

79. Cheng DT, Mitchell TN, Zehir A, et al. Memorial sloan kettering-integrated mutation profiling of actionable cancer targets (MSK-IMPACT): a hybridization capture-based next-generation sequencing clinical

assay for solid tumor molecular oncology. J Mol Diagn 2015;17:251–64.

80. Cottrell CE, Al-Kateb H, Bredemeyer AJ, et al. Validation of a next-generation sequencing assay for clinical molecular oncology. J Mol Diagn 2014;16:89–105.

81. Ananda G, Mockus S, Lundquist M, et al. Development and validation of the JAX Cancer Treatment Profile for detection of clinically actionable mutations in solid tumors. Exp Mol Pathol 2015;98:106–12.

82. Pritchard CC, Salipante SJ, Koehler K, et al. Validation and implementation of targeted capture and sequencing for the detection of actionable mutation, copy number variation, and gene rearrangement in clinical cancer specimens. J Mol Diagn 2014;16:56–67.

83. Nikiforov YE, Carty SE, Chiosea SI, et al. Highly accurate diagnosis of cancer in thyroid nodules with follicular neoplasm/suspicious for a follicular neoplasm cytology by ThyroSeq v2 next-generation sequencing assay. Cancer 2014;120:3627–34.

84. Beadling C, Neff TL, Heinrich MC, et al. Combining highly multiplexed PCR with semiconductor-based sequencing for rapid cancer genotyping. J Mol Diagn 2013;15:171–6.

Printed and bound by CPI Group (UK) Ltd, Croydon, CR0 4YY

03/10/2024

01040381-0003